ORTHOPEDIC
BOARDS REVIEW II
A Case Study Approach

ORTHOPEDIC
BOARDS REVIEW II
A Case Study Approach

Timothy S. Loth, M.D.
Department of Orthopedics
Iowa Medical Clinic, P.C.
Cedar Rapids, Iowa

with 239 illustrations

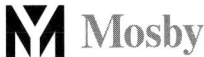 Mosby

St. Louis Baltimore Boston Carlsbad Chicago Naples New York Philadelphia Portland
London Madrid Mexico City Singapore Sydney Tokyo Toronto Wiesbaden

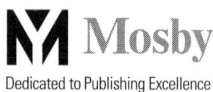

Mosby
Dedicated to Publishing Excellence

A Times Mirror
Company

Publisher: Anne Patterson
Editor: Robert Hurley
Developmental Editor: Lauranne Billus
Project Manager: Dana Peick
Production Editor: Dottie Martin
Designer: Amy Buxton
Electronic Production Coordinator: Pamela Merritt
Manufacturing Manager: Betty Richmond
Cover Designer: Scott Tjaden/GW Graphics and Publishing

Printed in the United States of America
Composition by Mosby Electronic Publishing
Printing/binding by Maple-Vail Book MFG Group

Mosby–Year Book, Inc.
11830 Westline Industrial Drive
St. Louis, Missouri 63146

Library of Congress Cataloging-in-Publication Data
Orthopedic boards review II : a case study approach / [edited by]
    Timothy S. Loth
        p.   cm.
    Includes index.
    ISBN 0-8151-5322-8 (hard cover)
    1. Orthopedics—Examinations, questions, etc.
  2. Orthopedics—Outlines, syllabi, etc.
  3. Orthopedics—Case studies—Examinations, questions, etc. I. Loth, Timothy S.
    [DNLM: 1. Orthopedics—examination questions. WE 18.2 0765 1996]
  RD732.6.0772   1996
  617.3'0076—dc20
  DNLM/DLC
  For Library of Congress   95-32367
                                    CIP

95 96 97 98 99 / 9 8 7 6 5 4 3 2 1

To my wife, Lisa, and my children, Renée and Karl

Contributors

J. Kenneth Burkus, M.D.
The Hughston Clinic, P.C.,
Eufaula, Alabama

Grant A. Dona, M.D.
Orthopedic Clinic of Monroe,
Monroe, Louisiana

Stanley H. Dysart, M.D.
Marietta Orthopaedics, P.A.,
Marietta, Georgia

Richard C. Fisher, M.D.
Associate Professor,
Department of Orthopaedics,
University of Colorado Health
  Sciences Center,
Denver, Colorado

Keith R. Gabriel, M.D.
Department of Orthopaedic
  Surgery,
St. Louis University;
Department Director,
Pediatric Orthopaedics,
Cardinal Glennon Children's
  Hospital,
St. Louis, Missouri

LTC D. E. Casey Jones, M.D.
Chief of Orthopaedics,
Chief of Hand Surgery,
Director, Orthopaedic Residency,
Madigan Army Medical Center,
Tacoma, Washington;
Clinical Assistant Professor,
Department of Orthopaedic
  Surgery,
University of Washington,
Seattle, Washington

Kenneth J. Koval, M.D.
Chief, Orthopaedic Fracture
  Service,
Hospital for Joint Diseases,
Orthopaedic Institute,
New York, New York

Timothy S. Loth, M.D.
Department of Orthopedics
Iowa Medical Clinic, P.C.,
Cedar Rapids, Iowa

Douglas J. McDonald, M.D.
Associate Professor,
Department of Orthopedic
  Surgery,
St. Louis University School of
  Medicine,
St. Louis, Missouri

Michael H. McGuire, M.D.
Professor and Chairman,
Department of Surgery,
Creighton University School of
  Medicine,
Omaha, Nebraska

Howard M. Place, M.D.
Chief, Spine Surgery Section,
Orthopedic Surgery Service,
Fitzsimons Army Medical Center,
Aurora, Colorado

James J. Sferra, M.D.
Associate Staff,
Section of Lower Extremities,
Department of Orthopaedic
  Surgery,
The Cleveland Clinic Foundation,
Cleveland, Ohio

Michael J. Shereff, M.D.
Director,
Division of Foot and Ankle
  Surgery;
Associate Professor,
Department of Orthopaedic
  Surgery,
Medical College of Wisconsin,
Milwaukee, Wisconsin

Theodore C. Yee, M.D.
Orthopaedic Surgery Resident,
Creighton-Nebraska Universities
  Health Foundation,
Division of Orthopaedic Surgery,
Omaha, Nebraska

Preface

Although this book is somewhat similar to our first book, *Orthopedic Boards Review*, there are several important differences. Ten new contributors were selected to author chapters in *Orthopedic Boards Review II: A Case Study Approach*. The content of these chapters is consequently distinct, offering fresh, different perspectives on orthopedic surgery. The format has also been changed to place a greater emphasis on clinical case studies. We have continued to offer the same "user friendly" question-and-answer format developed for the first book, which proved so popular.

Timothy S. Loth, M.D.

Acknowledgments

I am deeply grateful to the contributors, whose expertise and enthusiasm made this project possible. I also thank: Robert Hurley, Executive Editor, and Lauranne Billus, Developmental Editor, Mosby–Year Book, for encouragement and technical assistance; Caryl Rammelsberg, the transcriptionist who typed the text and its countless revisions; my colleagues at Iowa Medical Clinic, P.C., for their insightful criticisms and suggestions during the book's preparation. Special thanks to Drs. Fred Pilcher, Mark Mehlhoff, Warren Verdeck, Teri Formanek, James Johns, James Pape, Behrooz Akbarnia, Mitchell Rotman, David Strege, Urban Lingren, and many others who took time from their busy schedules to critically evaluate the manuscript.

Timothy S. Loth, M.D.

How to Use this Book

The goal of this book is to better prepare orthopedic surgeons and residents for the Orthopaedic Board Exams, Orthopaedic In-Training Examination, and recertification examinations. The book's essay-question format simulates the oral examination of the Orthopaedic Board Exams and provides more rigorous test preparation than the multiple-choice format used in most other review books. In addition to identifying deficiencies in knowledge and conceptualization, our format provides short discussions of grouped topics to better prepare reviewers for both written and oral examinations.

Although some will think it an undesirable omission, I have deleted references from this text. A text peppered with references can be distracting. They are not in the text of this book because most of the information in these questions and answers represent "common" knowledge found in standard orthopedic texts. Anyone preparing for the boards, the in-training exam or recertification should be familiar with and have access to the appropriate texts (which have tremendous reference lists), thereby eliminating the need for references in this one.

No attempt has been made to comprehensively review all of orthopedic surgery in this book. This would clearly be impossible. We have, however, attempted to discuss many current clinical topics as well as some of the esoteric ones that are recurrently encountered during examinations. We attempted to present "accepted" approaches to orthopedic problems and have not sought to present every option for treatment. We have not avoided controversial areas, and instead, we have attempted to identify these areas and to give short explanations for each advocated approach. All of the questions and answers contained within this text have been verified through multiple peer and editor reviews.

I would suggest that this book be used in the following ways: first, to review and reinforce concepts and information, and second, to determine areas of deficiency or vague concept development. To be most efficient in the review, I suggest that the book be used in close proximity to a personal or departmental library. If expansion of topics or concepts is needed, these sections can be easily looked up in the appropriate orthopedic surgery texts.

This book was written to dovetail with my first book, *Orthopedic Boards Review* (OBR) with each book emphasizing different aspects of examination preparation. OBR presents a core of knowledge intended to serve as a basis for orthopedic decision making and patient care. *Orthopedic Boards Review II: A Case Study Approach* intensifies the review by using clinical case studies that provide interpretive-type questions in order to further challenge the reviewer's understanding of each topic. When used in conjunction with OBR, this book will impart a greater depth of understanding of orthopedics and an improved test performance than if either were used alone.

Please allocate enough time to go through the book at least twice before the exams. On the first time through, identify those questions that were answered incorrectly or in which concept development was weak. I would then recommend going through the same section with attention to the incorrectly answered questions several days later to assure that the information has been retained. Finally, I would review everything once again just prior to the exam to assure that the information is reinforced and easily retrievable.

I invite you to send me your impressions (positive or negative) regarding this book. I shall use these suggestions to improve subsequent editions.

I believe that mastering this book will give you a core of knowledge that will serve you well in your short-term goals of board certification and success on the in-training exams, as well as the more important pursuit of excellence in patient care. Best of luck.

Timothy S. Loth, M.D.

Contents

CHAPTER 1

Pediatric Orthopedics

Keith R. Gabriel

QUESTIONS

1   A 10-year-old girl is brought to your office with complaints of increasingly high arches. Her parents state that she seems to be walking on the outside edges of her feet. What might be included in your initial differential diagnosis?

2   What specific information would you seek in the family history?

3   What skin findings will you seek when performing the spinal examinations?

4   The family of the patient in Q1 reports that she has had an increasingly clumsy, "staggering" gait over the past year. Your lower extremity examination finds diminished deep tendon reflexes and bilateral up-going Babinski responses. You should be especially aware of what spinal condition in this patient?

5   Your diagnostic suspicions from Q4 are confirmed. A radiograph shows the patient has a 20-degree right dorsal curve. Your thoughts about management of the scoliosis include:

6   A family has recently immigrated from southeast Asia. Their 10-year-old child has unilateral atrophy of the calf musculature and a cavus foot. The foot is remarkable in that the heel is in extreme calcaneus: it almost looks to you like a "pistol grip." The patient's foot was previously normal, and the deformity developed after a severe febrile illness. Your diagnosis is:

ANSWERS

1   This may be a developing cavus, or cavovarus, foot. Think of a possible neurologic etiology: neuropathy, such as Charcot-Marie-Tooth disease; spinal cerebellar degeneration, such as Friedreich's ataxia; structural spine problems such as diastematomyelia.

2   Many of the peripheral neuropathies are inherited. You need to know whether there have been other family members with such neurologic disorders. You also need to know whether other family members have similar foot deformities (i.e., a cavus foot) or suggestive hand deformities, such as wasting of the intrinsic muscles.

3   Hairy patch or skin dimple over the spine or hyperpigmented midline nevus. These findings may be associated with occult spinal dysraphism.

4   The description suggests Friedreich's ataxia. Most of these patients develop scoliosis.

5   Bracing is poorly tolerated and not effective for control of scoliosis in Friedreich's ataxia. If this curve progresses, surgery may be necessary. Your eagerness to treat must be tempered by the reality that Friedreich's ataxia is a progressive neurologic disorder with death usually occurring before age 40 years.

6   Polio. Worldwide, polio is the most common cause of a calcaneocavus foot deformity.

QUESTIONS

7 You are asked to see an infant in the nursery who has a foot deformity. The dorsum of the foot is lying nearly against the anterolateral distal tibia, yet the heel seems to be rigidly in an equinus posture (*Figure 1-1*). You suspect:

Fig 1-1

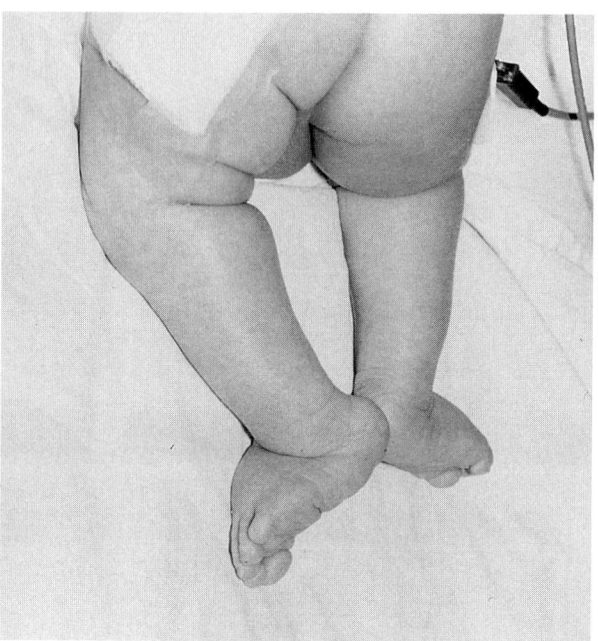

8 As you continue your examination, you carefully but persistently massage and manipulate the foot. Will you be able to reduce the position to neutral?

9 The nursery staff has already obtained a "clubfoot series" for your review. Are these radiographs helpful?

10 What do you plan to tell the parents about the success of nonsurgical treatment?

11 You are asked to see an infant in the nursery who has a foot deformity. The dorsum of the foot is lying nearly against the anterolateral distal tibia, and the heel is quite prominently in calcaneus posture. You suspect:

12 Will you be able to reduce this foot deformity to the neutral position by gentle manipulation as you perform the physical examination?

ANSWERS

7 Congenital vertical talus (CVT); also known as rocker bottom foot, Persian slipper foot, congenital convex pes valgus.

8 Probably not. CVT is almost always rigid. In fact, if you can reduce the foot to a true neutral position, you are probably not dealing with CVT.

9 Minimally. A clubfoot is usually evaluated with a maximum dorsiflexion lateral radiograph. For CVT, a maximum plantar flexion lateral view is preferred (*Figure 1-2*). In CVT, a line projected through the talus will extend plantarward of the navicular, even with the foot held in maximum plantar flexion. Because the navicular is not ossified in the newborn, the line projected through the talus may be referenced to the cuboid; in CVT this line will be plantarward.

Fig 1-2

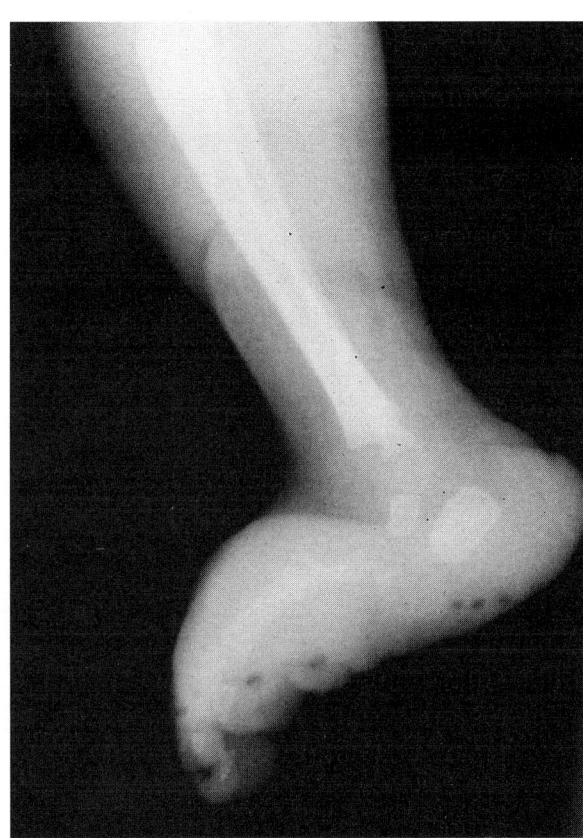

10 Passive stretching and sequential casting may help stretch soft tissues, but this is almost never a sufficient treatment. A true CVT will virtually always require surgical correction.

11 Calcaneovalgus foot deformity. The key is that the heel is in calcaneus, actually aligned with the forefoot. The entire foot has dorsiflexed through the ankle. There is no midfoot breach as seen with a CVT.

12 At least to neutral, although perhaps not into plantar flexion at the ankle. The ability to correct the hindfoot to neutral is an important discriminator when assessing the severity of a foot deformity.

QUESTIONS

13   What radiographs would you request?

14   Assume your patient has an associated posteromedial angulation of the tibia. How do you propose to treat the tibia?

15   You are asked to see an infant in the nursery who has a unilateral foot deformity. There is adduction and perhaps some varus of the forefoot, but the heel is in a valgus posture. You cannot fully correct the forefoot position by gentle manipulation. The ankle moves freely. You suspect:

16   How do you propose to treat this problem?

17   The infant in the next bed has a similar adduction of one midfoot, but the heel is in neutral position. As you gently manipulate the foot, you are able to manually correct the forefoot to hindfoot relationship. You suspect:

18   You carefully examine the patient described in Q17. As you stroke the lateral border of the foot, the peroneal muscles strongly contract. The adduction of the midfoot corrects to neutral. Your treatment plan is:

19   Suppose the infant has the foot deformity as described in Q17 but bilaterally. What commonly associated anomaly should you radiographically exclude?

20   A 3-year-old child has rigid MTA, perhaps more correctly "congenital metatarsus varus," resistant despite casting and "corrective" shoes (*Figure 1-3*). What surgical options would you suggest?

Fig 1-3

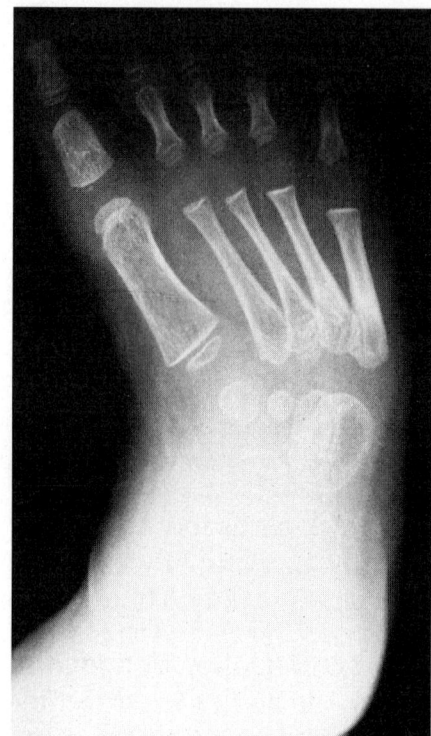

ANSWERS

13 First, the foot; also, the tibia. Calcaneovalgus foot is often associated with kyphoscoliotic tibia (posteromedial bowing of the tibia). The hips should be evaluated, either with radiographs or ultrasound imaging, because of a reported relationship between calcaneovalgus foot and developmental dysplasia of the hip.

14 The natural history of posteromedial bowing of the tibia is spontaneous improvement. Therefore consideration for corrective osteotomy should be deferred for several years. Early orthotic management (bracing) is recommended. Leg length discrepancy sometimes results; consequently periodic monitoring is needed to completion of growth. Length equalization procedures may be necessary.

15 This is probably a "skewfoot" or serpentine foot. Some authors use the term "congenital metatarsus varus." The point of distinction is that the rigidity of the tarsometatarsal articulation, together with the tendency for heel valgus, makes this deformity more problematic than the usual metatarsus adductus.

16 Casting will probably be needed. The difficulty lies in correcting the forefoot adductus without exacerbating the hindfoot valgus. Improperly performed exercises and most braces will tend to evert the entire foot without supporting the heel in neutral (or even slightly varus).

17 Because the heel is not in valgus and given the flexibility of the tarsometatarsal area, this condition is the more common metatarsus adductus (MTA).

18 The active correction should reassure you and the infant's parents of a good prognosis. Simple observation should be sufficient.

19 An association between bilateral MTA and hip dysplasia has been described. Either radiographs or an ultrasound examination of the hips should be considered.

20 In this age group the tarsometatarsal (TMT) release (Heyman, Herndon, Strong procedure) might be recommended. One variation of this procedure includes release of TMT joints 1, 3, 4, and 5 with osteotomy of the base of the second metatarsal (MT). Some investigators have reported a high incidence of late midfoot stiffness and pain with TMT release and therefore have preferred multiple metatarsal osteotomies. Release of the abductor hallucis and lateral transfer of the tibialis anterior, either in its entirety or as a split transfer, could be considered to maintain correction.

QUESTIONS

21 A 7-year-old child is referred for a unilateral midfoot deformity (*Figure 1-4*). The heel is neutral, but the forefoot remains adducted. When she was a toddler, the parents were told that this deformity would correct with normal growth. It has not. Shoe wear is a significant problem. You should now consider:

Fig 1-4

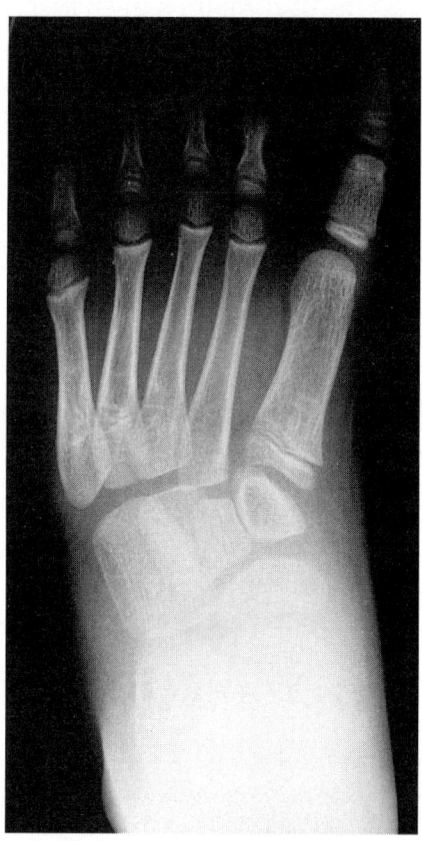

22 You are asked to see an infant in the nursery who has a unilateral foot deformity. The heel is in equinus and varus, and the midfoot is in adductus. The foot is not supple. How will you initiate treatment?

23 Can you speculate about the sex of the child and the side of the deformity in Q22?

24 A infant has bilateral clubfeet, but your physical examination has not disclosed any other abnormality. Surgical correction of the feet is indicated. What radiographs do you want? Why?

25 A infant has bilateral rigid clubfeet. Your examination also shows severe symmetrical limitation of motion, both passive and active, at multiple other joints. There is a striking absence of the expected flexion creases, and the skin has a stretched, leathery feel. The infant does not seem "paralyzed." What are the implications for treatment of the feet?

ANSWERS

21 Surgical correction with several possible procedures: multiple MT osteotomy; simultaneous closing wedge osteotomy of the cuboid and opening wedge osteotomy of the medial cuneiform to equalize lengths of the medial and lateral columns; opening wedge osteotomy of the medial cuneiform with osteotomy of the minor MTs.

22 This description sounds as though the child has a clubfoot (talipes equinovarus). Initial management should begin as soon as possible and include sequential passive manipulation and application of a holding device. Taping or casting are the usual holding devices, although some braces have been described.

23 Clubfoot is more common in boys and more common on the right side.

24 The usual "clubfoot series" should include simulated standing anteroposterior (AP) and maximum dorsiflexion lateral views of the feet. Search for the talocalcaneal relationship in each projection. In bilateral cases, also study the spine. Some patients with bilateral clubfeet have spinal dysraphism, either overt or occult.

25 The description seems consistent with arthrogryposis multiplex congenita. These clubfeet are notoriously resistant to treatment. Some authors have obtained reasonable results with soft-tissue releases, but others have advocated primary talectomy.

QUESTIONS

26 A small infant has bilateral rigid clubfeet. Your examination also discloses bilateral "hitch-hiker" thumbs (abducted at the MC-P joints) and "cauliflower" ear deformities. What are the implications for treatment of the feet?

27 A 7-year-old has developed an equinovarus foot deformity. He also has hyperextensible elbows, subluxing patellae, and a progressive flexion contracture of the right long finger proximal interphalangeal joint. The skin is easily bruised and seems flimsy and elastic. What are the implications for treatment of the foot?

28 An otherwise normal 3-year-old has an asymptomatic, bilateral toe deformity in which the second toe curls laterally and lies underneath the third toe. Father and paternal grandmother have similar deformities. What operation has been suggested for this situation?

29 A 2-year-old refuses to walk or bear weight on his lower extremities. You are surprised by his reasonably good hip motion bilaterally; yet the child protests vigorously when a parent simultaneously elevates both lower extremities while changing a diaper. The abdomen is benign. You begin to suspect:

30 Symptoms have been present for only 18 hours. Blood and urine specimens have been sent to the laboratory, and are pending. Radiographs of the spine, pelvis, and both lower extremities are normal for age. What might be your next imaging study?

31 The child's erythrocyte sedimentation rate (ESR) is 35 mm per hour (nl 0 to 20). The peripheral white blood cell (WBC) count is 8500; there has been no fever. Blood and urine cultures have been obtained and are pending. The bone scan does suggests discitis. Should you begin antibiotic therapy?

32 This same patient complains of some posterior thigh pain, and hamstring tightness is evident during physical examination. You think:

33 A 14-year-old girl is referred with a tentative diagnosis of a septic knee and contralateral septic wrist. As you examine her, you find that the appearance of the wrist is more compatible with tenosynovitis rather than joint sepsis. Your differential diagnosis must include:

34 The infant of a diabetic mother is referred for treatment of bilateral clubfeet. You see that the feet are relatively rigid; but you also note that there is striking bilateral calf atrophy, with little or no active motion in any of the muscle groups below the knee. You cannot stimulate activity in the gluteus maximus. What radiographs do you request?

35 Suppose that radiographs confirm your suspicion. What other investigations should be requested at this point?

ANSWERS

26 The description of the child seems consistent with diastrophic dwarfism. These clubfeet are exceptionally difficult to treat; essentially, the feet are similar to those described in Answer 25.

27 This patient may have Ehlers-Danlos syndrome. The joint (and foot) deformities tend to be recurrent. Operative interventions are complicated by frequent wound dehiscence and high infection rates. This patient should be evaluated by a geneticist or dysmorphologist to establish the diagnosis of the underlying disorder before initiating treatment.

28 "Curly toes" can be an autosomal dominant condition. Usually no treatment is required. Taping and bracing can help control local complaints such as ingrown nails or dorsal callouses, but these treatments do not correct the deformity. Surgical release of the long flexor tendon or transfer to the extensor hood has been recommended. Syndactylization can also be an effective treatment.

29 A bilateral straight leg raise, as when changing the diaper, causes the lumbar spine to flex. Pain on this maneuver should direct your thoughts to the spine. Discitis in this age group often presents as a refusal to bear weight or walk.

30 Bone scan is recommended. Magnetic resonance imaging (MRI) is more sensitive early in the course of a discitis but is usually more expensive. Bone scan has the additional advantage of offering information about other parts of the body.

31 This is controversial. Some authors would not give systemic antibiotics unless there were some systemic signs of sepsis such as fever or an elevated WBC count. Bed rest or cast immobilization may be tried first. Other authors recommend that antistaphylococcal drugs should be given immediately.

32 The picture can still be consistent with discitis. The inflammatory mass at the level of the intervertebral disk can produce nerve root irritation.

33 Sexually transmitted disease; specifically, gonorrhea.

34 Spine films are needed. You should suspect sacral agenesis.

35 Renal and cardiac anomalies are associated with sacral agenesis and should have ultrasonographic evaluations. Spine radiographs must show the entire spine, including the cervical area, because other vertebral anomalies may be present. It is prudent to consult a developmental pediatrician whenever you encounter a child with these potentially multisystem anomalies.

QUESTIONS

36 Suppose that spinal radiographs of the infant from Q34 show truncation of the sacrum, as well as multiple vertebral anomalies throughout the lumbar spine. The renal ultrasound showed only one kidney. The nursery staff reports that the infant has been having difficulty swallowing. You may be dealing with:

37 Suppose a child has absence of the lumbar spine and sacrum. At age 5 the resulting spinopelvic instability is causing severe functional problems. What might you offer?

38 A family is interested in overseas adoption. A photograph shows a child with apparent unilateral quadriceps atrophy and mild ipsilateral hip flexion contracture. Medical records have not yet been translated. The agency spokesperson says that the child was ill approximately 2 years ago and now walks by pushing the involved knee with the hand. You suspect:

39 As an adult, what systemic symptoms might this patient develop many years later?

40 A 12-year-old girl is referred because of repeated ankle sprains. The referring physician has already obtained routine ankle radiographs and stress films of the ankle, all of which are normal for her age. You suspect:

41 What special radiographic views might you request?

42 Suppose that the special plain radiographs are inconclusive. What other imaging study might you consider?

43 A 14-year-old boy has a rigid flat foot. His parents believe that the cosmetic "flat" appearance of the foot is worsening. His neurologic examination is normal. You suspect:

44 You evaluate a 6-year-old boy with a painless limp, which has been noticed by the parents for the last 3 months. You characterize the limp as a gluteus medius lurch. Which condition is first in your differential diagnosis?

45 The bench examination of the child described in Q44 shows equal thigh length with painless limitation of internal rotation and abduction of the involved hip. Radiographs of the hips confirm your suspicion. What would be your initial goal in management of this process?

46 What interventions might help achieve this goal?

47 Your initial goal has been achieved. Assume that the extent of the pathologic process is such that active intervention, rather than observation, is indicated. The family declines surgery; consequently, you discuss:

ANSWERS

36 A variation of the VATER syndrome. Again, multisystem anomalies deserve multisystem evaluation.

37 Amputation of the nonfunctional lower extremities, using the long bones as graft to fuse the truncated spine to the pelvis.

38 Polio. Quadriceps weakness is a classic sequelae.

39 Postpolio syndrome with early fatigue, new weakness in either previously affected or unaffected muscles, new atrophy, cold intolerance, muscle and joint pain.

40 Tarsal coalition. Repeated ankle sprains in an adolescent is a classic presentation.

41 The Harris axial view of the calcaneus provides visualization of the posterior and middle facets of the subtalar joint. The Slocum oblique of the midfoot effectively shows the calcaneonavicular area.

42 Computed tomography (CT) scan of the hindfoot and midfoot. The MRI is less precise for bone structure.

43 Peroneal spastic flatfoot: this diagnosis presumes tarsal coalition. Other causes (e.g., stress fracture, unicameral cyst of calcaneus) must be excluded.

44 This is a classic presentation for Legg-Calvé-Perthes (LCP) disease.

45 Restoration of full range of motion of the hip is always the initial goal.

46 Bed rest, with or without traction in abduction; physical therapy; serial Petrie abduction casts. Sometimes surgical release of the adductor longus is necessary to facilitate these nonoperative methods.

47 Nonoperative containment methods include serial Petrie abduction casts and various types of braces. The most commonly used brace is probably the Atlanta Scottish Rite.

QUESTIONS

48   You continue to manage the patient from Q44. Six months go by. The pathologic process is now clearly defined on radiographs as the affected portion of the femoral head has entered the "fragmentation" stage. Assume a Catterall IV situation. The family now reconsiders surgery. What options do you discuss?

49   You diagnose LCP in a 4-year-old boy. Later that same day, you diagnose LCP in a 9-year-old boy. In both cases, radiographs show a Catterall Group 2 involvement of the femoral head. How does your counseling differ for these two families?

50   You are managing a case of Perthes' disease. The 5-year-old patient has been doing well with only observation. The femoral head is now radiographically in the "fragmentation" stage. What radiographic findings might make you change your strategy?

51   An obese 10-year-old has Perthes' disease. Despite an adductor tenotomy, repeated periods of traction and sequential Petrie ("broomstick") casts, the patient has not maintained hip abduction. The radiographs are shown (*Figure 1-5*). What options will you consider now?

Fig 1-5

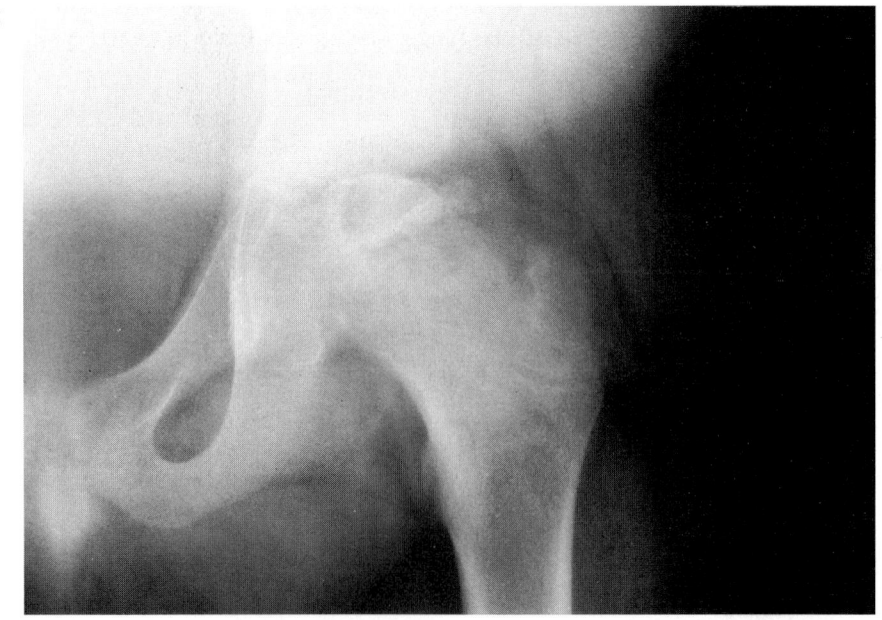

52   An obese 12-year-old black girl is brought to your office because her mother has noticed that the patient has been walking with a limp for the past 3 months. You observe a gluteus medius lurch and an outward foot progression angle on the affected side. Your thoughts turn to:

53   Some would say that the patient in Q52, as a result of race and gender, might be at an increased risk of a particular complication or adverse outcome. That secondary pathologic process is:

ANSWERS

48 Varus osteotomy of the proximal femur or Salter innominate osteotomy of the pelvis are the most commonly used techniques. Shelf acetabular augmentation or the Chiari pelvic osteotomy are usually considered salvage techniques in this age group, although in an older age group these options may be used primarily.

49 In general, patients of less than 5 years of age with Catterall Group 2 head involvement will have a good result with little or no intervention. Those patients older than 8 years of age have a guarded or even poor prognosis. You will want to recommend some form of intervention for the 9-year-old child, rather than simple observation.

50 Consider the "head at risk" signs described by Catterall. They include (1) lateral extrusion of the femoral head, (2) calcification in the femoral head lateral to the ossific nucleus of the epiphysis, (3) metaphyseal rarefaction, (4) Gage's sign (rarefaction of the lateral epiphysis and adjacent metaphysis), and (5) horizontal orientation of the physis or actual growth disturbance of the physis.

51 The femoral head deformity (i.e., collapse of the avascular weight-bearing dome) has created joint incongruity. At this age there is not much potential for acetabular remodeling with growth. This is the patient who may need a salvage procedure such as the Chiari osteotomy or a shelf acetabular augmentation.

52 Slipped capital femoral epiphysis.

53 Chondrolysis.

QUESTIONS

54 An obese 14-year-old boy has unilateral "knee pain." You check range of motion of the knees and hips and suspect slipped capital femoral epiphysis (SCFE). What findings lead you to that diagnosis?

55 The father of the patient in Q54 is a mechanic. He asks you why SCFE should cause a change in hip range of motion (ROM).

56 Six months ago, a 14-year-old boy was treated for severe SCFE by fixation in situ. The involved physis has closed. He complains of a persistent inability to sit with his legs straight at his school desk; that is, he has to cross the affected leg over the unaffected leg. Your advice is:

57 Suppose a situation identical to that in Q56, except that the patient was treated 24 months ago. Your advice is:

58 A patient underwent fixation of acute SCFE 6 months ago. Three pins were directed just slightly superior to the center of the femoral head. There was no pin protrusion. The patient now complains of a new onset of pain in the same hip. Your examination documents crepitance throughout the range of motion. You suspect:

59 The patient described in Q52 was treated for her SCFE by pinning in situ. A few weeks later you suspect that she has developed chondrolysis. Her physical examination shows:

60 The patient from Q59 has an ESR of 50 mm per hour (lab nl to 20 mm per hour). You must worry about:

61 A 3-year-old girl is sent for evaluation of a painless limp. Her mother says the patient has "always walked that way" and cannot understand why her new pediatrician insisted on referral. On the girl's left, you notice the combination of a gluteus medius lurch with short leg "bobbing." At the top of your differential diagnosis is:

62 You request a standing pelvis radiograph. To your surprise, the hips are both concentrically located. However, on the affected side you see a femoral neck-shaft angle of 85 degrees. There is a triangular fragment of metaphysis at the inferior neck surrounded by a radiolucent area shaped like an inverted letter Y. Treatment of this condition will almost certainly require:

ANSWERS

54 Knee examination will be unremarkable with full ROM. The hip on the affected side will have decreased internal rotation and decreased flexion, compared with the unaffected hip. You should specifically see decreased internal rotation of the affected hip in flexion compared with extension; that is, there will often be an obligatory external rotation of the hip as you passively move it from extension toward flexion.

55 You explain that the capital femoral epiphysis has remained in the acetabulum, but that the femoral metaphysis (neck) has moved anteriorly and superiorly. As you attempt to flex the hip, the edge of the metaphysis impinges on the anterior lip of the acetabulum. With external rotation of the thigh, the impingement is relieved so that further flexion is possible.

56 Wait. There is literature evidence that some improvement in ROM will occur over 18 months following fixation of SCFE. There is some disagreement as to whether this improvement is actual change of bony alignment or simply accommodation of the patient to the altered ROM.

57 At this point it may be reasonable to consider corrective osteotomy to improve the ROM. The subtrochanteric osteotomy of Southwick would be one example.

58 You must worry about avascular necrosis of the femoral head. "Nesting" the tips of multiple pins, especially toward the anterolateral part of the epiphysis, has been implicated in interruption of the intraosseous blood supply (the artery of Brodetti).

59 A limp with both an antalgic pattern and a hip flexion pattern on the involved side. Bench examination confirms restriction of hip motion in all planes.

60 An infection. Chondrolysis, in and of itself, should not cause ESR elevation.

61 Hip dysplasia. Despite various screening programs, late diagnosis of a congenitally or developmentally dislocated hip is still a problem.

62 Best results in treatment of developmental coxa vara have been reported with derotation valgus producing osteotomy of the proximal femur, including concomitant adductor release.

QUESTIONS

63 A 5-year-old boy is referred because of excessive lumbar lordosis and a bilateral Trendelenburg lurch. Radiographs are shown (*Figure 1-6*). You advise:

Fig 1-6

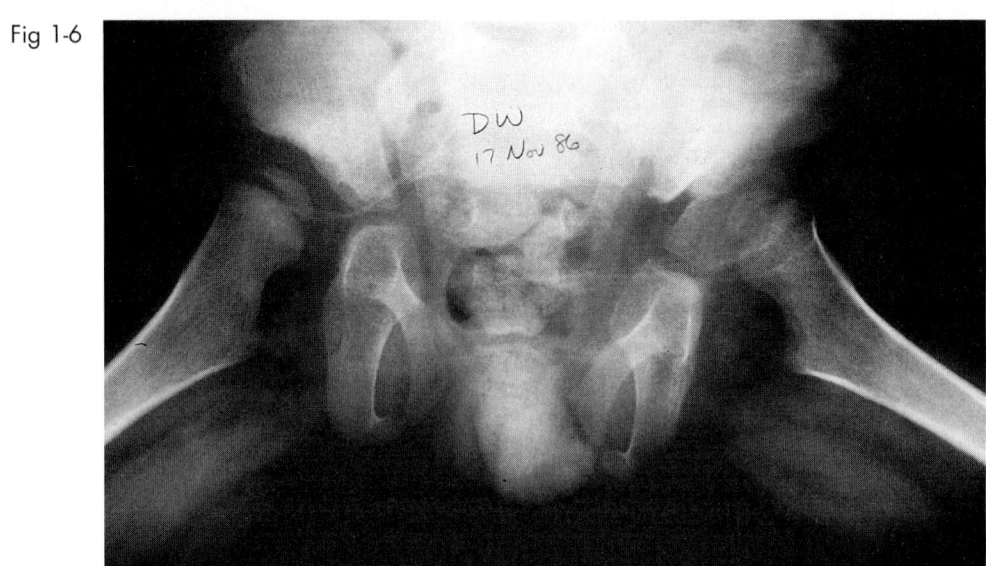

64 Suppose the patient described in Q61 has a unilateral hip dislocation. Your recommended treatment will include:

65 Again, suppose the patient described in Q61 has a unilateral hip dislocation. The parents ask you if the pediatrician who performed the child's newborn examination has been negligent. You answer:

66 A family is considering adoption of an infant with congenital shortening of the entire right lower extremity. The shortening is distributed among the femoral, tibial, and foot segments. No other abnormalities are present. What can you tell the prospective parents about expected growth of that limb?

67 You evaluate a 5-year-old child who has hypertrophy of one lower extremity. The proportions of the limb are somewhat distorted. You see at least six macular areas of light brown skin discoloration on all parts of the body. One parent has multiple similar areas on the visible parts of the body. You should think of:

68 You evaluate a 2-year-old child who has hypertrophy of one lower extremity. The limb is well proportioned and functions normally; radiographs are normal. You find no other orthopedic abnormalities. The skin is clear. What ultrasound study should you recommend?

ANSWERS

63   Observation. For all practical purposes, the true acetabuli have ceased to exist. The abnormal ossification pattern of the left ilium confirms that this condition is not a "typical" hip dislocation. In this "terato-genic" bilateral dislocation, at age 5 years, attempts to reduce the joints should be avoided.

64   Open reduction with femoral shortening. Rotational correction and varusization of the proximal femur will certainly be a part of the shortening osteotomy. A concomitant procedure for acetabular redi-rection or augmentation is not always needed.

65   Not necessarily. There is substantial literature supporting the concept that some hips are stable at birth but dislocate later with growth. This possibility has been officially acknowledged by the trend to change the terminology to "developmental dysplasia of the hip," or DDH.

66   In many of these congenital shortening situations, growth of the limbs will proceed at a relatively constant ratio. That is, if the affected limb is 85% of the length of the unaffected side, it will probably grow at approximately 85% of the length of the unaffected side and will be approximately 85% of that length at maturity.

67   Neurofibromatosis (NF) type I and the Albright's syndrome with polyostotic fibrous dysplasia.

68   The adrenal glands and kidneys are conveniently imaged by ultra-sound. You are concerned because of the association between Wilms' tumor and lower extremity hypertrophy.

QUESTIONS

69 Several days before a scheduled new patient office visit, you receive this single radiograph in the mail (*Figure 1-7*). Other records have not yet arrived. What subject might you review before you see this patient?

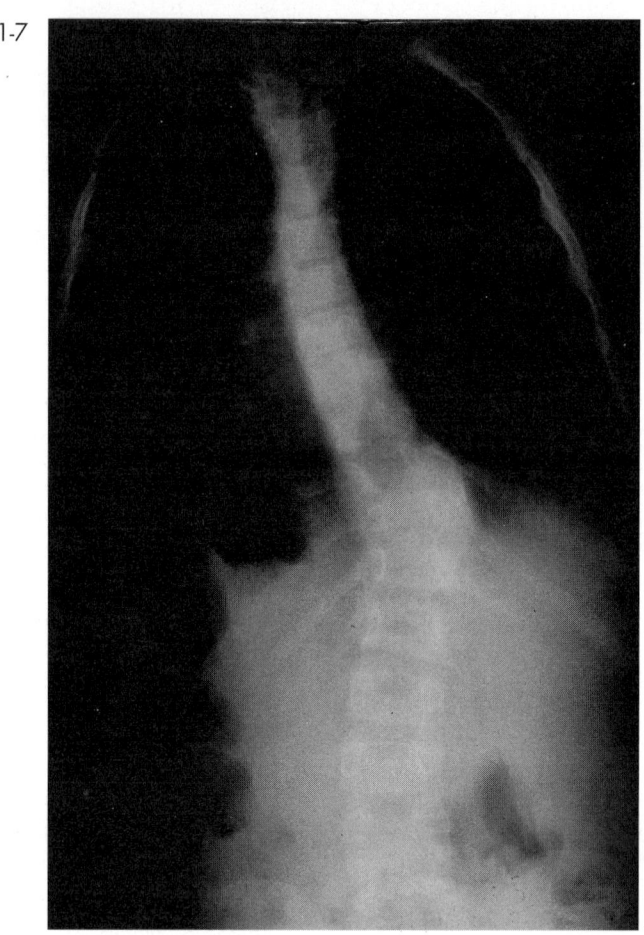

Fig 1-7

70 The patient in Q69 is a 6-year-old girl. How do you think the scoliosis might best be managed?

71 When you see the patient, it becomes obvious that the family had no previous knowledge about the possibility of an underlying disorder. Your letter to the referring physician should suggest that the patient be referred to specialists in what other fields?

72 The patient described in Q70 has a bowing deformity of her right tibia. Her referring physician has suggested that the family should ask you about an operation to straighten the leg, since you will be evaluating the child's spine. You reply:

73 An 11-year-old boy falls from his bicycle, sustaining a knee injury with immediate effusion. The anterior drawer test is positive. You suspect:

ANSWERS

69 This sharply angulated curve, spanning only approximately four segments, should remind you of the dysplastic scoliosis associated with neurofibromatosis type 1.

70 NF dysplastic scoliosis has never been shown to respond to bracing. If the curve progresses, surgical management should be advised.

71 NF can have manifestations in any organ system; neurology, ophthalmology, and genetics consultation should be obtained. Audiology, psychology, plastic surgery, and other subspecialty consultation may be needed. Multidisciplinary clinics are available at some centers; listings of those clinics can be obtained from the Neurofibromatosis Foundation.

72 This deformity represents the least severe variation of tibial pseudarthrosis associated with neurofibromatosis. Osteotomy is contraindicated; as the condition will likely never heal, but will convert the situation into a frank pseudarthrosis. The usual recommendation is to support the tibia with an orthosis until skeletal maturity, after which the incidence of fracture is much less.

73 This history is absolutely classic for tibial spine avulsion. This injury is the childhood equivalent of an anterior cruciate ligament rupture. No one knows why so many of these injuries happen with a fall from a bicycle.

QUESTIONS

74 A 9-year-old boy sustains a twisting injury to the knee. He describes repeated buckling, which is associated with brief sharp pain. On examination you can reproduce the pain by extending the knee from a fully flexed position with the tibia internally rotated. A similar test, but with the tibia externally rotated, does not cause pain. You suspect:

75 A 10-year-old soccer player sustains knee trauma with immediate effusion. On examination you find an extensor lag; available active extension is weak. The radiograph is shown (*Figure 1-8*). This injury is:

Fig 1-8

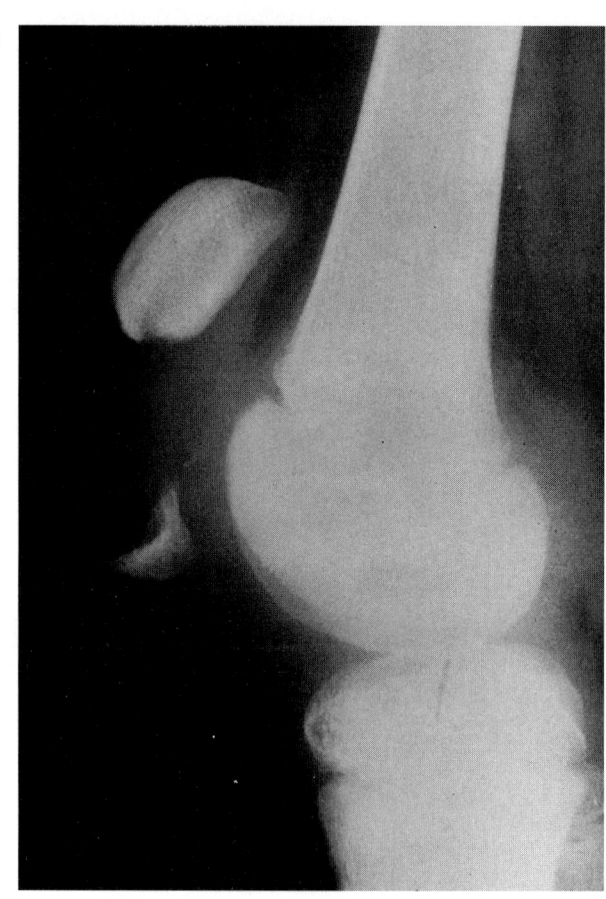

ANSWERS

74 This positive Wilson's test is suggestive of an osteochondritis dissecans lesion.

75 A patellar "sleeve" fracture. The patellar ligament (tendon) avulses a sleeve of cartilage with a small rim of subchondral bone. During surgery the amount of cartilage avulsed is often surprisingly large.

QUESTIONS

76   A 4-year-old girl is struck on the leg by a falling table. The radiograph is shown (*Figure 1-9*). As this fracture heals, what deformity might occur?

Fig 1-9

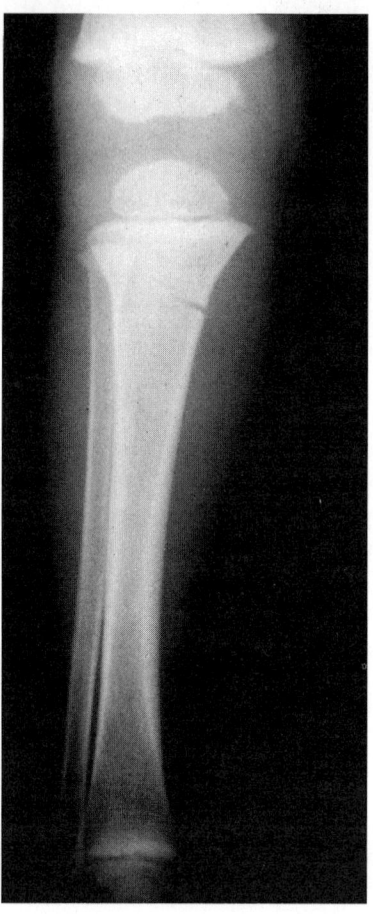

77   How do you propose to manage the deformity?

ANSWERS

76 Progressive valgus at the proximal tibia.

77 Most of these deformities will spontaneously correct over approximately 5 years. Osteotomy in this young age group may precipitate recurrent valgus deformity and should be deferred.

QUESTION

78 A 14-year-old is beginning her first season of cross-country running. She complains of activity-related pain at the proximal tibia. The radiograph is shown (*Figure 1-10*). You advise:

Fig 1-10

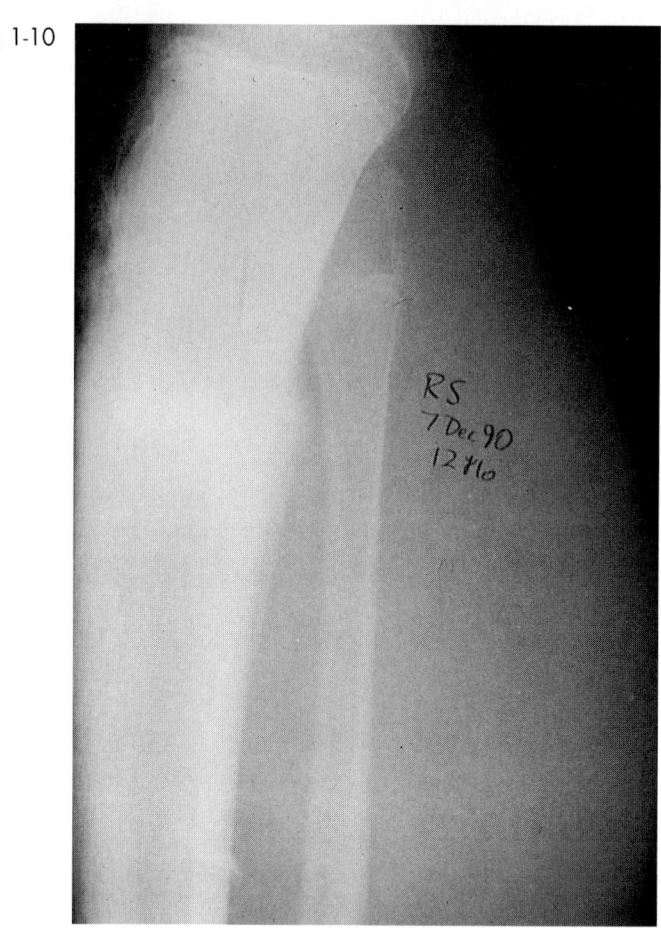

ANSWER

78 Healing of this stress fracture will occur if the patient can be maintained pain free for approximately 6 weeks. This may simply require avoidance of running. Sometimes crutches or a brace (knee immobilizer) are necessary. Casting is rarely needed, other than as an "anchor" to enforce rest in the adolescent.

QUESTIONS

79 A 10-year-old complains of medial pain, popping, and repeated buck-ling of the ankle. The radiograph is shown (*Figure 1-11*). You advise:

Fig 1-11

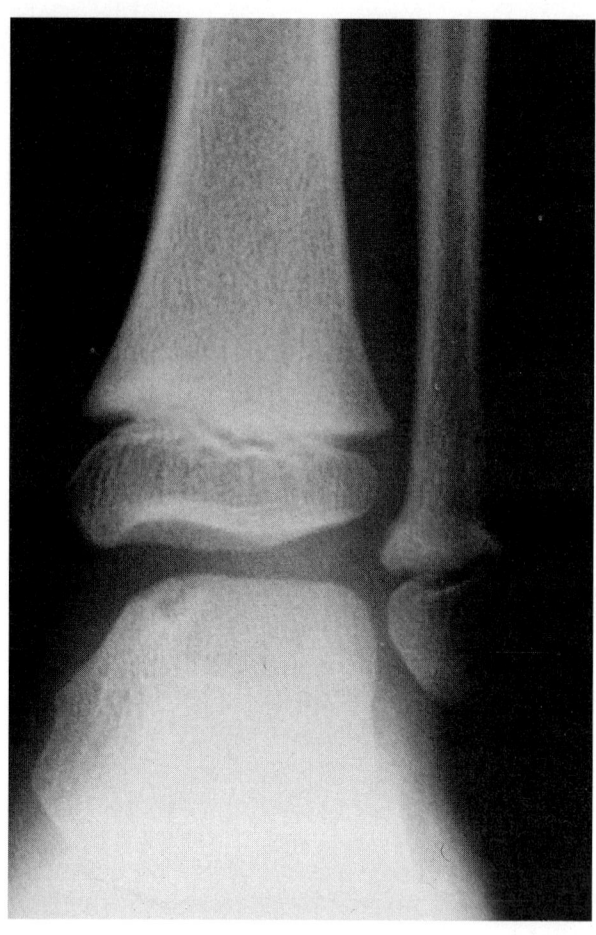

80 An 8-year-old sustains an inversion injury to the ankle. The patient complains of lateral foot pain. You suspect:

81 Suppose the patient from Q80 was complaining of lateral ankle pain?

82 A 14-year-old girl is beginning her first season of cross-country run-ning. She complains of pain at the proximal tibia that awakens her from sound sleep. The radiograph is almost identical to that shown for Q78. You advise:

83 A 4-year-old boy, first child for this family, is evaluated because of a new difficulty walking up stairs; his parents say that he "hangs on the bannister." His preschool teacher has reported that he is the slow-est runner in the class: last year he was usually in the middle of the group. You begin to think of:

84 As you interviewed this patient's parents, the boy was playing on the examination room floor. You ask him to "stand up" for examination. You watch for:

ANSWERS

79   Often a nondisplaced osteochondritis dissecans of the talus will heal with cast immobilization. Those that do not and displaced lesions need surgical management.

80   Avulsion of the base of the fifth MT, or an actual fracture of the fifth MT.

81   In this age group a Salter I separation of physis of the distal fibula would be more common than an "ankle sprain." The exact location of the tenderness should be your guide, even if the radiograph is unremarkable. Treatment should include immobilization with a cast. Because physeal injuries, especially if nondisplaced, heal rapidly, 3 weeks of immobilization with a short leg walking cast is usually sufficient.

82   Spontaneous pain that awakens the patient from sound sleep should make you worry about neoplasm. This patient needs careful evaluation and appropriate imaging studies. Unless you regularly manage bone tumors, you should refer the patient before biopsy.

83   Progressive neuromuscular disorders, such as muscular dystrophy or spinal muscular atrophy.

84   Gowers' sign (or maneuver), indicating pelvic girdle muscle weakness. A positive Gowers' sign is present if the child cannot rise to the standing position without using his hands, but must use his upper extremities to push or "climb" his legs to stand.

QUESTIONS

85 Your suspicions are increased as you complete the physical examination. The parents ask if there is a blood test you could order to diagnose the problem.

86 The blood test agrees with your suspicions. You and the child's neurologist now request a specimen of another tissue. What changes might you see on that sample?

87 Four years pass. Despite physical therapy and bracing, the boy from Q83 has developed contractures at the ankle and hip that are interfering with walking. How might you help?

88 The patient from Q83 has spinal muscular atrophy. At age 10, he uses a wheelchair as his primary means of ambulation. He has developed a long, sweeping scoliosis measuring 30 degrees. You recommend:

89 You are called to the nursery to see an infant who is not spontaneously moving her right upper extremity. As you wait for the elevator, you think about a differential diagnosis that includes:

90 The infant in Q89 has normal radiographs. As you observe her, you see that she does, in fact, move her fingers into flexion and extension. She does not abduct or externally rotate the shoulder and does not flex her elbow. She has a/an:

91 You meet the parents of the infant in Q90. Your treatment recommendation at this point should be:

92 The parents of the infant in Q89 ask about the chances for recovery. You tell them:

93 Consider a situation as in Q89. As you examine the infant you see that she seems a bit "cross-eyed," her right pupil is a bit small, and the right eyelid is lower than the left. What does this tell you about the prognosis?

ANSWERS

85 Major elevation of the creatine phosphokinase (CPK) level is very suggestive of a muscular dystrophy. Acutely, this enzyme may be elevated to 200 times laboratory normal.

86 Muscle biopsy is frequently requested. If the child has a primary muscle disorder, presumably muscular dystrophy, classic findings would include fiber size variation, fiber type disproportion, branching of fibers, necrosis of fibers or groups of fibers, phagocytosis, and replacement of muscle fibers by fat.

87 Patients having muscular dystrophy frequently develop ankle equinus contractures. Tendo Achilles lengthening is usually considered. Because of relative preservation of the tibialis posterior, some authors have advocated rerouting the tibialis posterior tendon through the interosseus membrane to the dorsum of the foot. At the hip, contracture of the tensor fascia/iliotibial band creates flexion and abduction. Percutaneous release of the origin of the tensor fascia muscle, along with percutaneous section of the iliotibial (IT) band distally, can relieve the contracture. Percutaneous technique is preferable to formal open Ober and Yount procedures because the patient must be rapidly mobilized—SAME DAY!—after surgery to prevent loss of strength.

88 Once the patient becomes confined to the wheelchair, progression of the scoliosis is essentially inevitable. The primary disease also causes a decline in respiratory function. Bracing may be used to delay surgery but is not effective as definitive management of the scoliosis. Spinal fusion should be considered relatively early, before the concomitant deterioration in pulmonary function poses an unacceptably high surgical risk.

89 Brachial plexus palsy and various birth fractures, such as clavicle or humerus break or rupture.

90 Erb's palsy (upper brachial plexus palsy).

91 Passive exercises to maintain the range of motion of all right upper extremity joints. Prolonged splinting in abduction and external rotation is not favored because of possible secondary shoulder dislocation.

92 The majority of brachial plexus palsies (approximately 80%) will resolve spontaneously. The majority of the recovery will take place in the first 3 to 6 months, although continued spontaneous improvement may be seen up to 18 months.

93 Horner's syndrome implies a proximal (root level) nerve injury with poor prognosis for spontaneous recovery. Phrenic nerve paralysis is similarly a poor prognostic sign.

QUESTIONS

94 An infant identical to Q89 is brought to you. This time, consider that the initial radiographs show a right midshaft humerus fracture. You recommend:

95 You are asked to see an infant with multiple fractures. Radiographs are shown (*Figure 1-12*). How do you plan to advise treatment?

Fig 1-12

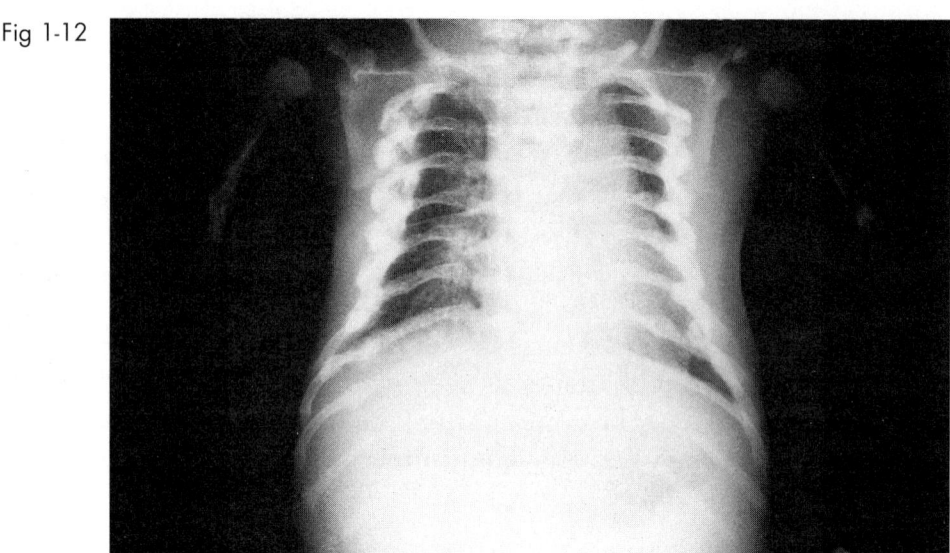

96 What is the molecular defect in this condition?

97 A 4-month-old infant has three long bone fractures. The skull films are normal. Sclerae are of normal hue. Inflicted trauma is suggested. You are asked if there is any other laboratory test that might help rule out a genetic brittle bone disorder.

ANSWERS

94 Birth fracture of the humerus is second only to clavicle fractures in frequency. Treatment is gentle splinting of the arm against the child's chest for approximately 2 weeks. Examples might be strapping with cast padding, reinforcing with a piece of burn netting, or an Ace wrap. Associated nerve palsy invariably resolves spontaneously in 6 to 8 weeks. Fracture angulation corrects with growth.

95 The radiograph is consistent with a severe, congenital form of osteogenesis imperfecta. The infant can be managed on an "egg crate" or similar soft mattress. Rigid cast immobilization of all the fractures is impractical and unnecessary. Gentle splinting of selected fractures, such as cast padding and an elastic bandage, may be helpful for pain control. Deformity is inevitable in these severe cases.

96 Failure of maturation of collagen with inadequate progressive crosslinking.

97 It is possible to analyze collagen produced by fibroblasts obtained from a skin punch biopsy. Failure of these fibroblasts to produce collagen polypeptide would help with a diagnosis of osteogenesis imperfecta.

QUESTIONS

98   You are asked to evaluate an infant who has a fractured humerus. This family's previous child died in infancy; presumably of sudden infant death syndrome (SIDS), although an autopsy was never performed. Social Services now suspects inflicted trauma in the current case, also with the obvious questions about the previous child's death. As you look at the radiographs (*Figure 1-13*), can you help the distraught parents?

Fig 1-13

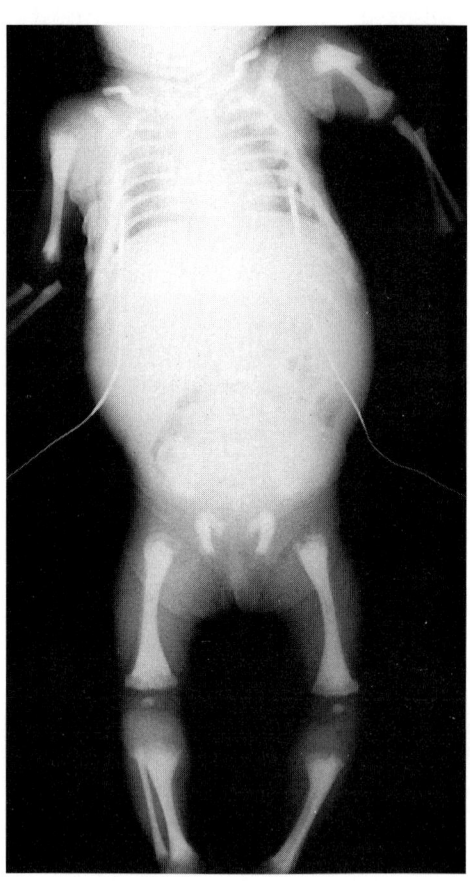

99   Beyond fracture treatment, what may be more important in treatment of this infant's underlying condition?

100   A 1-year old infant is brought to your office for evaluation of a "bow-leg" deformity. The child reportedly began walking early, at age 9 months. You find mild bilateral internal tibial torsion. The knees are stable and painless. You measure approximately 15 degrees of genu varum bilaterally. A recent abdominal radiograph, taken for complaints of constipation, shows the hips to be normal for age. Do you need more radiographs?

101   The child from Q100 returns to see you at age 24 months. Now you measure 20 degrees of genu varum bilaterally. Do you need to see radiographs now?

ANSWERS

98 This infant probably has the congenita (autosomal recessive, sometimes called "malignant") type of osteopetrosis with abnormally brittle bones. The current fracture may have indeed occurred with normal handling. The previous child might well have had the same disorder, accounting for the early death.

99 Bone marrow transplantation may be curative.

100 Probably not. Mild physiologic genu varum is normal at this age.

101 Yes. By now there should have been some spontaneous correction, sometimes even overcorrection into valgus.

QUESTIONS

102 The radiograph is shown (*Figure 1-14*). How will you treat this condition?

Fig 1-14

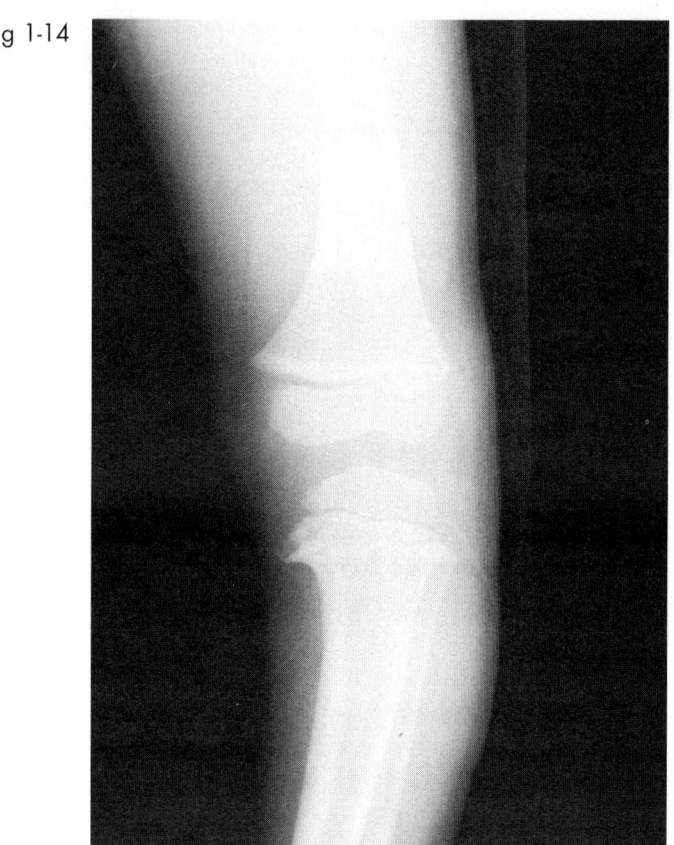

103 The parents are horrified at the idea of having their child's legs braced, and they leave. About 3 years later they return. With this new radiograph (*Figure 1-15*), how will you treat this condition?

Fig 1-15

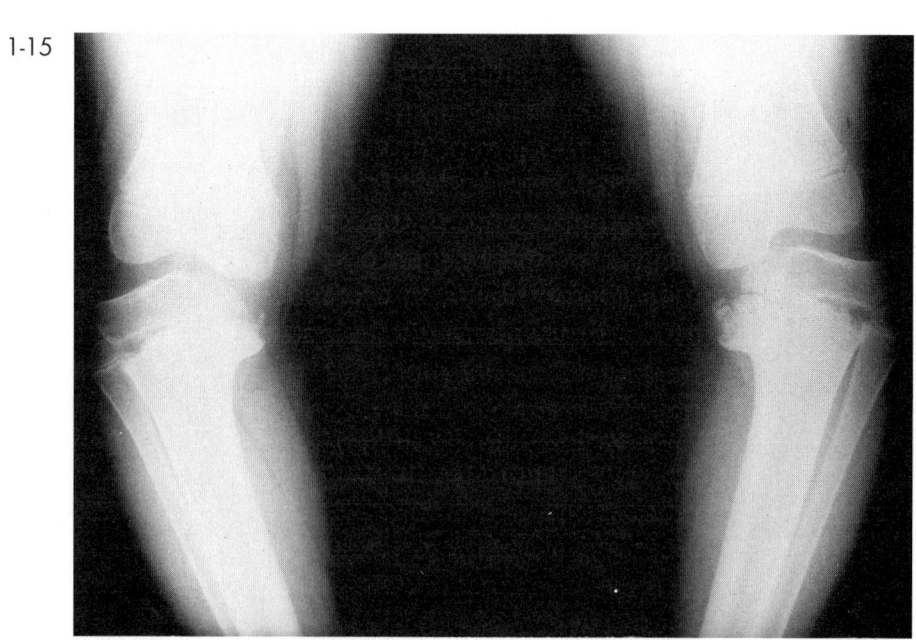

ANSWERS

102 In this age group at this stage of Blount's disease, bracing is appropriate. Bracing is appropriate in the 24- to 36-month age group, when the process is radiographically in Stage I or Stage II. Surgery is generally reserved for cases in which the disorder progresses despite bracing, for patients of age 4 years or more, and for radiographic Stage III and beyond.

103 At this point, surgical intervention is indicated. The usual recommendation is for valgus producing osteotomy of the proximal tibia. A single osteotomy has an excellent chance (83%) of providing lasting correction if performed before the age of 5 years.

QUESTIONS

104 Suppose a case similar to Q103 except that the child returns at age 8 years. The "stage" of the disorder is as you might expect for this age group. What additional situations must you consider as you plan corrective surgery?

105 You are asked to evaluate an infant who has a unilateral foreshortened thigh with mild limitation of adduction and extension at the ipsilateral hip. A radiograph shows a markedly dysplastic acetabulum. The femoral diaphysis is much shorter than the contralateral femur and tapers to a point proximally. What do you expect on ultrasound examination of the hip?

106 The patient from Q105 has associated hypoplasia of the ipsilateral fibula with ankle instability. The foot is hypoplastic with absence of the two lateral rays. The overall shortening of the affected limb places the foot at the level of the contralateral knee. Your long-term ideas for definitive management would include:

107 The patient from Q105 has an adequate ipsilateral fibula so that the ankle is stable. The foot is essentially normal. The shortening is such that the foot is at the level of the contralateral knee. In this scenario, what additional option is available for definitive management?

108 Consider the more severe case where the acetabulum and femoral head are absent and the femur is represented only by a distal tuft of metaphysis. For definitive management, how might you compensate for the resulting instability at the hip?

109 Consider the situation described in Q108, except that the deformity is bilateral. Your thoughts for definitive management now include:

110 A 12-year-old spina bifida patient complains of occasional back pain and has scoliosis measured at 32 degrees. Six months ago the curve measured only 20 degrees. Your thoughts:

111 A 1-year-old spina bifida patient, with high lumbar functional level, has a congenital vertical talus deformity of one foot. Stretching and casting have been ineffective. Your treatment team agrees that surgical correction is desirable to facilitate standing the child in braces. Your operation might include:

112 A 6-year-old patient who has trisomy 21 asks for evaluation of neck pain. What studies will you request? Why?

113 The patient from Q112 has 7 mm of atlantoaxial motion documented on the flexion and extension radiographs. You recommend:

ANSWERS

104 The medial tibial physis may have fused. In addition to corrective angular osteotomy, it may be necessary to either resect the medial physeal bar or actually perform epiphyseodesis of the lateral proximal tibia and the fibula. Linear tomograms, computerized axial tomography (CAT) scanning, MRI, or single photon computed tomography (SPECT) scan may give the critical information.

105 This is proximal femoral focal deficiency, Aitken Type C. Given that the femoral diaphyseal shaft is present and tapered, even though short, you would expect a cartilaginous femoral head to be present within the dysplastic acetabulum. Sometimes it may be absent. When present, it would not be expected to move with the femoral shaft. If the femur were represented only by the most distal tuft of metaphysis, as in Aitkin type D, then you might not find any femoral head.

106 Ablation of the foot (Syme's amputation), fusion of the knee, and prosthetic fitting as a knee disarticulation or an above-knee amputation.

107 The van Ness rotation plasty of the tibia could allow the ankle to function as a knee for more efficient prosthetic fitting.

108 In some cases the stump of femur has been flexed 90 degrees and fused to the pelvis for stability. The anatomic knee then substitutes as a hip.

109 No intervention. Patients with bilateral deformity are often quite agile and function well, despite the shortening and cosmetic appearance.

110 The rapid increase in the curve with pain should alert you to possible problems in the neural axis: shunt malfunction, Arnold-Chiari deformity, syringomyelia, or tethered spinal cord.

111 Excision of the navicular to shorten the medial column of the foot. In the paralytic situation, this is often simpler to perform with less risk to soft tissue than other corrective procedures.

112 It will be necessary to obtain cervical spine radiographs, specifically to include lateral views in maximum flexion and in maximum extension. Between 15% to 20% of patients having the Down syndrome may have C1-C2 instability. Additionally, occipitoatlantal instability has been described in the Down syndrome population.

113 Normal motion should be 4 mm or less. Most authors would consider C1-C2 fusion if motion is 10 mm or more, even in asymptomatic patients. Between 5 mm and 9 mm seems to be a "gray area," and asymptomatic sedentary patients may be observed. Because the patient from Q112 has symptoms of neck pain, fusion should be offered at 7 mm of motion.

QUESTIONS

114 A 4-year-old patient who has trisomy 21 comes to you with presenting symptoms that include an increasing limp, intermittent refusal to walk, and a frequent audible "pop" at the left groin. You should suspect:

115 An 8-year-old boy comes to you with symptoms of intermittent neck pain. On his cervical spine radiographs you see a hypoplastic dens. There is an ossicle above the dens that seems to move with the anterior arch of C1 on lateral flexion and extension films. What will you recommend?

116 The parents of the patient in Q115 ask what might have caused this condition. You would answer:

117 A 1-month-old infant has held her face turned toward the right since birth. There has been no trauma. She has not been systemically ill. You notice her facial asymmetry. In addition to limited motion (rotation), what do you expect to find as you examine her neck?

118 Yes, but on which side is the affected muscle located?

119 Do you need to biopsy this mass?

120 You are called to the phone before you finish examining this child. The family leaves the office. Because of unfortunate social situations, the patient from Q117 is not evaluated again until age 3 years. She still holds her head with the face turned toward the right. Your treatment recommendation now is:

121 As you evaluate the child from Q120, you find that she walks with a painless limp. The bench examination confirms asymmetry of the thighs and unilateral limitation of hip abduction. She probably has:

122 A 7-year-old boy has a 1-week history of a neck deformity. He holds his head turned with the chin toward the left shoulder and the right ear depressed toward the right shoulder. Two weeks ago he was treated for a severe sore throat. Radiographic studies do not show any anterior shift at C1-C2. Your initial orthopedic treatment should include:

123 A 7-year-old boy has come to you with the same clinical deformity as in Q122. This patient's wryneck began 2 months ago, after a fall. Radiographic studies show approximately 25% anterior shift of C1 on C2. Your treatment plan is:

ANSWERS

114   Spontaneous, or "habitual," subluxation of the hip. Some (perhaps 4% or 5%) Down syndrome patients can truly dislocate the hip, presumably as a result of generalized ligamentous laxity.

115   C1-C2 fusion. If there is any question about the competency of the posterior arch of C1, fusion to the occiput may be necessary.

116   Most authorities believe that the os odontoideum is caused by trauma. This is mildly controversial, in that some argue in favor of a congenital etiology.

117   A localized firm mass (the "olive") in the substance of the sternocleidomastoid muscle.

118   If the patient's face is turned toward the right, then the left sternocleidomastoid muscle is expected to be abnormal.

119   With such a typical presentation, no. It can be observed. The patient should be treated by positioning to encourage her to turn toward the left (toys, bottle, etc.). Gently passive stretching exercises for the neck should be advised.

120   Surgical release or lengthening of the left sternocleidomastoid muscle. Nonoperative methods generally do not work in this age group.

121   A hip dislocation. Approximately 20% of infants with congenital muscular torticollis will also have hip dysplasia.

122   Peritonsillar abscess must be considered in this setting. Assuming that has been excluded, orthopedic management may include hospitalization for traction, analgesics, and muscle relaxants. After reduction, a cervical brace may be continued until all symptoms subside.

123   Traction may be tried, but when the deformity has been present for this long, there is a low success rate from nonoperative methods. A C1-C2 fusion will probably be necessary.

QUESTIONS

124 A high school football player is evaluated for persistent anterior thigh pain several weeks after an especially violent tackle. His radiograph is shown (*Figure 1-16*). Should you biopsy this lesion?

Fig 1-16

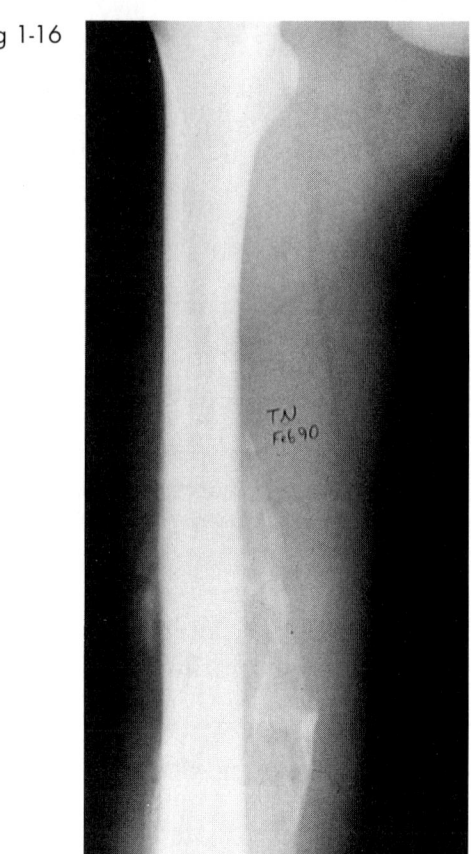

125 Three months later the patient can still feel the mass in his thigh and occasionally complains of local pain. He requests excision. You advise:

ANSWERS

124 This is a typical history and a typical radiograph for posttraumatic myositis ossificans. One typical finding is that the outer circumference of the mass is radiographically more mature than the center. A biopsy is not necessary and, in fact, might be mistaken for a malignancy.

125 Excision at this point might simply lead to a recurrence of the process. These lesions typically require nearly a year to mature sufficiently to permit successful excision. Activity seen on a technetium 99m bone scan is a good guide; the area of myositis should show no greater uptake than the adjacent normal bone.

QUESTIONS

126 A junior high school athlete competes in the hurdles. He complains of a sudden "pop" and then persistent pain in the groin. A radiograph is shown (*Figure 1-17*). Do you need to surgically repair this lesion?

Fig 1-17

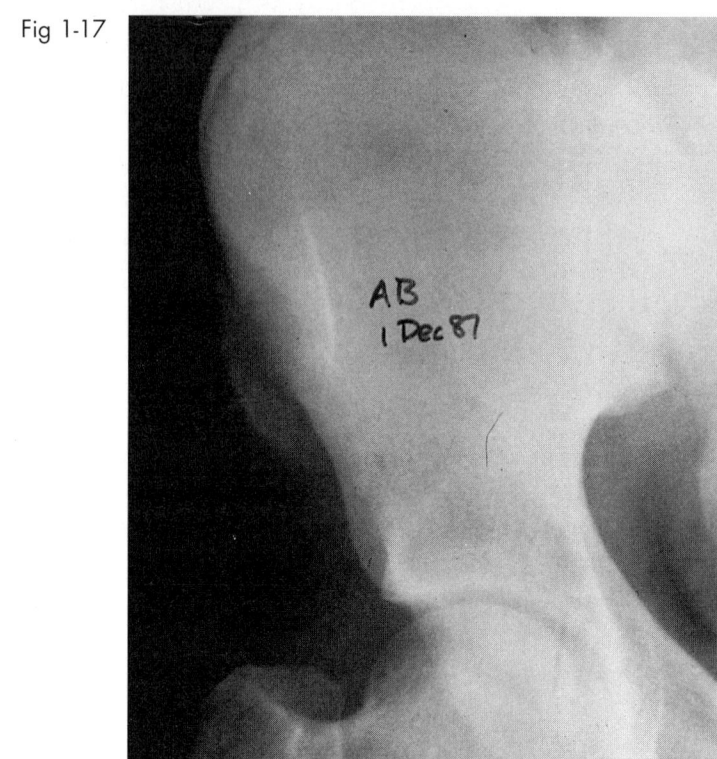

127 You are planning a hip reconstructive procedure for a severely involved, institutionalized patient with spastic quadriplegia. Postoperatively, 4 to 6 weeks of immobilization in a spica cast will be needed. Discuss some of your concerns about this patient's preoperative nutrition.

128 You perform a hip stabilization procedure for a patient who has spina bifida. Approximately 6 hours later you are called by the nurse who reports that your patient is complaining of a severe headache with nausea. What do you suspect is happening?

ANSWERS

126 No. The customary treatment of avulsion fractures of the pelvis is relative rest for approximately 2 weeks, followed by functional rehabilitation.

127 Most of these patients may be said to have a "pentaplegia" in that their cerebral palsy affects the musculature of the head and neck, as well as the rest of their body. Feeding difficulties may be caused by an inability to effectively chew or swallow. There may be incompetent gastroesophageal (GE) sphincter function with chronic reflux. Barium swallow or upper gastrointestinal (GI) studies can be helpful, as can pH studies of the GE junction. Constipation is a common problem. Body weight and general appearance should be assessed. Poor healing and higher complication rates have been associated with serum albumin less than 3.5 mg% and absolute neutrophil count less than 1500. A nutritional and dietary consultation should be considered.

128 You should call the neurosurgeon immediately. Almost all spina bifida patients have some degree of hydrocephalus, and most have indwelling ventricular shunts. Even with a normal preoperative screening, cerebrospinal fluid (CSF) flow may be marginally sufficient. The changes in CSF dynamics, which occur during and after general anesthesia, can precipitate acute hydrocephalus.

QUESTION

129   A 7-year-old comes to you with bilateral worsening genu valgum (*Figure 1-18*). Your differential diagnosis should include:

Fig 1-18

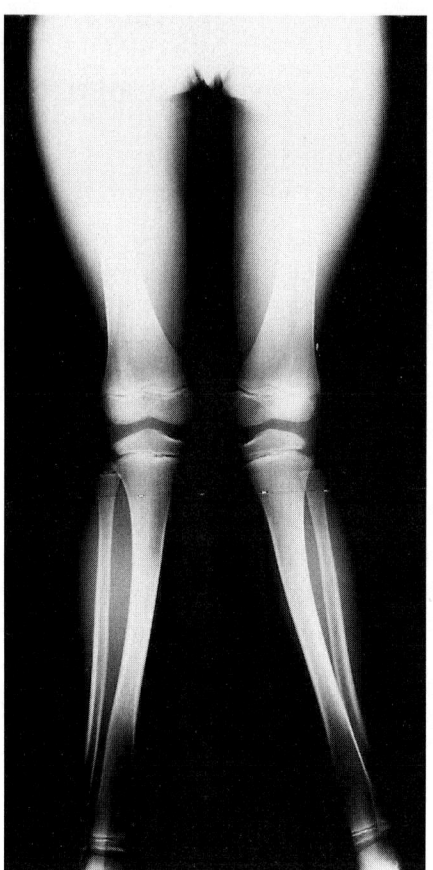

ANSWER

129   By age 7, the angular alignment of the lower extremities should be stable. Progressive genu valgum should alert you to the possible rachitic syndromes. In this country the most common type would be secondary to renal abnormalities.

QUESTIONS

130 A 6-year-old patient is referred with a 3-week history of vague neck pain. There has been no trauma. His neurologic examination is totally normal. He is not febrile, his peripheral WBC count is normal, and his ESR is not elevated. The referring physician sends along radiographs (*Figure 1-19*) and an MRI study (*Figure 1-20*). At the top of your mental list of differential diagnoses is:

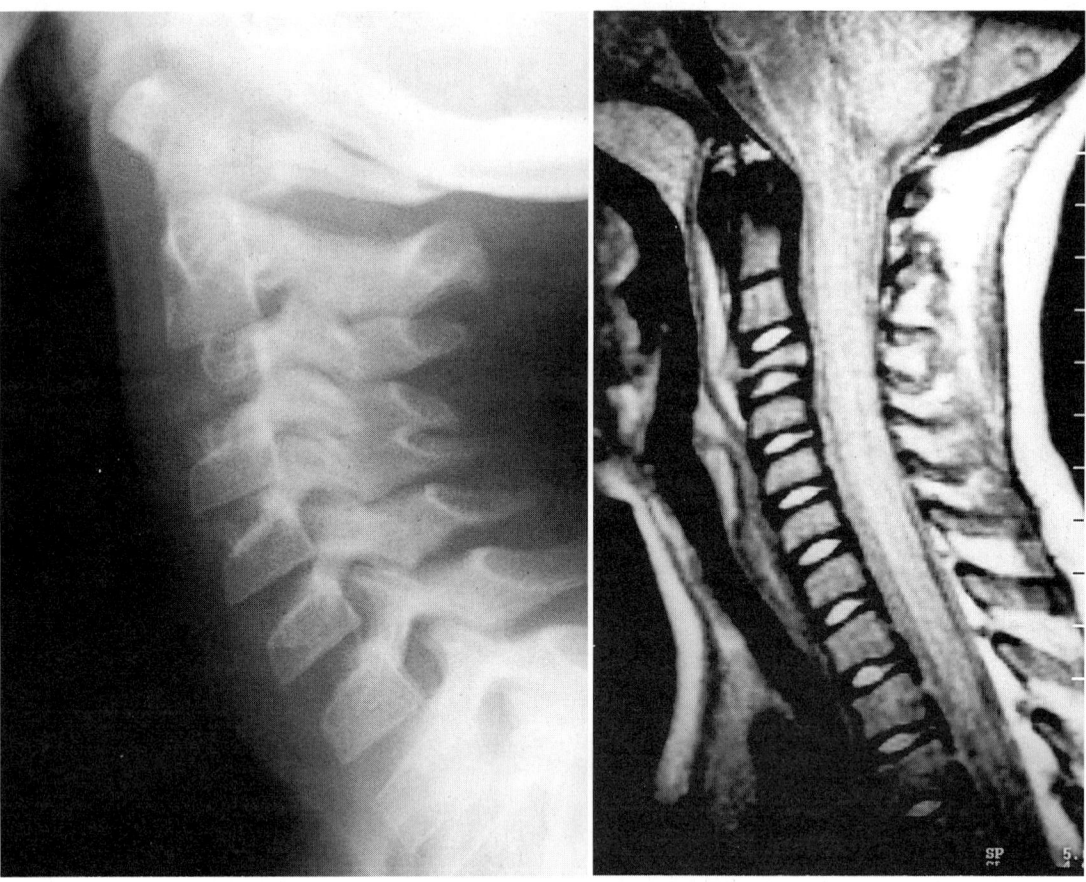

Fig 1-19   Fig 1-20

131 You request a skeletal survey for this patient. The insurance company objects. You explain your rationale:

132 An 8-year-old girl has recently joined a summer soccer league and has purchased her first pair of soccer shoes. She now complains of heel pain. The tenderness is at the posteroinferior aspect of the calcaneal tuberosity. The lateral radiograph shows only that the calcaneal apophysis is irregular and sclerotic. You tell the family:

ANSWERS

130 The vertebra plana at C3 is probably due to eosinophilic granuloma (EG).

131 EG is not always an isolated process. Other occult lesions should be sought. EG classically does not show increased uptake on technetium 99m bone scan, so that multiple plain radiographs are needed.

132 This is a repetitive stress injury, typically exacerbated by the low heel of a soccer shoe. Clinically this can be called Sever's disease. The radiographic irregularity of the apophysis may be a normal finding, and the greatest value of the radiograph is to rule out other abnormalities. Treatment should include activity modifications, heel cord stretching, and ankle dorsiflexor strengthening. Shoe modifications such as a semi-rigid heel pad or a heel cup are often helpful.

QUESTIONS

133 You performed reconstructive surgery a few weeks ago for a patient with severe cerebral palsy and chronic painful hip dislocation. Soft-tissue releases and open reduction were performed, along with pelvic and femoral osteotomy. Now your patient seems to have new onset of severe pain with any attempted motion of the operated hip. The area is indurated and slightly warm. The patient is not febrile, and the peripheral WBC count is not elevated. The radiographs are unchanged. Possibilities include:

134 This is, in fact, HO. How will you manage the patient?

ANSWERS

133 Infection certainly must be at the top of your differential list. However, the onset of heterotopic ossification (HO) can be clinically identical.

134 Gentle physical therapy and nonsteroidal antiinflammatory medications are indicated. As with any HO the process must fully mature before excision can be performed without an unacceptable recurrence rate.

CHAPTER 2

Tumors

Theodore C. Yee
Douglas J. McDonald
Michael H. McGuire

QUESTIONS

1 The patient is a 19-year-old man who complains of vague pain in his right shoulder. This pain has been present for several years. There is no history of trauma. His radiograph is shown (*Figure 2-1*). Is this likely to be a benign or malignant lesion?

Fig 2-1

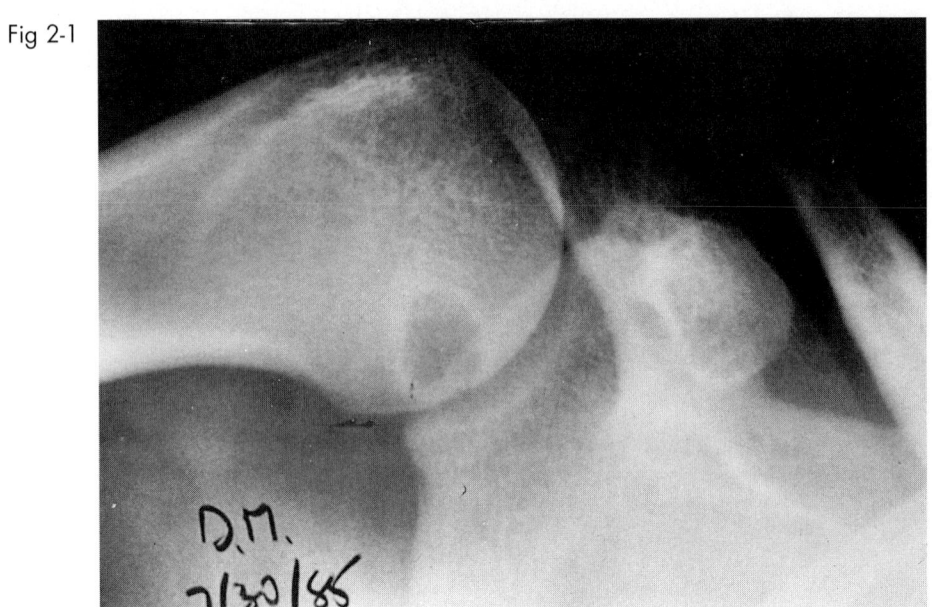

2 How can one differentiate a benign from a malignant lesion by viewing radiographs?

3 With what symptoms do patients with musculoskeletal tumors present?

4 How does the finding of a soft-tissue mass in association with a bone tumor affect the evaluation of the patient?

5 Which two clinical features lead most directly to the diagnosis in a patient with a bone tumor?

ANSWERS

1 Benign.

2 Conventional radiographs are best at predicting the diagnosis in patients with skeletal neoplasms. In a benign process the host bone responds by developing a rim of reactive bone around the neoplasm. This development results in a sharp margin between the lesion and the surrounding bone. Malignant lesions, however, have a broad zone of transition and cause permeative destruction of bone with little or no host bone response. When solid and dense, periosteal new bone-suggests a benign lesion. An expansile appearance with elevated periosteal new bone, as in a Codman's triangle, is suggestive of a more aggressive or malignant lesion.

3 The majority of patients have symptoms of pain or a mass. Occasionally the patient may have a pathologic fracture, which can occur through either a primary or metastatic lesion. The presence of symptoms for many years suggests a more benign lesion, although this is not always the case. For example, synovial sarcomas may be present for many years before being diagnosed.

4 A soft-tissue mass as part of a bone tumor usually suggests that the tumor is malignant. A tumor arising in a bone must destroy the cortex and elevate or transgress the periosteum to produce a soft-tissue mass. Destruction of a bony cortex is a remarkable cellular and biologic event consistent with or demonstrating the features of a malignant lesion. Therefore this finding demands a full staging work-up of the patient to define the local extent of the tumor and to rule out any evidence of systemic disease.

5 The age of the patient and location of the lesion in the bone. Many bone tumors tend to occur in well-recognized age groups. For example, solitary bone cysts, aneurysmal bone cysts, and osteochondromas are examples of lesions that occur almost exclusively in young persons, usually before skeletal maturity. Osteosarcoma and Ewing's sarcoma generally occur in the second or third decade of life. Giant cell tumors are rare before skeletal maturity. Chondrosarcoma and malignant fibrous histiocytoma are lesions of adulthood. Metastatic carcinoma and myeloma are rare before age 45. The site of the lesion is also helpful in the diagnosis. Giant cell tumor and chondroblastoma usually involve the epiphyseal region and subchondral bone. Ewing's sarcoma and adamantinoma have a predilection for a diaphyseal portion of bone. Osteosarcomas, as well as osteochondromas, aneurysmal bone cysts, and osteoblastomas, are generally metaphyseal in location. Some lesions, such as enchondroma, have a distinct distribution to the small bones of the hands and feet.

QUESTIONS

6 Discuss the imaging techniques that are available and used in the patient with a skeletal neoplasm.

7 What are the advantages of an MRI compared with a CT scan in evaluation of a musculoskeletal neoplasm?

8 How can laboratory tests assist in defining the diagnosis in a patient found to have a bone tumor by radiographs?

9 What skeletal lesions do not require biopsy?

10 A 16-year-old girl complains of pain in her proximal left leg. It wakes her at night and is relieved with aspirin. A CT scan of her tibia is shown. (*Figures 2-2A and 2-2B*). The corresponding histology is also shown. What is your diagnosis?

Fig 2-2 **A**

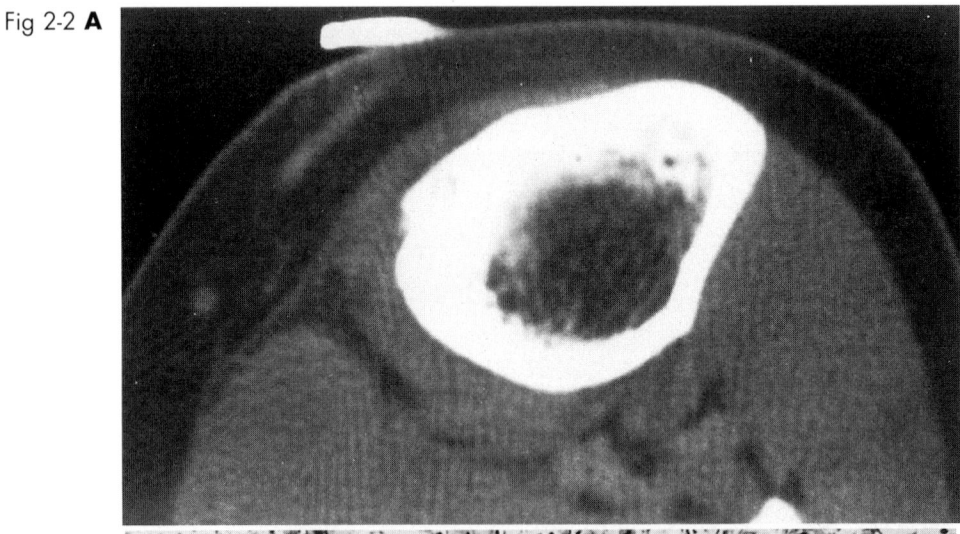

Fig 2-2 **B**

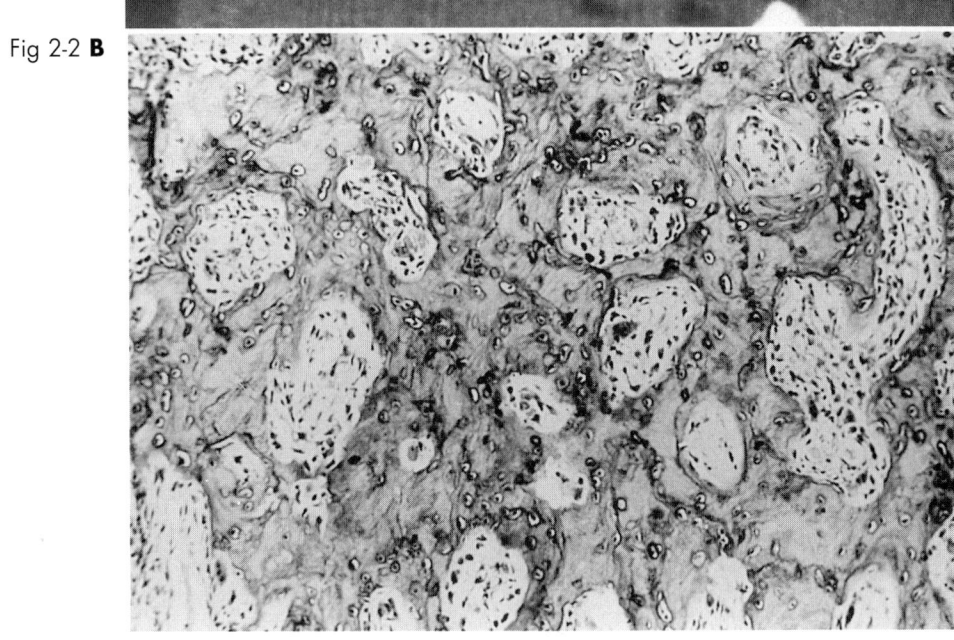

ANSWERS

6 Plain radiographs, computed tomography (CT), magnetic resonance imaging (MRI), and technetium 99m bone scanning are the most helpful imaging modalities. Bone scanning is used primarily to determine whether there are any other bony lesions and also to help determine a lesion's biologic activity. Lesions that appear benign by radiographs and have no increased uptake on bone scanning are most likely benign.

7 MRI is superior to CT in determining the intraosseous and extraosseous extent of a lesion. The intramedullary extent of the tumor can usually be seen in clear contrast to the high signal generated by normal marrow fat in a T1 weighted image. MRI is also superior to CT in illustrating soft tissue-lesions. Most soft-tissue masses, whether benign or malignant, will have a high signal on T2 weighted MR images. The signal for muscle, cortical bone, nerves, and vessels is low on T2 weighted images.

8 Most routine serum studies are normal in patients with skeletal lesions. The laboratory evaluation can rule out other categories of diseases that can affect the skeleton. Most infectious processes can be recognized when an elevated white blood cell (WBC) count and an elevated erythrocyte sedimentation rate (ESR) are present. A metabolic disease of bone would be unlikely in a patient with normal serum calcium, phosphorus, and alkaline phosphatase levels, as well as with normal renal function. In evaluating patients with metastatic disease or myeloma, laboratory tests can be helpful. Tumor specific antigens, such as a prostatic specific antigen, are elevated in patients with metastatic prostate cancer. Patients with myeloma have an abnormal serum or urine electrophoresis or may have hypercalcemia.

9 Lesions that may be observed include those that are discovered incidentally by x-ray films, those that are asymptomatic, those that do not predispose to pathologic fracture, and those that do not appear aggressive on radiographs. Such lesions include fibrous dysplasia, osteochondromas, enchondromas, fibrous cortical defects and nonossifying fibromas.

10 Osteoid osteoma. This is a clear example of when a CT scan is superior to MRI in evaluating a lesion. The CT scan shows excellent resolution of cortical and cancellous bony detail and demonstrates the nidus. Histologically, an osteoid osteoma is identical to an osteoblastoma (giant osteoid osteoma). The two lesions may be differentiated by size, with osteoblastomas greater than 1.5 cm in diameter. Both are characterized by a nidus of well differentiated osteoblasts and loosely arranged osteoid trabeculae. The margin of the nidus is well demarcated from the surrounding reactive bone. Osteoid osteomas can also occur in the spine and tend to involve the posterior elements.

QUESTIONS

11   How would you treat this patient?

12   A 16-year-old boy who injured his left knee 2 weeks ago while running complains of pain and swelling in the distal portion of his thigh. An anteroposterior (AP) radiograph is shown (*Figure 2-3A*). Is this lesion benign or malignant?

Fig 2-3 **A**

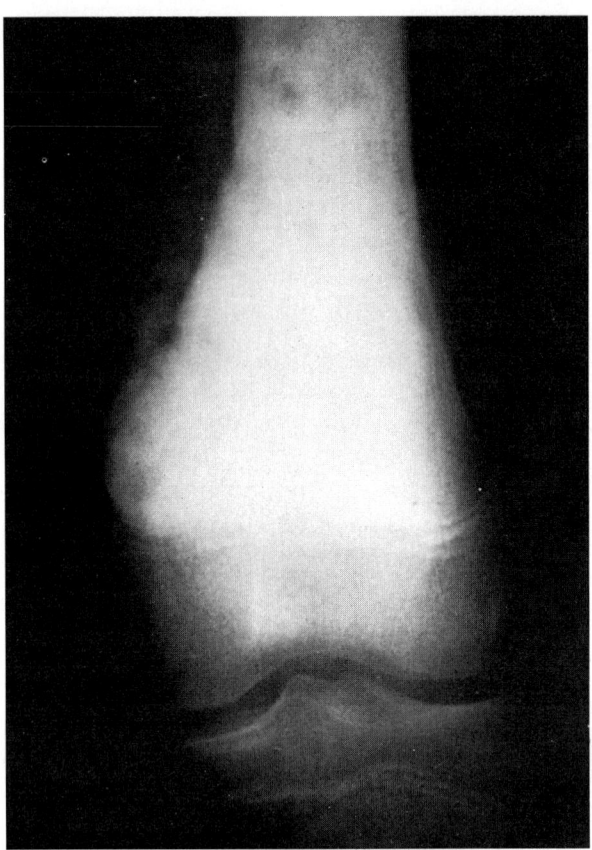

ANSWERS

11   Most symptomatic lesions deserve removal. The nidus must be completely resected. However, there have been reports of osteoid osteomas resolving spontaneously or with use of nonsteroidal, antiinflammatory medication.

12   Malignant. The radiograph demonstrates a radiodense lesion with a lack of reactive host bone suggesting an aggressive destructive lesion.

QUESTIONS

13 The histology is demonstrated (*Figure 2-3B*). What is your diagnosis?

Fig 2-3 **B**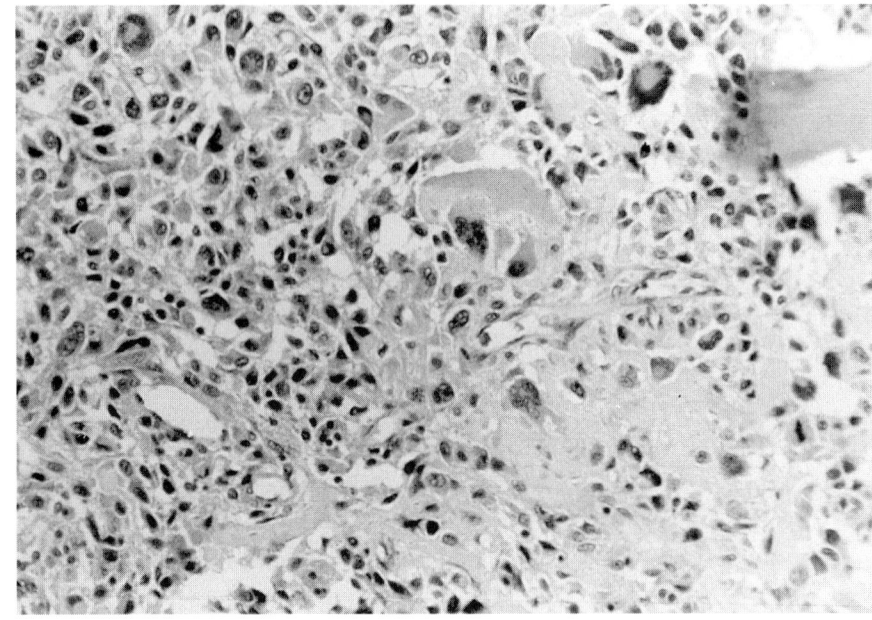

14 What is considered the appropriate management of this patient?

15 What is the expected local recurrence rate following surgical treatment of the osteosarcoma in this patient?

16 In addition to radiographs, a bone scan, an MRI of the lesion, and a chest CT scan, what other test is needed to stage this 16-year-old patient?

17 What biopsy techniques are appropriate in patients with bone tumors?

ANSWERS

13 Osteosarcoma. The histologic features demonstrate neoplastic new bone formation. The malignant cells are producing a matrix of osteoid. Osteosarcomas tend to be metaphyseal and occur at sites of rapid skeletal growth, which include the distal femur, the proximal tibia, the proximal humerus, and the proximal femur. The conventional intramedullary lesions are the most common and can be subclassified into osteoblastic, chondroblastic, or fibroblastic types depending on their predominant histologic pattern. In addition, a telangiectatic variant has been described. All of these high-grade lesions carry a similar prognosis. An important subset of osteosarcomas includes the surface

ANSWERS

lesions, examples of which are the parosteal, the periosteal, and the high-grade surface variants. Finally, a low-grade intramedullary lesion that can mimick fibrous dysplasia has been described.

14   Surgery plus chemotherapy. Historically, these tumors have been treated with ablative surgery of the affected limb, either with a wide or radical margin. In the last 20 years progress has been made in the area of limb sparing resection of the lesion. Limb salvage surgery represents a viable option (1) if a resection can be performed that achieves both a rate of local recurrence and a rate of patient survival equal to that of amputation, and (2) if a resection provides a superior functional result.

15   In the hands of experienced tumor surgeons, a local recurrence rate of approximately 5% occurs after a limb sparing resection with a wide surgical margin. This rate is comparable with that achieved with an amputation. The difference does not have a significant effect on overall patient survival. The functional results of a limb sparing resection compared with amputation and prosthetic fitting depend on the level of amputation required. For the distal tibia, a below knee amputation (BKA) with prosthetic fitting is preferred. However, for lesions of the proximal femur or pelvis requiring a hip disarticulation or hemipelvectomy, the results are significant functional loss; almost any reconstruction that preserves some limb function would be an improvement.

16   Biopsy. There are various ways to biopsy a tumor. Needle techniques, such as fine needle aspiration, and core devices, such as a Craig needle, are often appropriate. The closed needle techniques are useful for metastatic, spinal, and pelvic tumors, as well as for local recurrences or cystic lesions. Open incisional techniques are more likely to provide adequate tissue samples for accurate diagnosis.

17   The goal of the biopsy is to provide a histologic or tissue diagnosis. In a patient with a probable metastatic carcinoma, a needle aspirate and cytologic or cellular examination may be sufficient. Similarly, in a patient with an obvious osteosarcoma around the knee, sufficient tissue may be obtained with a core needle biopsy to confirm the diagnosis. An open biopsy may be incisional or excisional. An excisional biopsy removes the entire tumor as part of the biopsy and generally is used for benign tumors. An incisional biopsy creates a direct path from the skin to the lesion, hopefully without contamination of other tissue planes around the lesion. This is preferred for most malignant lesions and provides access to a sufficient amount of tumor tissue for whatever studies are needed.

QUESTIONS

18 When and how should an open biopsy be performed?

19 What is the most common staging system used for musculoskeletal tumors?

20 How are surgical margins classified in the management of tumors?

21 Can osteosarcomas arise on the surface of a bone?

22 What conditions of the skeleton predispose to the development of a sarcoma?

23 What is the role of chemotherapy in osteosarcoma?

24 What are the surgical indications for the use of an allograft bone transplant?

ANSWERS

18 A correctly placed biopsy is critical in the management of musculoskeletal neoplasms. A misplaced biopsy site may cause an unnecessary amputation. The biopsy tract must be placed so that it can be resected with the tumor. Transverse incisions on an extremity are contraindicated; they cannot be excised with longitudinal-directed segments of musculoskeletal tissue. In a bone lesion that contains a soft tissue extension, the extraosseous component should be biopsied because it provides the most rapidly growing and viable tissue. The soft tissue can be immediately cut with a frozen section technique.

19 The staging system developed by Enneking and the members of the Musculoskeletal Tumor Society. The system stages malignant lesions on the basis of their histologic grade and anatomic extent. Stage I lesions are low-grade malignant histologically and when confined to an anatomic compartment are stage I-A. If extracompartmental involvement is noted, they are stage I-B. Stage II lesions are high-grade malignant histologically and are either II-A or II-B, depending on their compartmental extent. Stage III lesions have regional or distant metastasis, regardless of their histologic grade or compartmental extent. A similar system exists for benign latent, active, and aggressive lesions.

ANSWERS

20 Surgical margins are classified as intralesional, marginal, wide, or radical. An intralesional margin occurs when surgical dissection is carried out within the substance of the tumor. A margin defined as marginal occurs when dissection is performed within the reactive zone adjacent to the tumor. A wide margin occurs through normal tissue outside the reactive zone of the tumor, generally one uninvolved tissue plane away. A radical margin occurs when excision of the entire compartment containing the tumor is performed.

21 Yes. Surface osteosarcomas can be parosteal, periosteal, or high-grade lesions. Parosteal are densely ossified lesions that characteristically are low grade and arise on posterior surface of the distal femur. Periosteal osteosarcomas are often cartilaginous in nature and are medium-grade malignancies. Occasionally, conventional high-grade lesions arise on the external surface of a bone.

22 Secondary osteosarcomas refer to lesions that have arisen at the site of a preexisting lesion, such as Paget's disease or fibrous dysplasia, or after radiation to a primary lesion. Similarly, chondrosarcomas arise frequently at the site of a pre-existing cartilage tumor. Sarcomas can also arise in a segment of bone affected by avascular necrosis.

23 Chemotherapy is now an accepted adjunct to surgical removal for all patients with high-grade conventional osteosarcoma. Methotrexate, cisplatin, doxorubicin, and ifosfamide have been found to be the most effective agents. Chemotherapy improves long-term survival in some groups of patients. Five-year survival rates of 60% are now reported, compared with the historical controls of 20% with surgical treatment alone. Neoadjuvant chemotherapy is a treatment regimen in which chemotherapy is initiated after histologic diagnosis but before definitive surgical removal of the tumor. Depending on the specific protocol, surgical resection is done approximately 6 to 15 weeks after initiation of treatment. Chemotherapy is then resumed as maintenance treatment. A good response to neoadjuvant therapy requires over 90% tumor necrosis.

24 The indication for the use of an allograft bone transplant following a tumor resection exists when a skeletal defect has resulted that cannot be ignored or adequately reconstructed with autograft. The disadvantages are that the surgery is technically more demanding than implanting a prosthesis. There is also a higher rate of early complications including infection and nonunion, and a longer period of protective weight bearing is required. There are also the risks of late complications including fracture, joint instability, and cartilage degeneration.

QUESTIONS

25 What are the contraindications to limb salvage?

26 What is the most common primary skeletal tumor?

27 A 48-year-old woman has a 1-month history of left upper extremity pain. The radiograph and histology are shown (*Figures 2-4A and 2-4B*). What is the diagnosis?

Fig 2-4 **A**

Fig 2-4 **B**

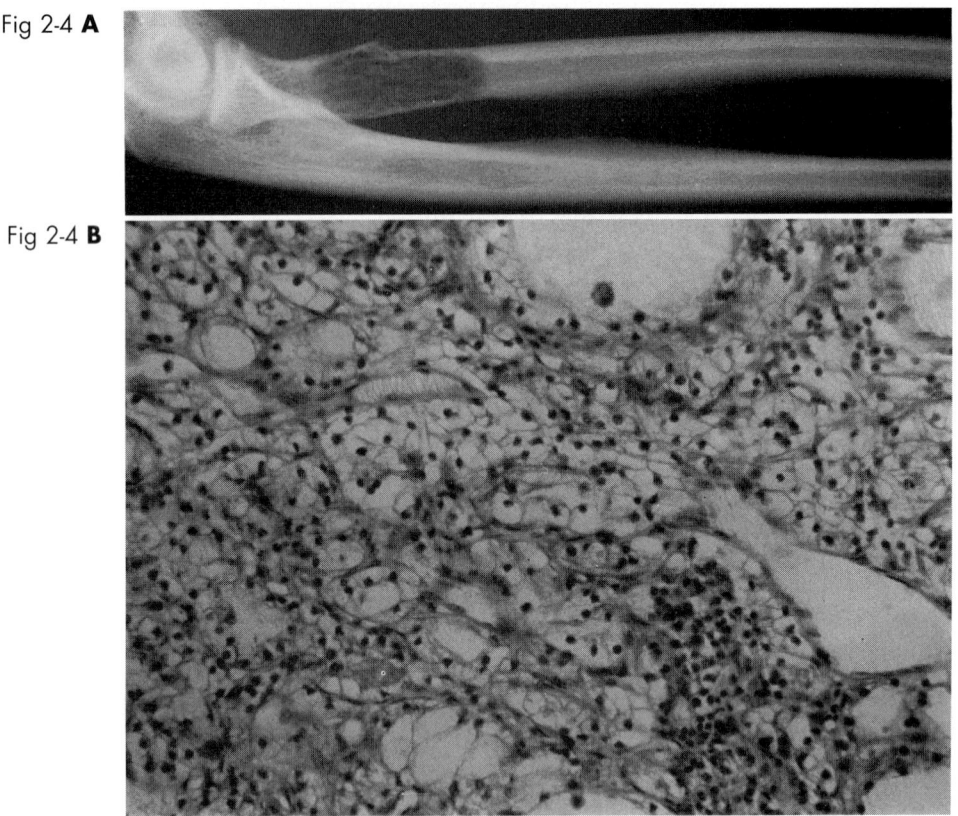

28 What is the most common site for metastatic tumor in women?

29 What is the most common site for metastatic tumor in men?

30 What are the most common sites for metastatic spread in the skeleton?

31 How much bone destruction must be present before a lesion is detectable by x-ray film evaluation?

32 What radiographic studies should be done in a metastatic work-up?

33 What radiographic criteria are used to determine the need for prophylactic stabilization of an impending pathologic fracture?

ANSWERS

25 The contraindications to limb salvage surgery include major neurovascular involvement by the tumor in an affected limb, pathologic fracture (the hematoma contaminates the surrounding muscle compartments), infection, improper placement of a biopsy, and extensive skin involvement by tumor.

26 Benign cartilage lesions are the most common primary bone tumors with osteochondromas making up a majority of the lesions. Myeloma is the most common malignant primary bone tumor; osteosarcoma is second.

27 Metastatic renal cell carcinoma. Metastatic lesions are more common than primary bone tumors.

28 Breast, followed by the lung, thyroid gland, and kidney.

29 Prostate, followed by the lung, thyroid gland, and kidney.

30 The spine, followed by the ribs, pelvis, proximal ends of long bones, sternum, and skull.

31 30% to 50%

32 Routine x-ray films of the most probable sites of involvement; a radionuclide bone scan can be helpful to detect other areas of bone metastases. Chest x-ray film, chest CT, and abdominal CT are helpful in determining involvement of other organs.

33 A destructive lesion involving greater than 50% of the diameter of the bone or measuring greater than 2.5 cm in diameter or a lesion in a patient with intractable bone pain deserve stabilization.

QUESTIONS

34 A 25-year-old man has multiple painless masses around his knees. A radiograph of both knees is shown (*Figure 2-5*). What is your diagnosis?

Fig 2-5

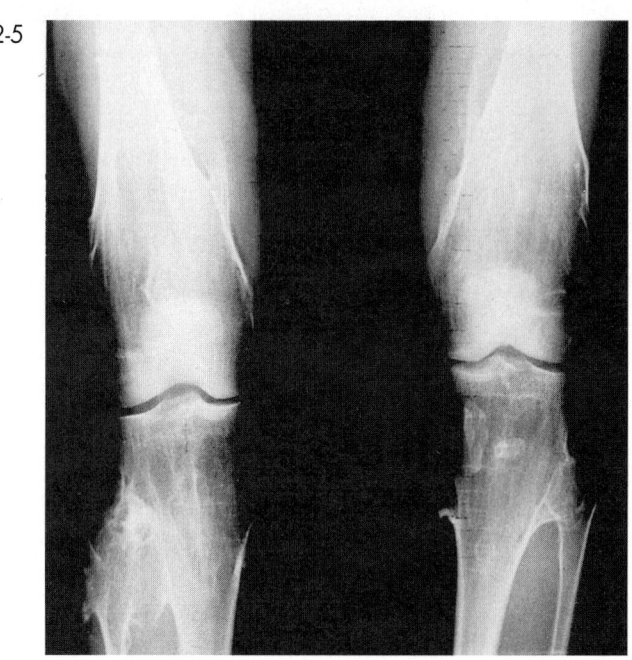

35 What are the chances of these masses becoming malignant?

36 The 19-year-old patient with shoulder pain described in Q1 underwent an open biopsy. The histologic specimen is shown (*Figure 2-6*). What is your diagnosis?

Fig 2-6

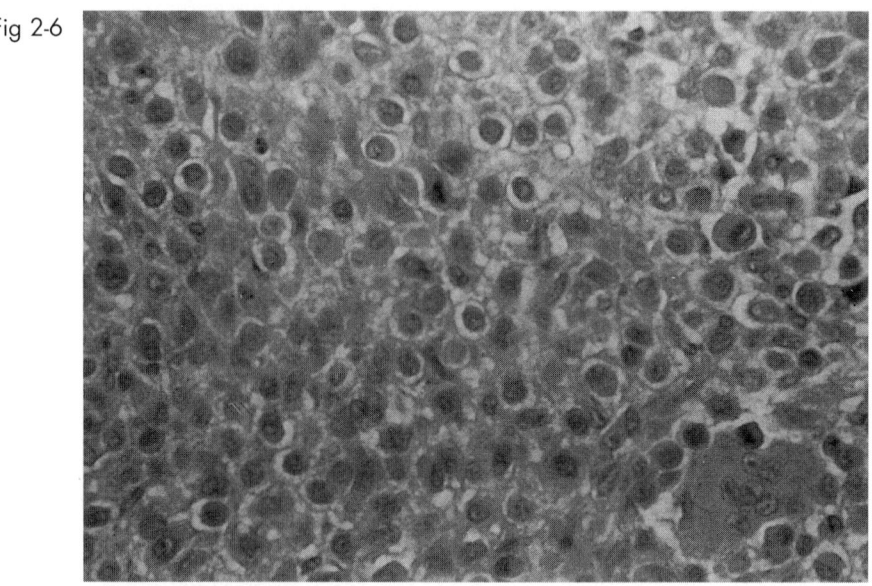

37 How would you treat this patient?

ANSWERS

34 Multiple hereditary osteocartilaginous exostosis. Radiographically, osteochondromas are seen as an exostosis on a bone. They may be either sessile or pedunculated and are characterized by direct continuity of trabecular and cortical bone of the host and the exostosis. As with most bone tumors, osteochondromas occur near the rapidly growing end of a bone. Therefore most will occur around the knee in the lower extremity and around the proximal humerus in the upper extremity. Osteochondromas result from an abnormality at the periphery of the physis during growth of the bone.

35 Malignant transformation is estimated to occur in approximately 10% of patients with multiple hereditary osteochondromas, but it is rare in patients with solitary osteochondromas. The development of pain or a lesion that is growing in size after skeletal maturity should raise the suggestion of malignancy.

36 Chondroblastoma. Chondroblastomas are generally radiolucent lesions with well-defined margins and seldom develop after the epiphyseal plates close. The tumor consists of sheets of chondroblasts. Chondroblasts are large cells with round nuclei, abundant cytoplasm, and well-defined cytoplasmic membranes. As the lesion matures, calcification of the matrix occurs, histologically giving it a "chicken wire" appearance.

37 Curettage and bone grafting.

QUESTIONS

38   What syndromes can occur with enchondromas?

39   What are the etiologies of benign cartilage lesions?

40   A 38-year-old man has a with 3-month history of right knee pain. Based on the radiograph (*Figure 2-7A*), what is your diagnosis?

Fig 2-7 **A**

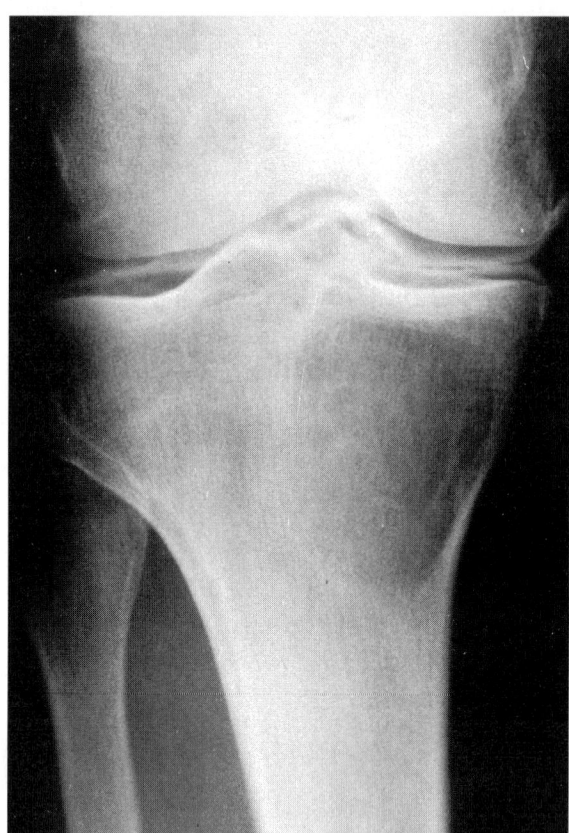

ANSWERS

38   Multiple enchondromas occur in a syndrome called Ollier's disease. This syndrome is characterized by widespread skeletal involvement that is often unilateral or even confined to one extremity. The lesions appear radiographically as a metaphyseal streak extending from the physis. The involved extremity may be short. Mafucci's syndrome is a disorder characterized by multiple enchondromas associated with angiomas of soft tissue. In the patient with solitary lesions, malignant transformation is rare. However, in the patient with multiple enchondromas, malignant transformation may occur in up to one third of the patients.

39   Enchondromas develop from failure of normal enchondral ossification below the growth plate centrally. Osteochondromas are formed by dysplasia of the peripheral portion of the growth plate. Dysplasia that occurs beneath the perichondrium results in a periosteal chondroma.

40   The radiolucent lesion is eccentric and at the end of the bone. There is no periosteal reaction. Giant cell tumor is typical for this age group and location.

QUESTIONS

41 The histology of the patient in Q40 is shown (*Figure 2-7B*). What is your diagnosis?

Fig 2-7 **B**

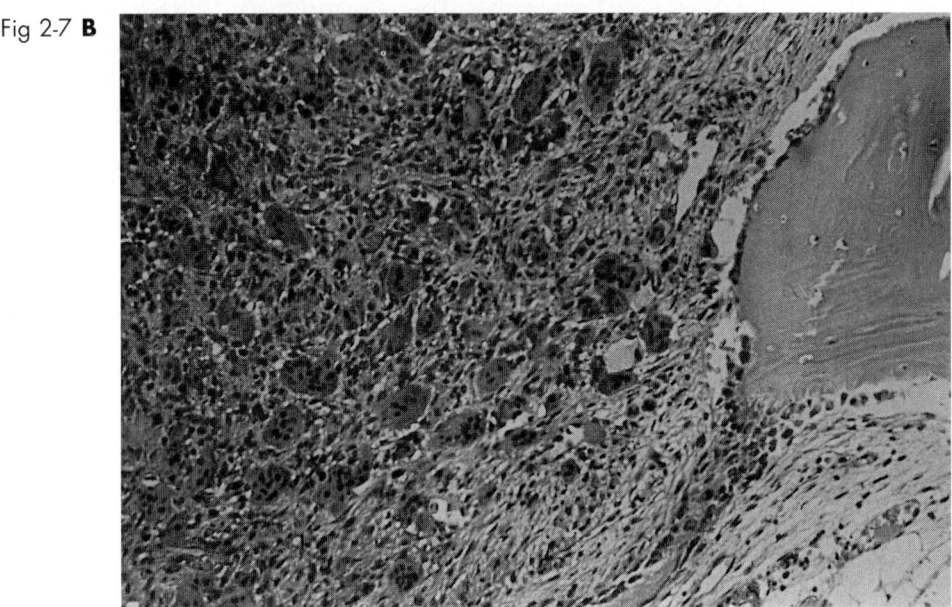

42 In what other disease processes can giant cells be found?

43 What is the appropriate treatment for a giant cell tumor?

44 How does the surgical management of giant cell tumors affect the local recurrence rate?

45 What is the malignant potential of this tumor?

ANSWERS

41   Giant cell tumor. Giant cell tumors are composed of multinucleated giant cells in a stroma of benign fibrous connective tissue with moderate vascularity. The giant cells contain between 5 and 100 nuclei. Almost all giant cell tumors occur in the skeletally mature patient with a peak incidence in the third and fourth decade. In addition to the usual locations, other areas of involvement include the spine (vertebral body and pedicle), sacrum, and occasionally the hands.

42   In both hyperparathyroidism and Paget's disease, multinucleated osteoclasts can appear as giant cells. In Paget's disease these cells can predominate in the early destructive phase with increased osteoclastic activity. In hyperparathyroidism, high levels of parathormone stimulate increased osteoclastic activity. The brown tumor of hyperparathyroidism may have both giant cells and osteoclasts. Occasional giant cells may be found in a number of lesions including chondroblastomas, aneurysmal bone cysts, and osteoblastomas.

43   Most surgeons agree that complete surgical removal through an aggressive curettage, supplemented by some surgical adjunct, is necessary. The curettage should be done through a wide cortical window so that the entire tumor cavity can be visualized. The tumor is removed with curettes, and the margin of removal is extended beyond the apparent cavity by use of a motorized burr. The use of surgical adjuncts include either chemical or thermal cautery to provide a further cytotoxic effect in the tumor cavity. Chemical agents commonly used include phenol, hydrogen peroxide, and alcohol. Thermal cautery can be achieved with liquid nitrogen. When the polymethylmethacrylate technique is employed, the heat of polymerization of the cement is believed to provide a cytotoxic effect.

44   The incidence of local recurrence is correlated with the degree of surgical removal. Simple curettage of giant cell tumors usually predicts approximately a 40% recurrence rate. The addition of surgical adjuncts (see Q43) lowers the recurrence rate to less than 20%. If an en bloc resection is achieved, the recurrence rate can be lowered 1% to 2%. Because the tumor extends to the subchondral bone, a wide surgical margin using an en bloc resection requires an allograft reconstruction.

45   The malignant potential is almost nonexistent as giant cell tumors are locally aggressive but benign lesions. However, malignancy in giant cell tumors is seen in two conditions. The most common is transformation after radiation of a benign giant cell tumor. On rare occasions one may find a high-grade sarcoma juxtaposed to an apparent benign giant cell tumor without any previous treatment. In either case the malignant portion represents high-grade sarcoma with little resemblance in appearance or behavior to routine giant cell tumors.

QUESTION

46   The patient is a 63-year-old man with sudden onset of severe low back pain following a fall at home. A radiograph and biopsy specimen are shown (*Figures 2-8A and 2-8B*). What is your diagnosis?

Fig 2-8 **A**

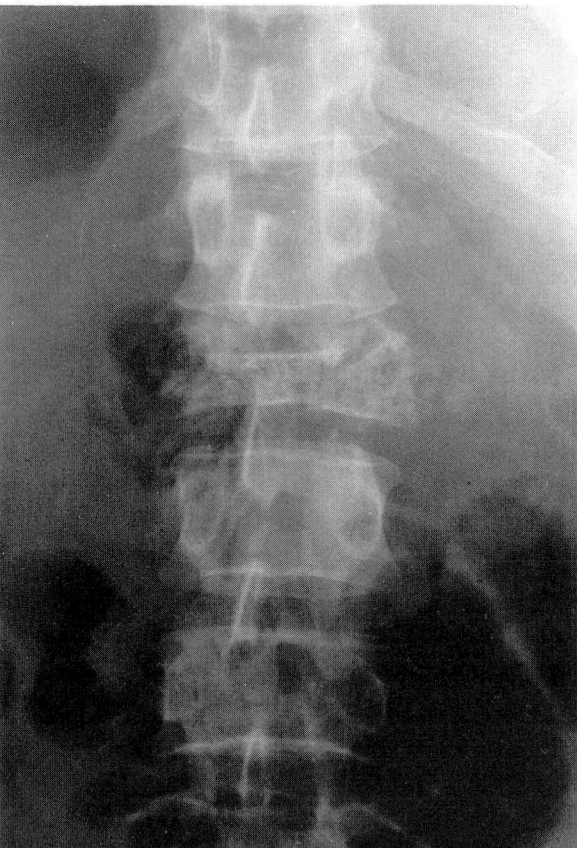

Fig 2-8 **B**

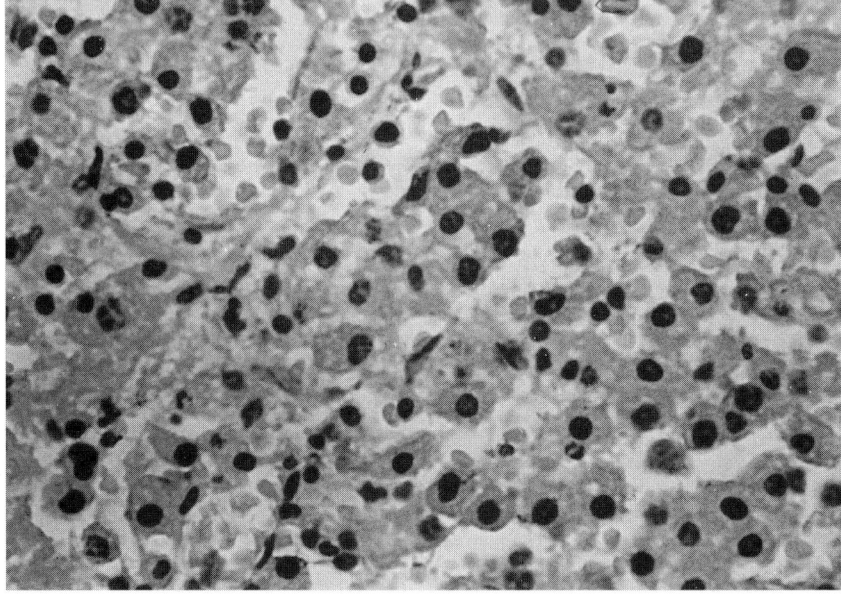

ANSWER

46   Multiple myeloma. This is the most common primary malignant lesion of the skeletal system. As a solitary lesion, it is known as a plasmacytoma. Radiographs show radiolucent, punched out lesions with no surrounding bony reaction. Occasionally the lesions show a more diffuse permeative pattern of bone loss. The plasma cell is the proliferating cell in myeloma. Multiple myeloma has a peak incidence in the sixth and seventh decades of life and is rare before the fifth decade.

QUESTIONS

47 What abnormal laboratory findings may be present in multiple myeloma?

48 How should patients with multiple myeloma be managed?

49 Is a technetium 99m bone scan an effective way to screen for this skeletal lesion?

50 A 4-year-old boy has a several month history of knee pain. An antero-posterior (AP) of his right knee is shown (*Figure 2-9A*). What is the differential diagnosis of the lesion in this child's bone?

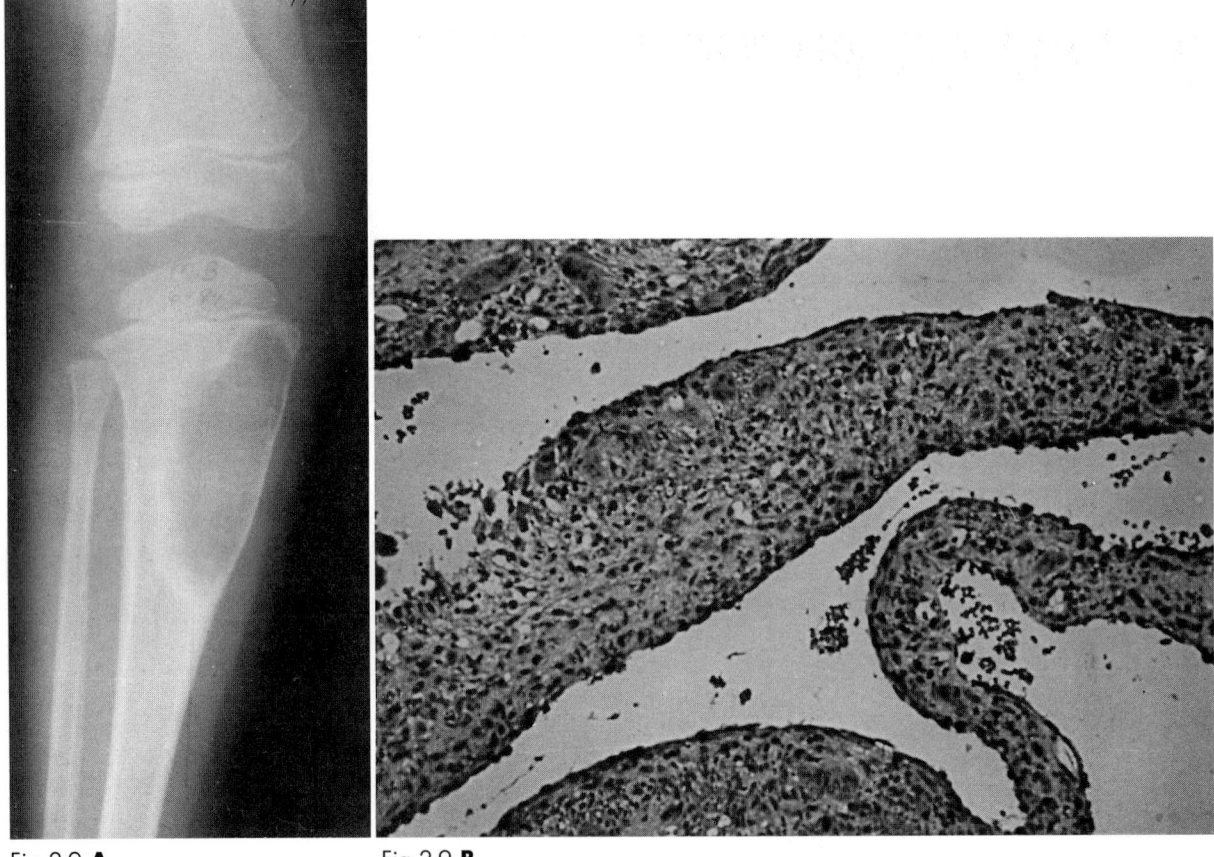

Fig 2-9 **A**   Fig 2-9 **B**

51 The histology is shown (*Figure 2-9B*). What is your diagnosis?

52 How does this lesion differ from a solitary bone cyst?

53 What is the most appropriate treatment for aneurysmal bone cysts?

54 What are fibrous cortical defects?

ANSWERS

47   Many patients will have anemia and the ESR is generally elevated. Bence Jones proteinuria is seen in approximately one half of patients. Serum immunoglobulin electrophoresis will show elevations in various globulin fractions in most of the patients. A monoclonal gamma globulin spike is the characteristic finding. With the onset of skeletal destruction, hypercalcemia is a frequent and dangerous feature of the disease.

48   Patients who have significant hypercalcemia must be hydrated and given diuretics. Occasionally, mithramycin is required. Chemotherapy regimens are used to control the systemic disease. Radiation therapy is administered to symptomatic skeletal lesions. Surgery is required to make a histologic diagnosis or for the management of an impending pathologic fracture. In addition, there may be an argument for more aggressive surgical management in the patient with a solitary myeloma or plasmacytoma. The patient with spinal involvement and neurologic compromise may require neurologic decompression and spinal stabilization.

49   No. A positive bone scan is present in only one half the patients with multiple myeloma. This is one example where a skeletal survey would be more helpful.

50   Osteomyelitis, eosinophilic granuloma, aneurysmal bone cyst, nonossifying fibroma, and simple bone cyst.

51   Aneurysmal bone cyst. Aneurysmal bone cysts are radiologically characterized by a thin expanding cortex of periosteal new bone that has replaced the cortex. These lesions are often eccentric. Histologically the lesion is composed of large cystic cavities containing red blood cells with a variable number of giant cells.

52   Solitary cysts (also called simple or unicameral bone cysts) appear as a fusiform widening of the metaphysis on x-ray film. The cortex may be thinned but is usually not expanded. The apparent widening of the bone is secondary to failure of metaphyseal remodeling. The inner wall of a solitary cyst is composed of a thin layer of fibrous tissue.

53   Curettage and bone grafting.

54   Fibrous cortical defects are a proliferation of benign fibrous tissue, usually located eccentrically in the metaphyseal portion of long bones in the skeletally immature. Other names for histologically identical lesions include fibroma, nonossifying fibroma, and metaphyseal fibrous defect. Characteristically these lesions are all eccentrically located in cortical bone. There is thinning or loss of the cortex with a well-demarcated rim of reactive bone along the inner margin. These defects are almost exclusively seen in childhood and adolescence and generally resolve spontaneously. They represent a failure of normal modeling of bone rather than a true neoplasm.

QUESTIONS

55 A 13-year-old girl has a several month history of left thigh pain. Her radiographs and biopsy are shown (*Figures 2-10A* and *2-10B*). What is your diagnosis?

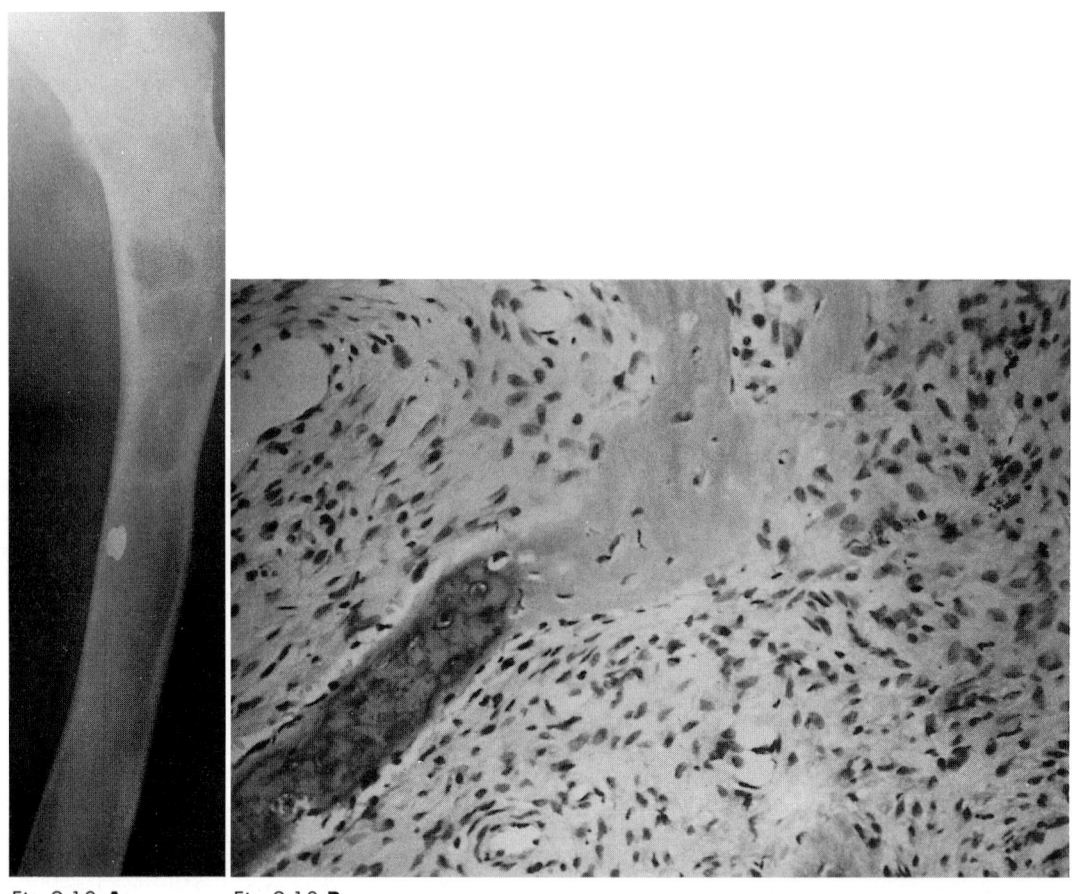

Fig 2-10 **A**   Fig 2-10 **B**

56 In what forms can this bony lesion occur?

57 What types of café au lait spots occur in fibrous dysplasia?

58 What is Albright's syndrome?

ANSWERS

55 Fibrous dysplasia. The radiographic appearance of fibrous dysplasia can be somewhat variable. Generally, fairly well-defined zones of rarefaction are surrounded by a rim of reactive bone. Typically these zones of rarefaction have a ground glass appearance. Expansion and thinning of cortical bone can occur, and bony deformity may develop. Histologically there is an abundant fibroblastic proliferation that surrounds rather bizarre and immature woven bone trabeculae. These trabeculae have a characteristic "Chinese lettering" appearance.

56 Monostotic and polyostotic. Monostotic involvement of the skeleton is commonly seen in the craniofacial bones and long tubular bones. Polyostotic disease is often associated with café au lait spots.

57 The café au lait spots found in fibrous dysplasia are coarse and irregular in appearance (coast of Maine) in comparison with the smooth appearing café au lait spots (coast of California) found in neurofibromatosis.

58 Albright's syndrome consists of polyostotic fibrous dysplasia, café au lait spots, and endocrine abnormalities including precocious puberty.

QUESTIONS

59 The patient is a 10-year-old girl with mild scoliosis noted on a school screening examination (*Figure 2-11A*). What primary bone lesions can give rise to a painful scoliosis in this age group?

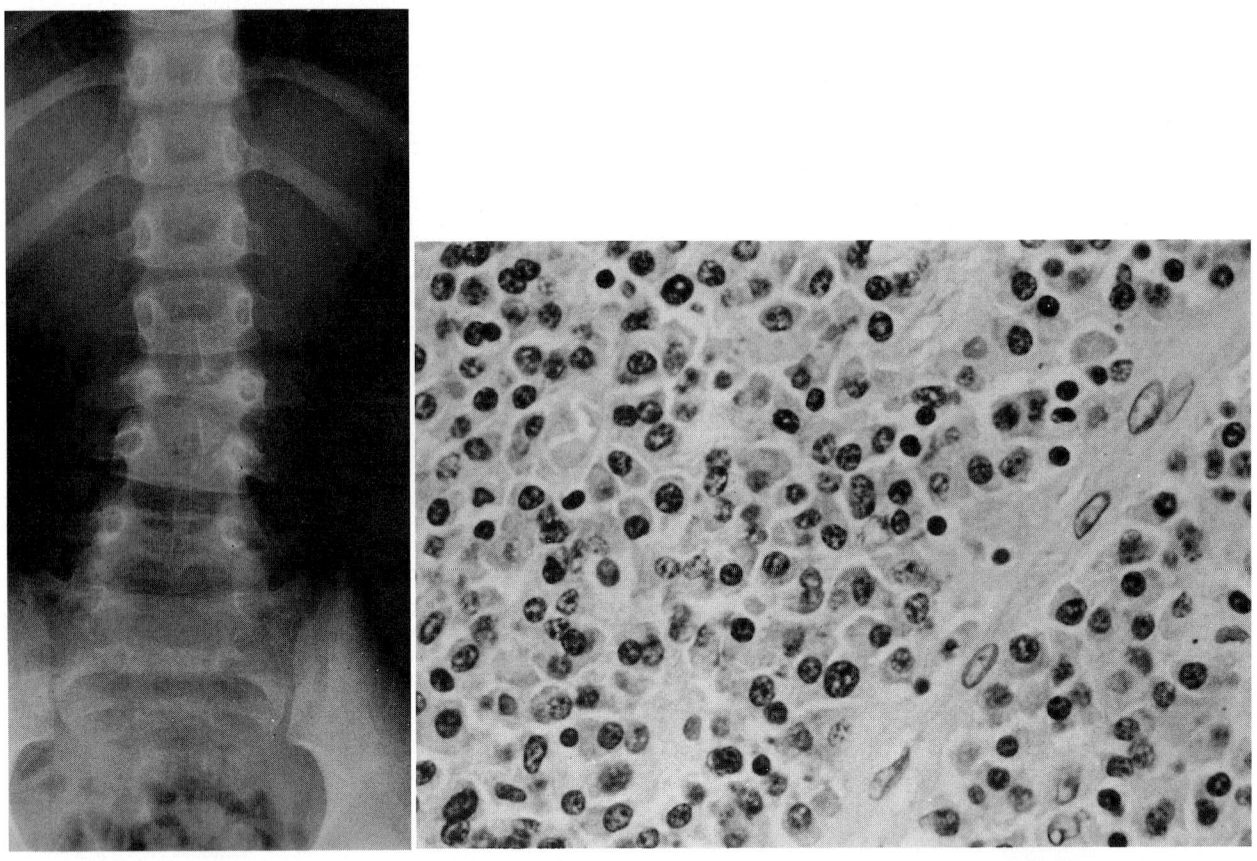

Fig 2-11 **A**   Fig 2-11 **B**

60 A biopsy of the lesion was performed (*Figure 2-11B*). What is your diagnosis?

61 In what syndromes can this lesion be manifest?

62 How would you treat an isolated lesion of eosinophilic granuloma?

ANSWERS

59   Osteoid osteoma, osteoblastoma, aneurysmal bone cyst, eosinophilic granuloma, or infection. All but eosinophilic granulomas and infection usually involve the posterior elements.

60   Eosinophilic granuloma (EG). On radiographs, eosinophilic granulomas appear as radiolucent "punched-out" lesions that are fairly well defined. When EG is located in a vertebral body, the body can be partly or completely collapsed (a vertebra plana). Histologically there is a proliferation of Langerhans' histiocytes with irregular nuclei. These cells are accompanied by eosinophils, lymphocytes, plasma cells, and occasional neutrophils.

61   There are two types of multifocal eosinophilic granuloma: Hand-Schüller-Christian syndrome and Letterer-Siwe syndrome. Hand-Schüller-Christian disease refers to the triad of skull lesions, exophthalmos, and diabetes insipidus. This syndrome has a chronic evolution and occurs in children over the age of 3 years. Letterer-Siwe disease is believed to represent a more acute manifestation of histiocytosis and generally has an age of onset of less than 3 years. In addition to bone lesions, clinical findings include recurrent bacteremia, diffuse lymphadenopathy, and skin lesions. Letterer-Siwe disease is commonly fatal.

62   If the diagnosis is established, no treatment is required in the absence of symptoms. A solitary lesion compromising the structural integrity of the bone is managed by curettage and bone grafting. Prophylactic stabilization may or may not be required.

QUESTIONS

63 A 21-year-old man has a 2-month history of left thigh pain and a mass. His radiograph is shown (*Figure 2-12A*). The histopathology is also shown (*Figure 2-12B*). What is your diagnosis?

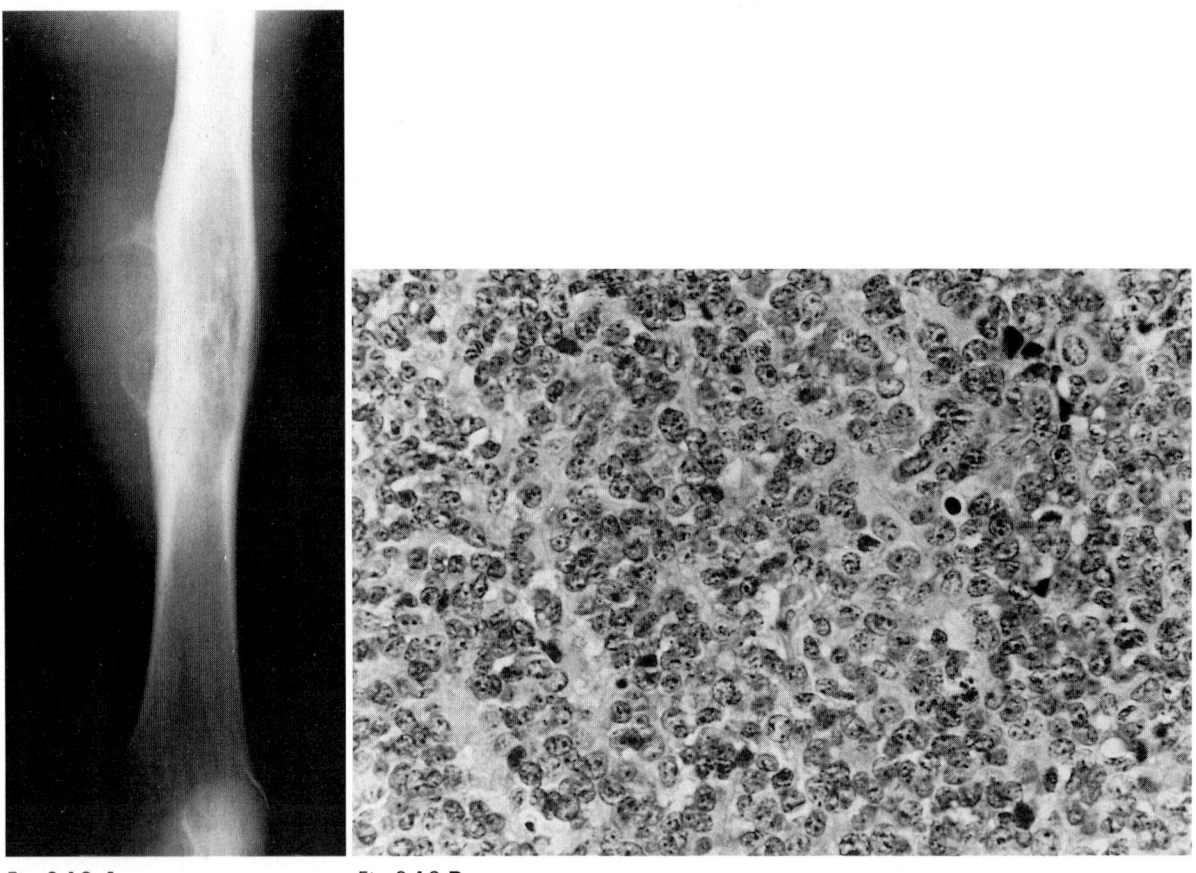

Fig 2-12 **A**   Fig 2-12 **B**

64 How would you treat this lesion?

65 What is the overall 5-year survival rate for these patients?

66 What specific chemotherapeutic agents are used?

67 What adverse effects can result from radiation treatment of a child?

ANSWERS

63 Ewing's sarcoma. Radiographically the lesion has a permeative pattern with cortical disruption. Ninety percent of these lesions occur before 21 years of age. The tumor usually originates in the medullary cavity of the bone in the metaphyseal and diaphyseal region of long bones. Many of the lesions arise in the pelvis and escape early detection. Histologically there are homogenous populations of densely packed cells. The origin of these cells is unknown but is thought to be from the pluripotent mesenchymal stem cell. Most cells stain positive for glycogen on periodic acid-Schiff (PAS) test.

64 Ewing's sarcoma is generally considered a radiosensitive tumor and often requires the combination of surgery, chemotherapy, and radiotherapy. The traditional approach to treatment has consisted of radiation for the primary lesion and chemotherapy as systemic treatment. The addition of a surgical excision (with a wide surgical margin) of the primary lesion leads to improved local control and improved survival.

65 The current overall prognosis for survival for patients with Ewing's sarcoma is 50%. In favorable sites where surgical resection is possible, the 5-year survival rate is 60% to 80%. In unfavorable sites, the rate is 20% to 30%.

66 Agents used in the chemotherapy of Ewing's sarcoma include vincristine, cyclophosphamide, doxorubicin, dactinomycin, ifosfamide, and etoposide.

67 Growth plate closure, joint stiffness, and the possibility of radiation-induced sarcomas in patients who survive.

QUESTIONS

68 The patient is a 50-year-old woman who has had a painful mass in her right shoulder for the last 8 months (*Figures 2-13A* and *2-13B*). What is your diagnosis?

Fig 2-13 **A**

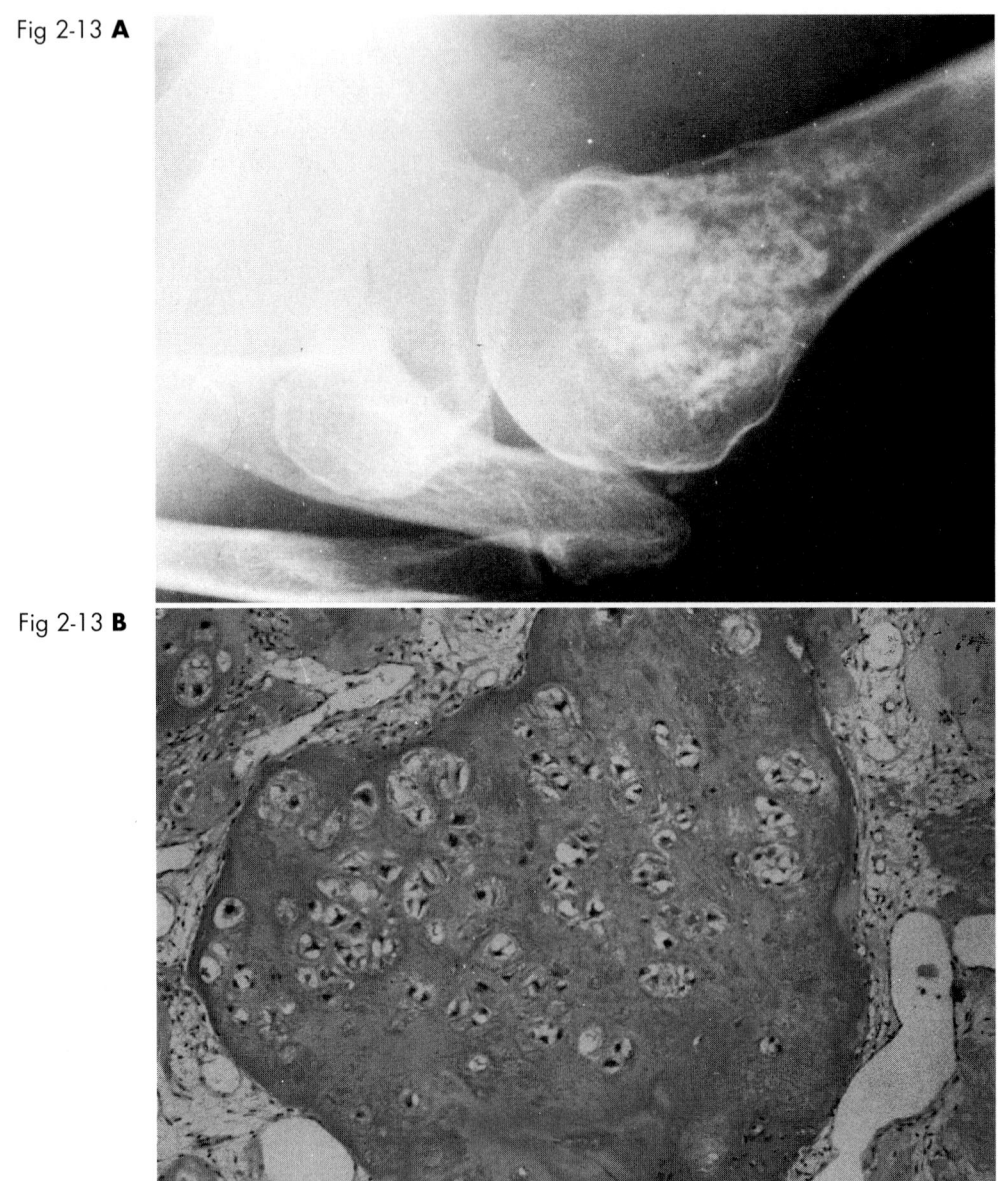

Fig 2-13 **B**

69 What are the different classifications for this lesion?

70 In general, are chondrosarcomas of a higher grade or lower grade than the typical osteosarcoma?

71 What histologic features are used to determine the grade of a tumor?

72 How do chondrosarcomas differ from osteosarcomas in terms of their age distribution and localization?

ANSWERS

68 Chondrosarcoma. The punctate, mottled densities attributable to calcification of a chondroid matrix are a characteristic finding. This pattern of mineralization with endosteal erosion, cortical thickening, and expansion suggests malignancy.

69 Chondrosarcomas can be divided into primary lesions, secondary lesions, which arise at the site of a previous osteochondroma or enchondroma, and dedifferentiated lesions. Two rare variants, the clear cell chondrosarcoma and the mesenchymal chondrosarcoma, have been described.

70 Lower grade. Approximately 90% of chondrosarcomas are grades I and II (based on Broder's method, which grades lesions from I to IV). Conventional osteosarcomas are Broder's grade III or IV.

71 The most important features are the degree of cellularity and the amount of cellular atypia. Cellular atypia includes variation in cell size and shape, variation in number or shape of nuclei, and the presence of mitoses. Other features considered are the presence of abnormal matrix production and areas of cellular necrosis.

72 Chondrosarcomas are tumors of adulthood and advanced age with a peak distribution in the fifth and sixth decades. Osteosarcoma has a peak distribution in the second decade. Most osteosarcomas occur around the knee, whereas chondrosarcomas frequently occur in the proximal limb girdles, including the pelvis and proximal femur. Chondrosarcomas also occur around the shoulder, both in the proximal humerus and the scapula.

QUESTIONS

73 What is the recommended treatment for this lesion?

74 Does chemotherapy or radiation contribute to the treatment of chondrosarcoma?

75 What is the survival rate for chondrosarcomas?

76 After surgery, what factors affect the local recurrence rate for chondrosarcomas?

77 The patient is a 55-year-old man with left shoulder pain of 3 months duration. His medical history is negative. His general physical examination is normal. Examination of his left shoulder demonstrates a large soft tissue mass and limited motion of the shoulder. What is your differential diagnosis based on the radiograph (*Figure 2-14A*)?

Fig 2-14 **A**

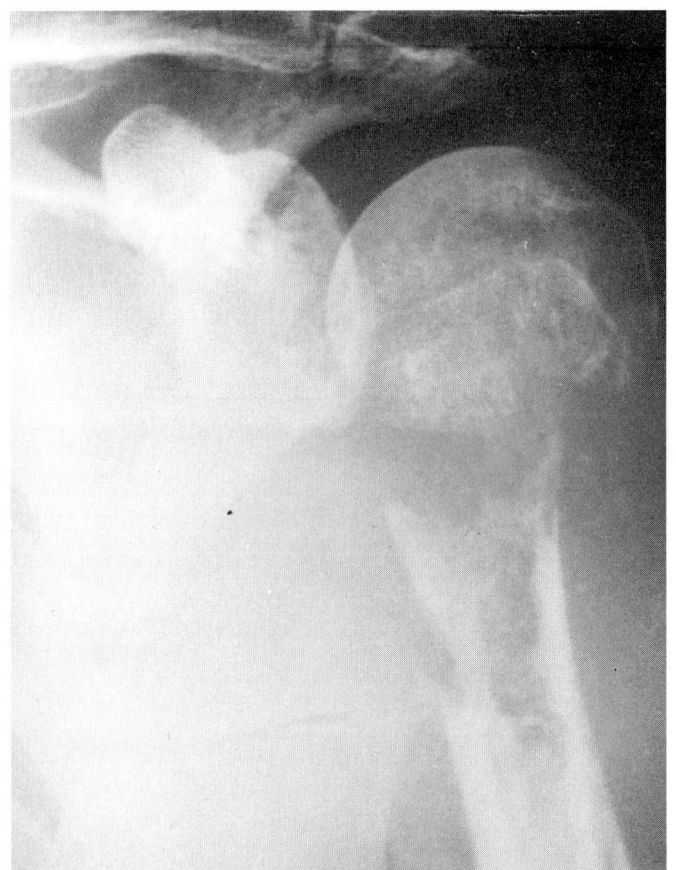

ANSWERS

73 Complete surgical removal with a wide surgical margin. This can be done either through amputation or limb sparing resection.

74 No. Chondrosarcomas are relatively chemoresistant and radioresistant.

75 The survival rate is dependent on the grade of the lesion. With high-grade lesions, the overall survival rate may be as low as 40%. This may be attributable, in part, to the ineffectiveness of current chemotherapy. For lower-grade lesions, the survival rate may be closer to 80%. The dedifferentiated chondrosarcoma carries a poor prognosis with a 5-year survival rate of less than 20%. Another variant with a poor prognosis is mesenchymal chondrosarcoma.

76 If adequate wide margins can be achieved, the local recurrence rate should be relatively low (approximately 10%). The often large size of these tumors and their locations in anatomically difficult areas, such as proximal limb girdles, make wide surgical margins difficult to achieve. The tumors are notorious for their implantability, and actual recurrence rates are closer to 30%. Because the tumors are relatively slow growing, these recurrences can also occur many years after the initial treatment.

77 The lesion has a destructive appearance that suggests a malignant lesion. The differential diagnosis would include a metastatic lesion, myeloma, malignant fibrous histiocytoma (MFH), or fibrosarcoma. There is no evidence of production of a bony or cartilaginous matrix.

QUESTIONS

78   A tissue specimen is shown (*Figure 2-14B*). What is your diagnosis?

Fig 2-14 **B**

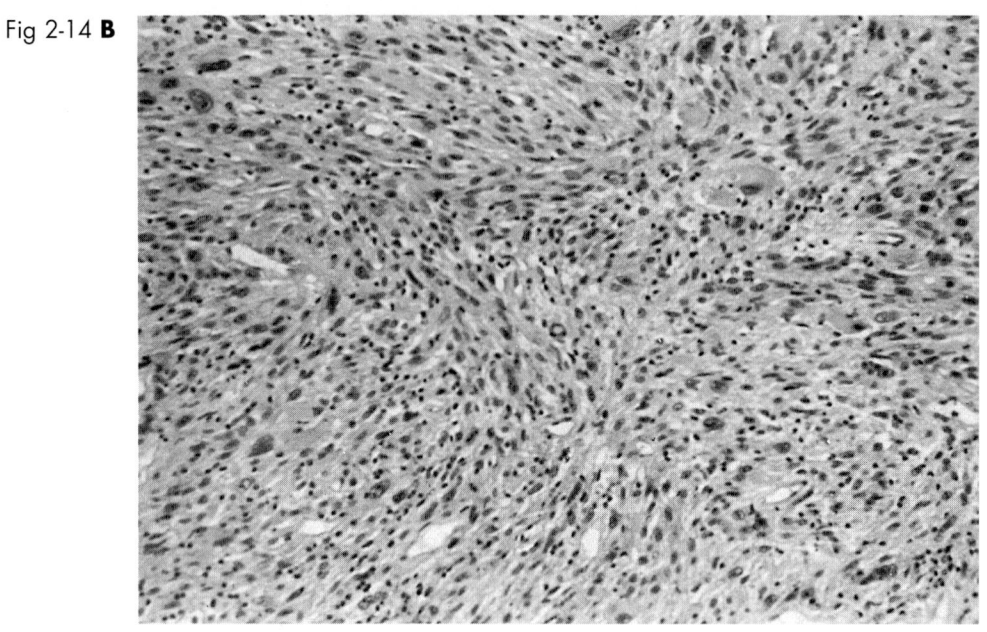

79   What preexisting lesion is associated with MFH of bone?

80   What is the role of chemotherapy in the treatment of MFH in either soft tissue or bone?

ANSWERS

78 MFH. MFH is the most common soft tissue sarcoma in adults older than 50 years of age. Less commonly, as in this case, MFH arises in bone. The histologic pattern of MFH is varied. In some areas, large histiocytic cells predominate; in other areas, a whirling pattern of spindle cells predominate in a storiform pattern. In fibrosarcoma the malignant spindle cells form a herringbone pattern.

79 Bone infarcts can be found in association with MFH.

80 Chemotherapy has not been shown to increase the survival rate of patients with MFH.

QUESTIONS

81 The patient is a 42-year-old man with a painful mass on the plantar surface of his right foot. The mass has increased in size over the past year. His radiograph and biopsy are shown (*Figures 15A* and *15B*). What is your diagnosis?

Fig 2-15 **A**

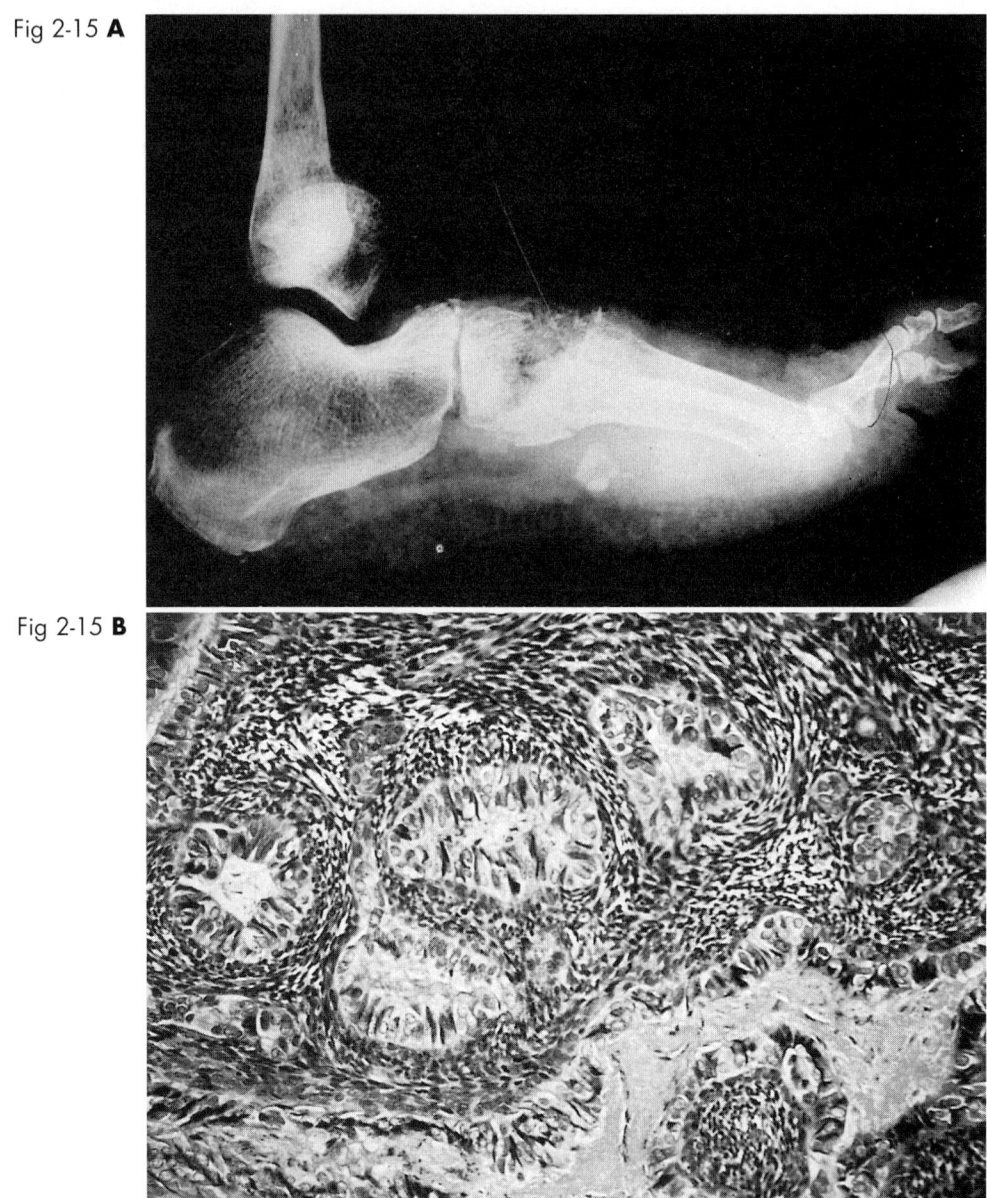

Fig 2-15 **B**

82 Where do these tumors arise?

83 What would be the appropriate treatment for this patient?

84 What physical findings suggest that a soft tissue mass is malignant?

ANSWERS

81 Synovial sarcoma. These lesions frequently show calcifications on x-ray film. Histologically they may have a biphasic pattern consisting of both a glandular and a fibrous component. These lesions may occasionally present with a single phase fibrous pattern.

82 These tumors are typically slow growing and are frequently found adjacent to joints. They arise from structures such as the bursa and tendon sheaths rather than directly from the joint.

83 Amputation followed by consideration of systemic chemotherapy.

84 Lesions that are greater than 5 cm in diameter and are deep to the fascia are more likely malignant than benign.

QUESTIONS

85 The patient is a 56-year-old woman who struck her sacrum on a counter 8 months ago and has had pain since. On physical examination, she is noted to have a palpable mass at the intergluteal fold. Her x-ray films and biopsy are shown (*Figures 2-16A* and *2-16B*). What is your diagnosis?

Fig 2-16 **A**

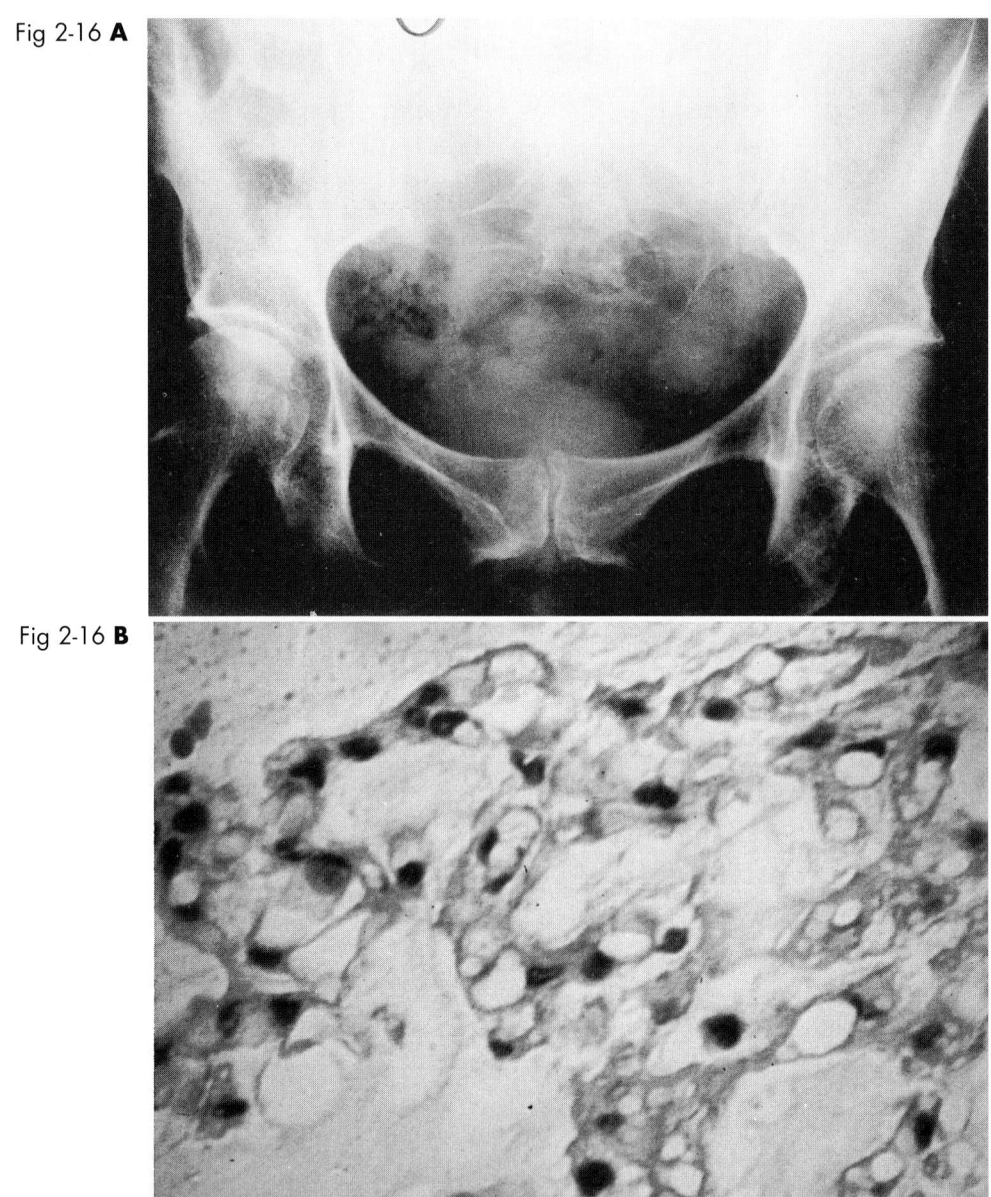

Fig 2-16 **B**

86 What is the treatment for this tumor?

87 Is there a role for radiation in the management of this tumor?

88 What neurologic dysfunction arises from sacrifice of sacral nerve roots?

ANSWERS

85   Chordoma. The traumatic episode is unrelated to the development of the tumor. Chordomas arise from notochordal remnants in the sacrococcygeal region and are also known to occur in the spheno-occipital area. Most tumors develop between the fifth and seventh decades. The most common clinical presentation is constipation with associated bladder and bowel dysfunction. Histologically the physaliferous cell is characteristic of this lesion. Abundant vacuolated cells are present in chords separated by fibrous septa.

86   Surgical resection with wide margins is the recommended treatment for this lesion. Lesions below S3 can be treated by a sacral amputation at this level from a posterior approach. Lesions involving the sacral nerve roots above S3 may require both an anterior and a posterior approach.

87   Chordomas have an unpredictable response, and radiation is generally reserved for unresectable lesions or lesions resected with less than a wide margin.

88   If the nerve roots through S3 can be preserved, on at least one side, patients will usually have minimal alteration in their bowel and bladder function. If both S3 roots are sacrificed, patients may have adequate bowel and bladder function, but they may need to employ some external maneuvers to empty their bladder.

QUESTIONS

89 A 59-year-old man who once injured his knee playing football now complains of pain, locking, and giving way in his left knee. The radiograph and histology are shown (*Figures 2-17A* and *2-17B*). What is the diagnosis?

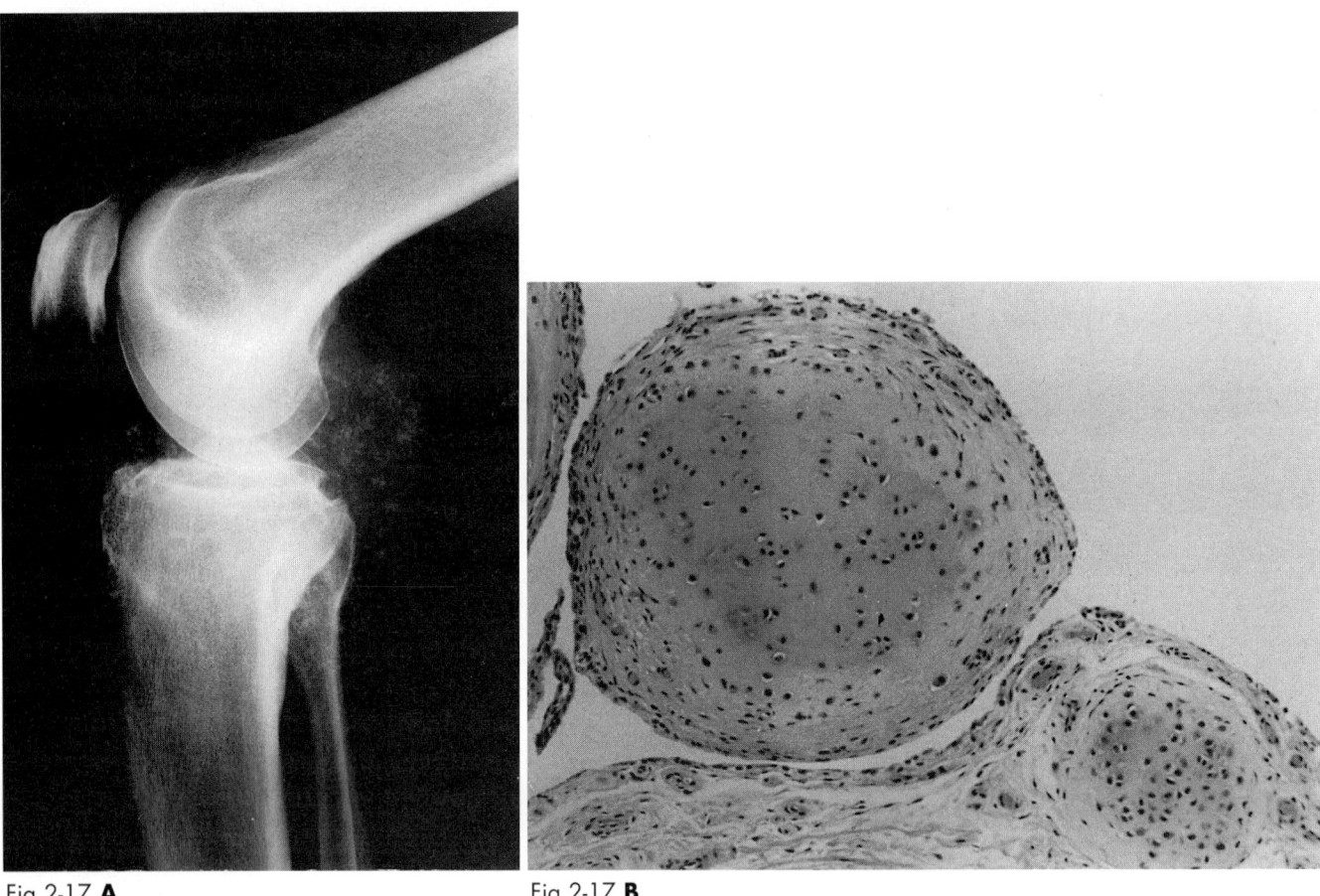

Fig 2-17 **A**   Fig 2-17 **B**

90 What is the treatment for this lesion?

91 What is the recurrence rate for this condition after loose body excision without synovectomy?

92 What is the incidence of malignant degeneration with this lesion?

ANSWERS

89 Synovial chondromatosis. Synovial chondromatosis results from metaplasia of cells in the synovium to cells that form masses of hyaline cartilage. The disease occurs mainly in the knees, hips, shoulders, and elbows.

90 Removal of the loose bodies from the joint and synovectomy.

91 If removal of loose bodies is performed without a synovectomy, recurrence is the rule rather than the exception.

92 Malignant degeneration is quite rare. There have been isolated reports of chondrosarcomas arising from this condition.

QUESTIONS

93 The patient is a 45-year-old man with massive swelling in his left shoulder, minimal pain, and multiple sores over both hands. From the radiograph (*Figure 2-18*), what is your diagnosis?

Fig 2-18

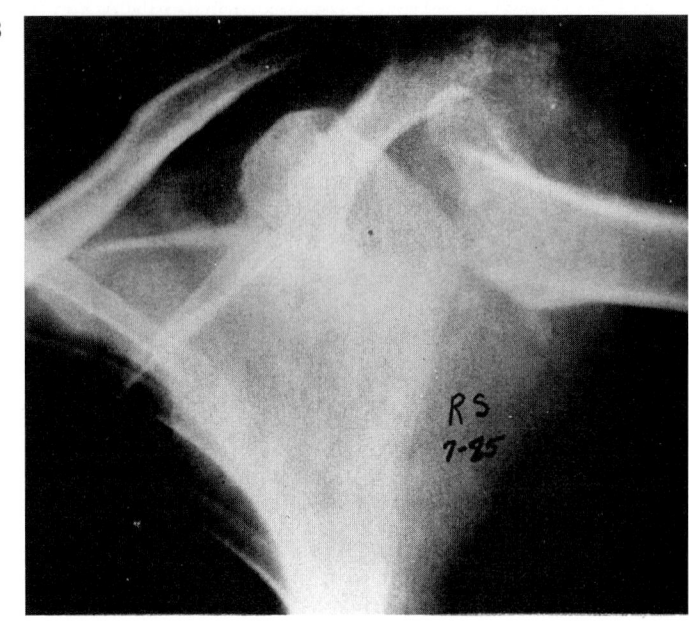

94 What disease entities can give rise to Charcot's joint?

95 What would be the most appropriate treatment for this patient?

ANSWERS

93 Neuropathic (Charcot's) joint. The gross destruction of the gleno-humeral joint with bone fragmentation in a patient with minimal pain suggests Charcot's joint arthropathy. The multiple sores on both hands suggests a loss of sensation. This patient was found to have a cervical syringomyelia.

94 Charcot's arthropathy is due to loss of joint sensation. Alcoholism, congenital indifference to pain, diabetes, syphilis, myelomeningocele, syringomyelia, and leprosy can all give rise to neuropathic arthropathy. In the upper extremity, syringomyelia is the most common cause of a neuropathic joint.

95 Nonoperative care of the joint would be the treatment of choice. Joint arthroplasty is contraindicated in Charcot's joint arthropathy.

QUESTIONS

96 A 46-year-old woman has a rapidly enlarging mass in her right thigh. A CT scan and biopsy are shown (*Figures 2-19A and 2-19B*). What is your diagnosis?

Fig 2-19 **A**

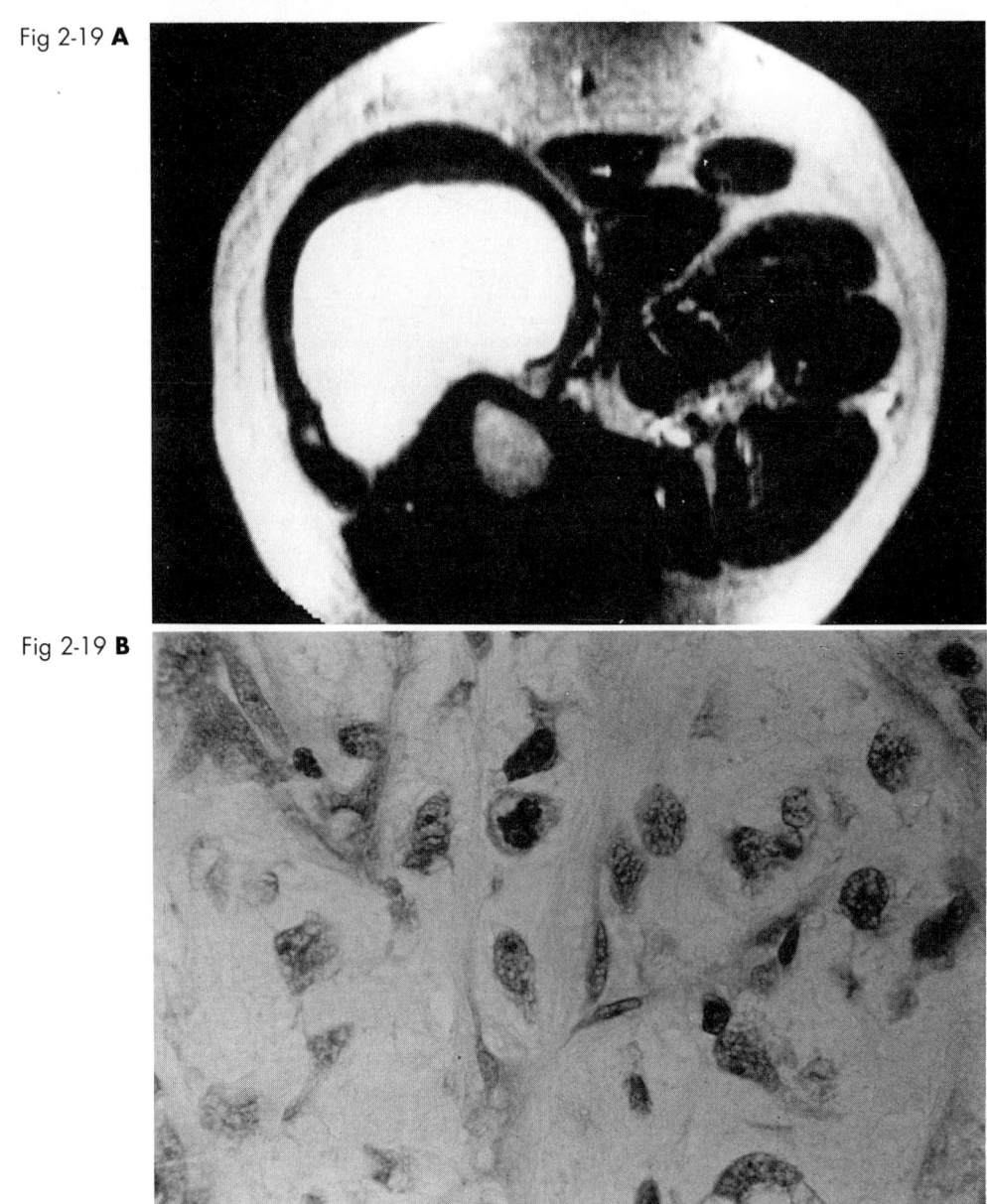

Fig 2-19 **B**

97 How are these lesions categorized?

ANSWERS

96   Liposarcoma. The CT scan shows a large tumor that is deep to the fascia. The most common malignant soft tissue tumors are liposarcomas, malignant fibrous histiocytomas, and synovial sarcomas. The photomicrograph shows a field of fat cells with characteristic clear cytoplasm, some with abnormal hyperchromic nuclei, and a number of mitotic figures. Liposarcomas usually occur in adults with a peak age between 50 and 60 years. They are generally found deep to the fascia in contrast to lipomas which are usually subcutaneous.

97   Liposarcomas are classified into four categories including the well differentiated (low grade), myxoid (low grade), and round cell and pleomorphic types (high grade). Myxoid, round cell, and pleomorphic types are richly vascular compared with the well-differentiated liposarcoma. Myxoid is the most common type.

QUESTION

98   An 83-year-old man complains of a painless mass in the anterior portion of his right thigh. The MRI scan (*Figure 2-20A*) and the histology (*Figure 2-20B*) are shown. What is the diagnosis?

Fig 2-20 **A**

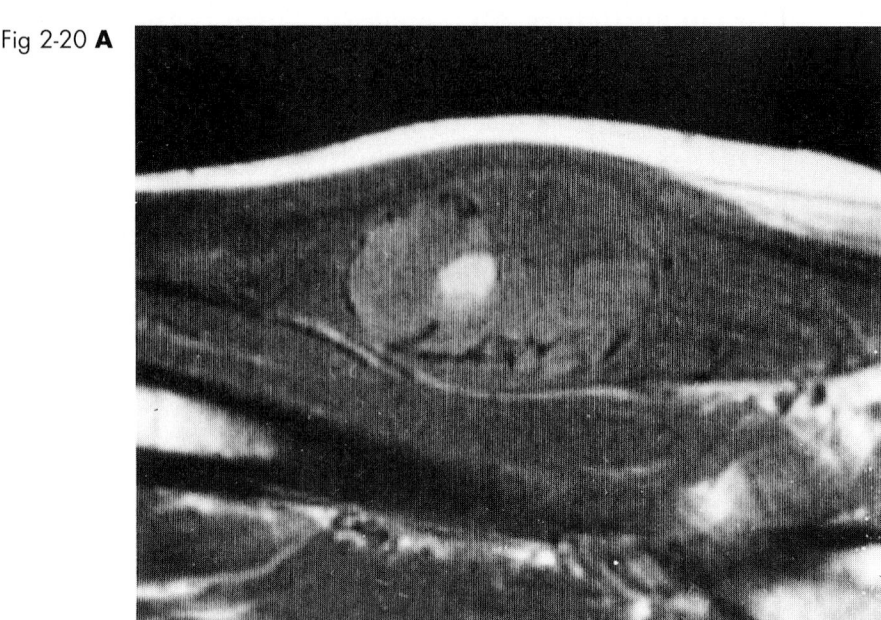

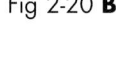

Fig 2-20 **B**

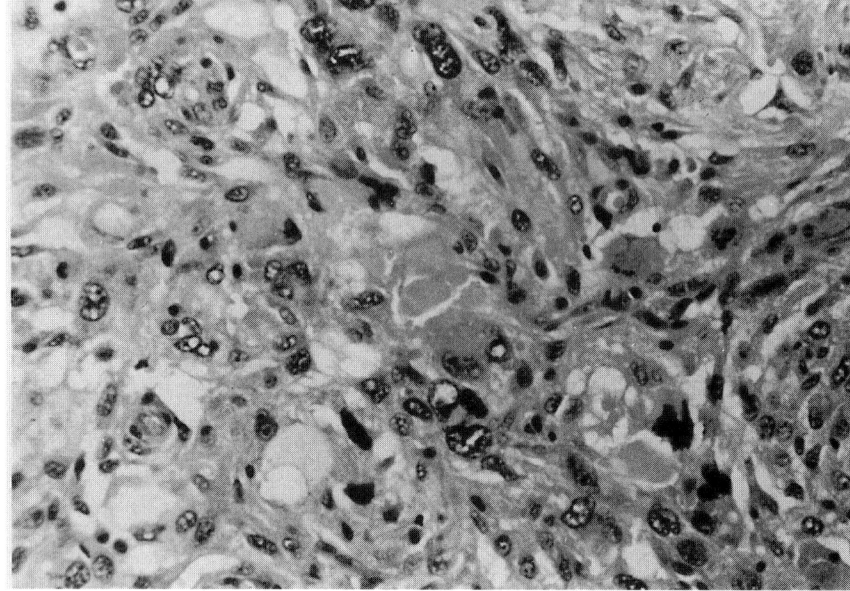

ANSWER

98   MFH. The MRI shows a lesion deep to the fascia. The tissue consists of malignant spindle cells and histiocytes in a storiform pattern.

CHAPTER 3

Metabolic Bone Disease

Richard C. Fisher

QUESTIONS

1 A 37-year-old woman complains of pain in her right hip and upper thigh region with walking. She has a history of a previous fracture of her left femur, which healed slowly, and two stress fractures in her feet. X-ray films of her hips and pelvis are shown (*Figure 3-1*). Which major category of metabolic bone disease would include this problem?

Fig 3-1
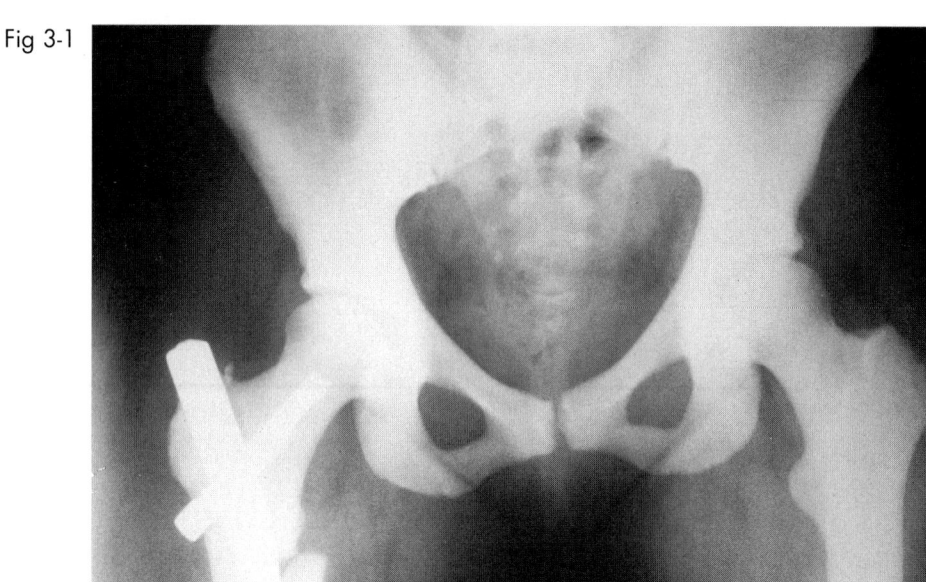

2 What are the clinical expressions of osteopetrosis?

3 Would you expect laboratory studies to help with the diagnosis?

4 The patient in Q1 had a tetracycline labeled iliac crest biopsy. Describe the expected findings from this study.

5 Bone marrow transplantation has been of some value in the severe infantile form. Why might this be expected?

ANSWERS

1 The sclerosing bone dysplasias. Although there are many types of osteosclerosis, osteopetrosis (first described by Albers-Schönberg) is probably the best known variety.

2 The common clinical manifestations include an autosomal recessive type that is usually fatal in infancy, a mild autosomal dominant form with few symptoms, and an intermediate autosomal recessive type that causes symptoms similar to the patient dscribed in Q1. A fourth type is associated with carbonic anhydrase II deficiency.

3 Generally not in the milder forms. In the severe infantile type, serum acid phosphatase and parathyroid hormone levels might be increased. Also, low calcium and high 1,25 vitamin D levels have been reported in these patients.

4 • Increased trabecular volume with marrow fibrosis.
• Islands of calcified cartilage remaining in the metaphyseal bone.
• Increased, normal, or decreased osteoclast numbers. These cells usually have an increased number of nuclei and a loss of their ruffled border.

5 The basic defect in most cases arises from abnormal osteoclast function. The osteoclast progenitor cell is derived from the monocyte line of marrow cells.

QUESTIONS

6 A 57-year-old man came to the emergency department with pain in his right leg after a fall from a height of one step while at work. He denied previous symptoms in his lower extremities and stated that he had been in good general health. Initial x-ray films and a bone scan are shown (*Figures 3-2A, 3-2B, and 3-2C*). What is your working diagnosis?

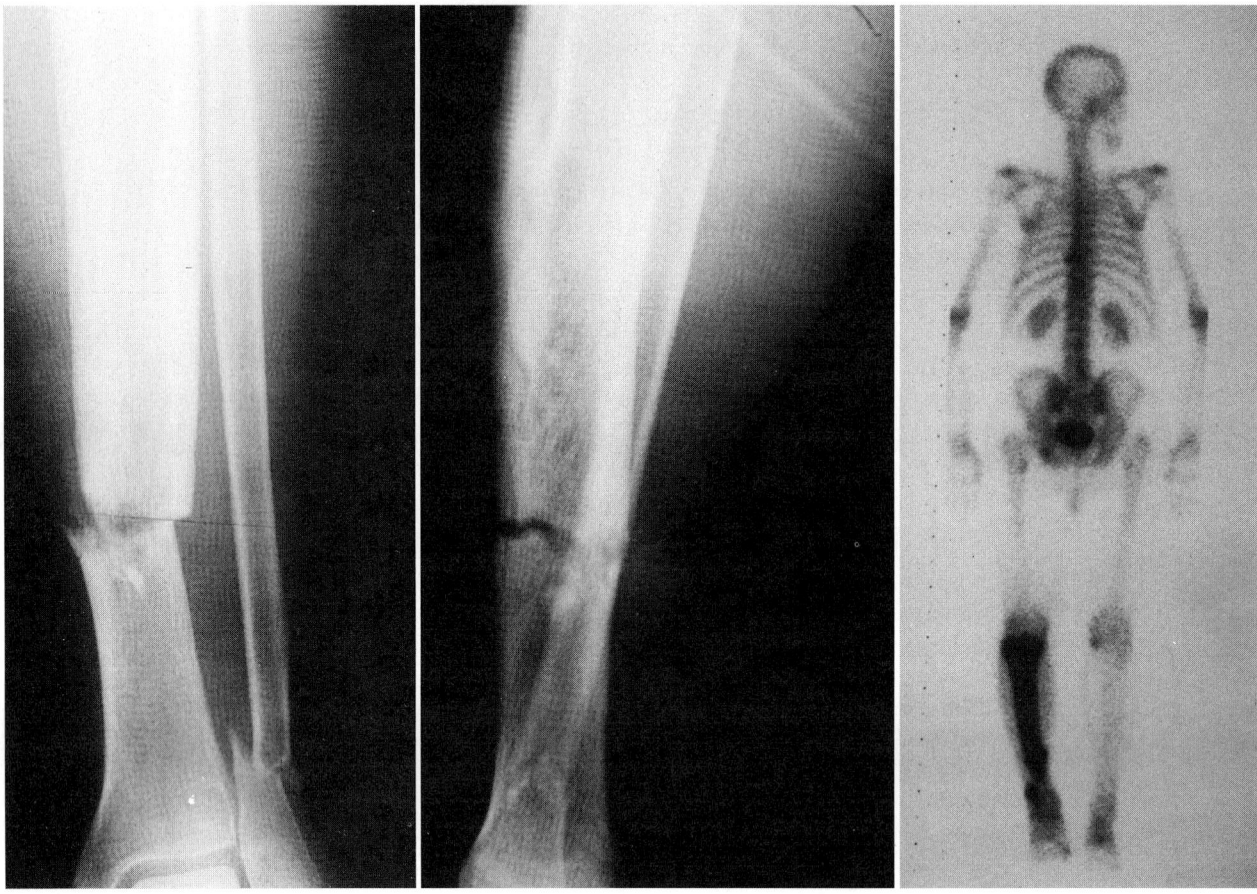

Fig 3-2 **A**   Fig 3-2 **B**   Fig 3-2 **C**

7 What are the typical diagnostic laboratory abnormalities seen in Paget's disease?

8 Describe the pathophysiology of Paget's disease, and relate it to the laboratory abnormalities noted in Q7.

9 Name the most common sites of fracture with Paget's disease.

ANSWERS

6   The fracture appears to be pathologic, and the bone changes are compatible with Paget's disease. X-ray film changes are usually pathognomonic for Paget's disease, showing a coarse trabecular pattern, general enlargement of the involved bone, and lytic and sclerotic changes. Occasionally, tumors are associated with the Pagetic process (prostatic carcinoma is the most common nonskeletal tumor). The incidence of sarcoma developing in Pagetic bone is about 1%.

7   Elevated serum alkaline phosphatase and elevated urinary hydroxyproline measured with a 24-hour urine collection.

8   Although Paget's disease has a blastic, lytic, and mixed phase, all are associated with an increase in the bone turnover rate. Bone formation and resorption are affected. Alkaline phosphatase is a marker of bone formation and probably bone resorption, whereas hydroxyproline is released from bone collagen with osteolysis.

9   The spine, tibia, humerus, and femur. In the femur, subtrochanteric fractures are the most difficult to treat. These fractures usually require surgical stabilization and have a high incidence of nonunion.

QUESTION

10 The x-ray films shown (*Figures 3-3A and 3-3B*) are from a patient with known polyostotic Paget's disease. Her chief complaints are right leg and left hip pain. What is the most likely etiology of her hip pain?

Fig 3-3 **A**

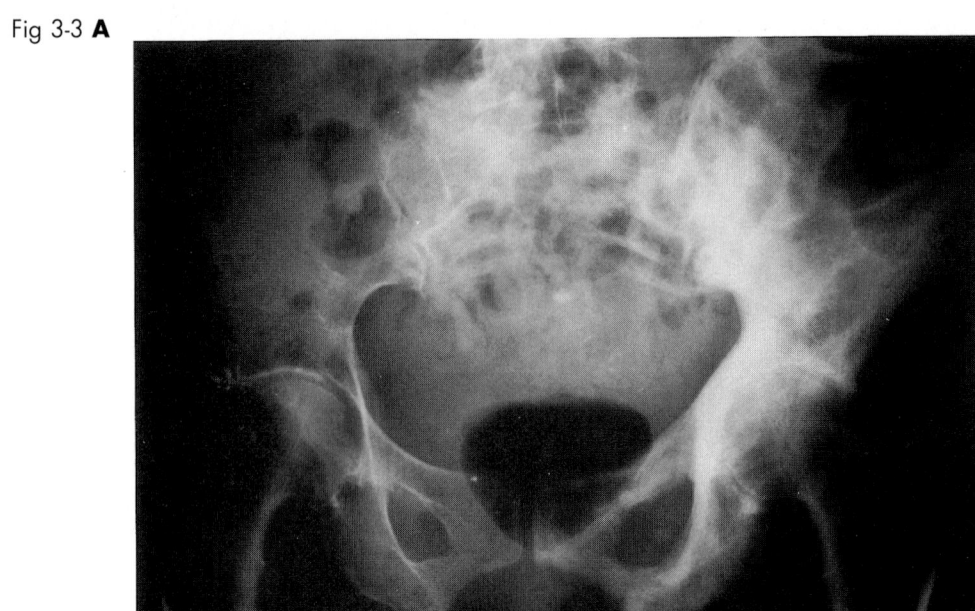

Fig 3-3 **B**

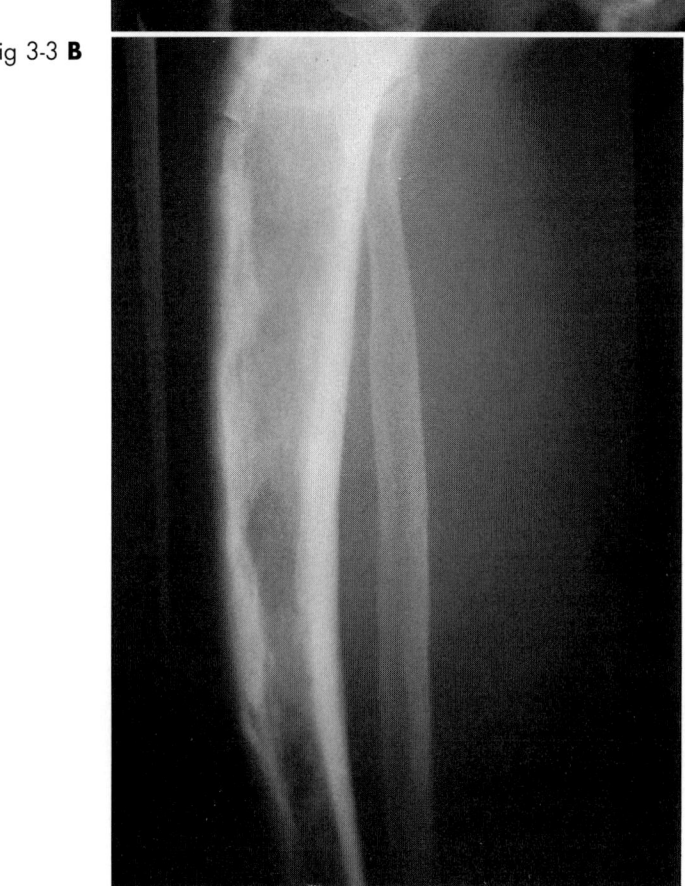

ANSWER

10   Osteoarthritis is one of the common causes of pain in patients with Paget's disease developing secondary to an enlargement of Pagetic bone in the periarticular region. Altered biomechanics associated with long bone deformity may also cause pain in the bone and associated joints.

QUESTIONS

11 When performing a total joint arthroplasty, what special precautions should be taken in these patients?

12 List the major complications of Paget's disease.

13 A 12-year-old girl is referred by her hematologist because of increased pain and decreased range of motion in her hips. She has been given a diagnosis of Gaucher's disease, and her neurologic examination is normal. Her hip x-ray films are shown (*Figure 3-4*). How can this diagnosis be established?

Fig 3-4
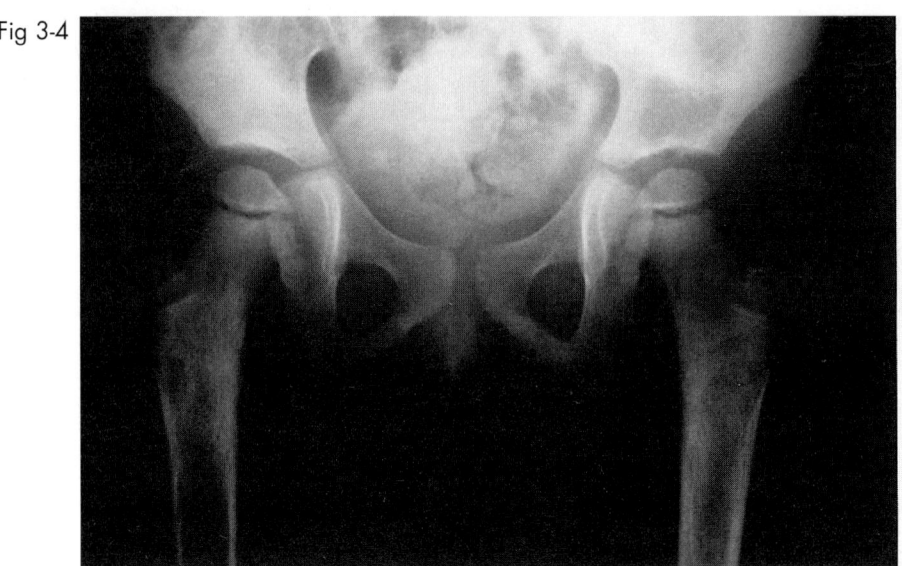

14 What are other manifestations of the disease?

15 Gaucher's disease has been organized into three types. To which type does this patient most likely belong?

ANSWERS

11 The prosthetic components should be cemented in place because there is a higher incidence of loosening of noncemented prostheses. The patient should be treated with calcitonin preoperatively to control the metabolic activity of the bone. Preparation should be made for replacement of excessive blood loss.

12 Skeletal complications are: fracture, deformity, secondary osteoarthritis, and sarcoma. Other complications are: high-output cardiac failure, hearing loss, headache and mental status change, and hypercalcemia.

13 Gaucher's disease is a lipid storage disease characterized by low levels of the enzyme leukocyte acid β-glucosidase. The test for this enzyme is reliable in establishing in the diagnosis. Visualization of Gaucher's cells on sternal marrow aspirate would confirm the diagnosis.

14 Splenic enlargement, bleeding disorders, hepatomegaly, thrombocytopenia, anemia, bone pain, and fractures.

15 Type I. Type I is the most common and the only type not associated with neurologic changes.

QUESTIONS

16 A new x-ray film is taken (*Figure 3-5*). What would you recommend for treatment of her current problem?

Fig 3-5

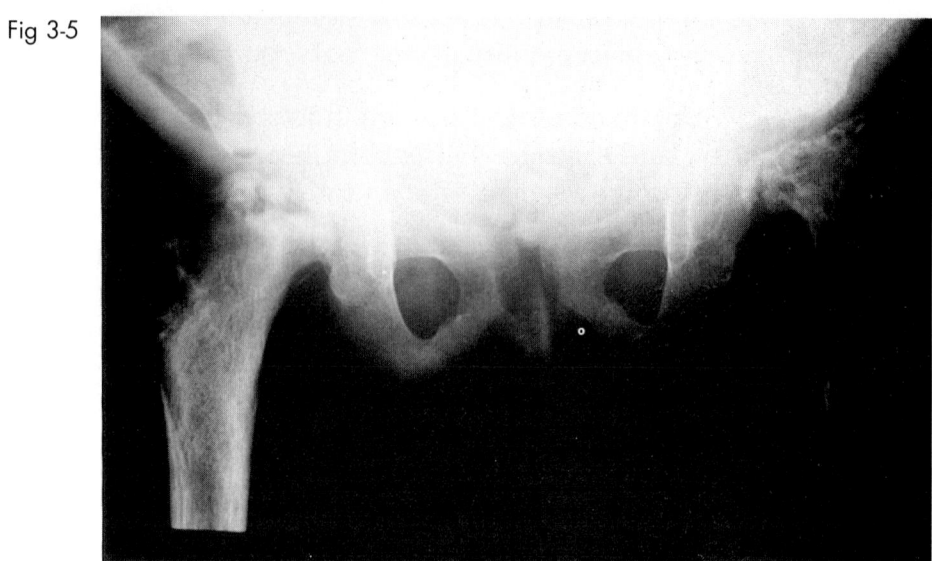

17 What other areas of the skeleton would you evaluate to further confirm the diagnosis and evaluate future problems?

18 The patient in Q13 returns one month later with extreme pain in her femur, which developed acutely and without known trauma. What is your differential diagnosis?

19 Are imaging techniques, other than routine x-ray film helpful in managing patients with this disease?

20 A 22-year-old man complains of pain in both upper thighs while standing or walking. His stature is unusually short, and he relates a history of taking medication most of his childhood. Current laboratory evaluation shows:

Calcium	9.6	(8.7-10.7)
Phosphorus	2.5	(2.7-4.5)
Alkaline phosphatase	184	(35-117)
Parathyroid hormone	123	(10-65)
Urine calcium	23	(100-300)
Urine phosphate	2644	(400-800)

What is his most likely diagnosis?

21 Describe this patient's primary metabolic defect.

ANSWERS

16 Avascular necrosis of the femoral heads is the second most common musculoskeletal problem affecting patients with this disease. In childhood it can be treated in a similar manner to Legg-Calvé-Perthes (LCP) disease. In adults total hip arthroplasty has been performed with success.

17 The most common skeletal abnormality is enlargement of the distal femurs (Erlenmeyer flask deformity). Other skeletal areas include avascular necrosis of the humeral head, endosteal scalloping of the distal humerus, and compression fractures of the thoracic and lumbar spine. The latter may be associated with neurologic impairment.

18 Pyogenic osteomyelitis versus Gaucher's "bone crisis" (pseudo-osteomyelitis).

19 The Technetium 99m bone scan is often positive in areas of bone involvement before changes are seen on routine x-ray films. The magnetic resonance imaging (MRI) is able to assess early bone marrow abnormalities and avascular necrosis of bone, but it is not reliable in differentiating pyogenic osteomyelitis from "bone crises." MRI is best done with clinical correlation.

20 Hypophosphatemic vitamin D-resistant rickets and osteomalacia have both acquired and hereditary forms. Most likely this patient has the hereditary type because his symptoms began in childhood. The classic triad includes hypophosphatemia, lower extremity deformity, and a decreased growth rate.

21 It is believed that there is a genetic defect affecting intracellular phosphate transport. The major target organs are the osteoblast and renal tubular cell and, secondarily, 1,25 (OH) 2 vitamin D synthesis.

QUESTIONS

22 Shown is an x-ray film of the patient's right proximal femur (*Figure 3-6*). Does this explain his pain?

Fig 3-6

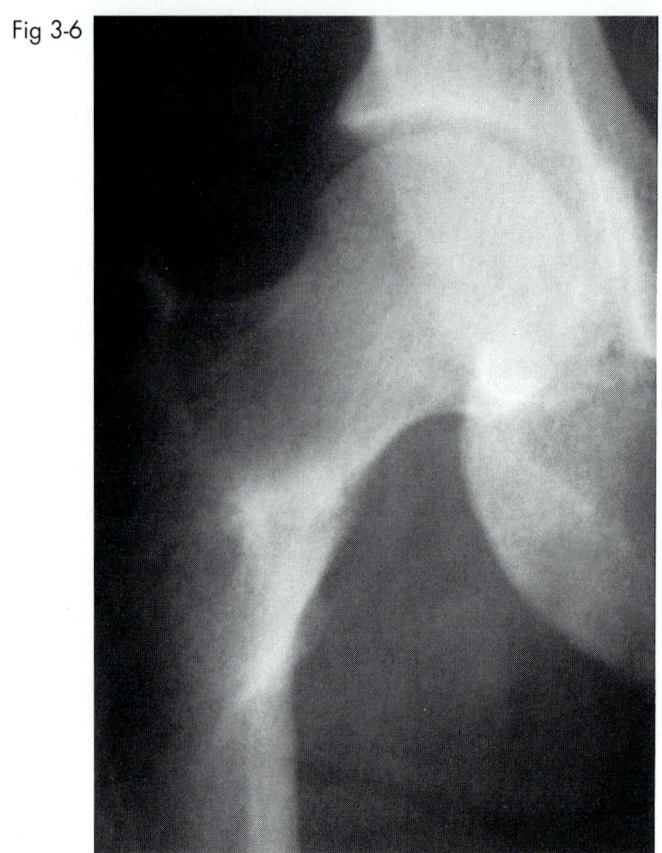

23 Should this patient receive medical treatment?

24 Describe what you would expect to find on a tetracycline-labeled iliac crest bone biopsy.

25 A 76-year-old woman is seen after sustaining bilateral nontraumatic fractures of her femoral necks. She has a history of surgery that included total-joint arthroplasty of a knee and shoulder and a gastric resection. She has lactose intolerance, and current medications include digoxin, Lasix, Os-Cal, and estrogen, which she has taken since menopause. Her initial laboratory values were:

Calcium	7.5	(8.7-10.7)
Phosphorus	2.6	(2.7-4.5)
Alkaline phosphatase	198	(35-117)
Parathyroid hormone	162	(10-65)
Urine calcium	60	(100-300)
Urine phosphate	365	(400-800)

What is her most likely diagnosis?

ANSWERS

22 Stress fractures, or Looser's transformation zones, occur in osteomalacia secondary to the mineralization defect. They are a common cause of pain and occur typically in the scapula, pubic rami, ribs, long bones, and metatarsals.

23 Before epiphyseal closure, treatment with phosphorus and calcitriol (1,25 vitamin D) has been shown to be beneficial in promoting growth and preventing deformity. In adults, similar treatment remains controversial but is indicated in symptomatic patients.

24 Increased osteoid content with wide osteoid seam covering the trabeculae, a moderate increase in osteoclast numbers, little or no tetracycline uptake, and an increased trabecular volume.

25 Osteomalacia secondary to malabsorption syndrome. In addition to her gastric surgery, she is taking Lasix, which is a calciuretic agent, and has a lactose intolerance that limits her calcium absorption.

QUESTIONS

26 Her vitamin D levels confirm your diagnosis: 25 vitamin D <5 and 1,25 vitamin D is 15 (normals are 16 to 37 ng/ml and 12 to 42 pg/ml, respectively). By what mechanism is she able to maintain her 1,25 vitamin D level near normal with such a low 25 vitamin D?

27 Which set of data from a tetracycline-labeled bone biopsy is most compatible with this patient?

	A	B	C
Osteoid surface (4-18)	12	60	65
Osteoid thickness (6-12)	28	10	25
Mineralization lag time (15-20)	42	32	99
Osteoclast number (0-2)	1.6	3.1	9.6
Aluminum stain (negative)	neg	pos	neg

28 How would you begin treatment in this patient?

29 What is the major complication from such treatment?

30 Which laboratory parameters would you follow to judge if your treatment is effective?

31 How is urinary calcium affected by serum calcium? By PTH? By 1,25 vitamin D? By thiazide diuretics?

32 Name the major etiologies of severe osteomalacia.

ANSWERS

26 The elevated parathyroid hormone (PTH) drives the alpha 1 hydroxylase to convert any available 25 vitamin D to the 1,25 form. The later will fall when the 25 vitamin D substrate is used up.

27 Column C represents the data from this patient. The abnormalities seen in overt osteomalacia include elevated osteoid surface and seam thickness as the osteoblasts continue to manufacture osteoid, but it cannot be properly mineralized. Thus the mineralization lag time is lengthened. The osteoclast number increases secondary to the compensatory increase in PTH.

28 The patient needs calcium and vitamin D supplementation. If there is evidence of impaired liver function or if she is unresponsive to vitamin D, 25 (OH) 2 vitamin D (calcidiol) should be given.

29 Hypercalcemia.

30 The serum calcium and phosphorus should move into the normal range. However, the most sensitive test is the PTH level, which will return to normal when there is no longer a need to compensate for inadequate calcium absorption. The urinary calcium should return toward normal with adequate treatment.

31 Urine calcium varies in direct proportion to serum calcium. PTH increases tubular reabsorption of calcium and tends to lower urine calcium. The effect of 1,25 vitamin D on urine calcium is secondary to its effect on serum calcium. The thiazide diuretics increase tubular reabsorption of calcium and lower urine calcium.

32
- Vitamin D deficiency: dietary
  - related to gastrointestinal (GI) disorders
- Medication induced: anticonvulsant therapy
  - antituberculous drugs
- Hypophosphatemic syndromes
- Renal failure
- Tumor induced (oncogenic osteomalacia)

QUESTIONS

33 A 47-year-old man is seen in a busy orthopedic clinic with a 4-month history of pain in the right hip and difficulty with ambulation. He has a history of a 10-pound weight loss over the past 2 months and complains that he is constantly thirsty but has had increasing nocturia. He has a history of nephrolithiasis and has had a peptic ulcer. His chest x-ray film is normal and his pelvic x-ray film (*Figure 3-7*) is shown.

Initial laboratory data:

serum calcium	12.2
phosphorus	2.6
alkaline phosphatase	396

Fig 3-7

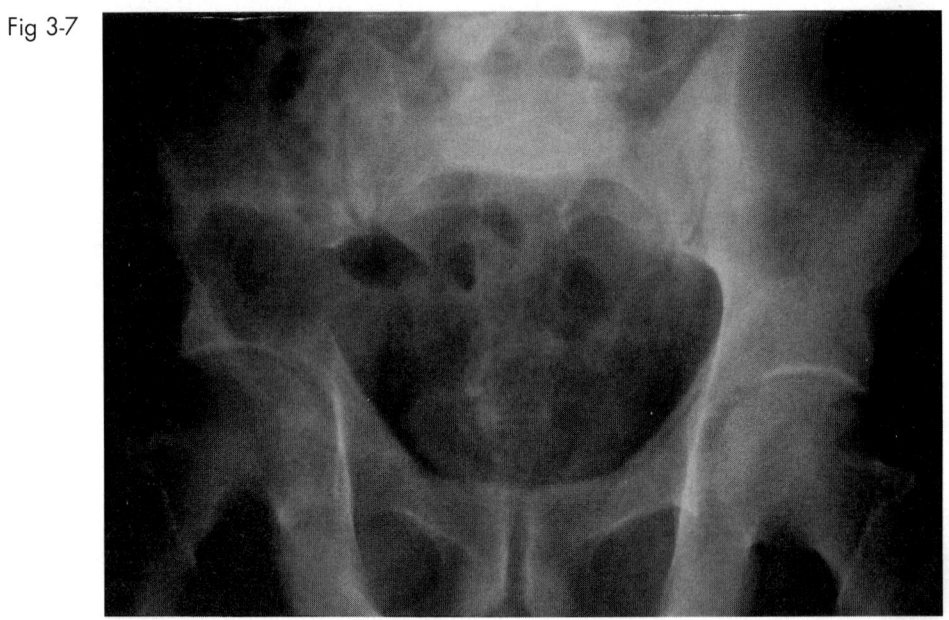

Outline your differential diagnosis.

34 Would additional tests be confirmatory?

35 The PTH level is markedly elevated. What would you suggest his urinary calcium and phosphate excretion to be?

36 What is the most likely etiology of this patient's pelvic lesion?

37 Describe the usual presentation of a patient with primary hyperparathyroidism. Does this patient fit this model?

38 Is the patient's history compatible with the diagnosis of hyperparathyroidism?

39 Describe the usual skeletal changes seen by x-ray film in this disease.

ANSWERS

33   The most common causes of hypercalcemia are primary hyperparathyroidism and hypercalcemia of malignancy. Other less common causes include thyrotoxicosis, granulomatous diseases, immobilization, certain drugs, and renal failure.

34   A PTH level would be elevated in primary hyperparathyroidism and depressed if his hypercalcemia is secondary to malignancy.

35   Both will be elevated. PTH causes increased phosphate excretion and increased calcium reabsorption at the renal tubule. A high serum calcium will eventually spill calcium into the urine, whereas the near normal serum phosphate allows the increased excretion to continue under the influence of increased PTH. This patient's urine values were:

Calcium	648	(100-300)
Phosphate	1015	(400-800)

36   Osteitis fibrosa cystica (brown tumor).

37   Most patients now have few presenting symptoms, and the diagnosis is made by abnormal laboratory tests (elevated serum calcium and PTH). This patient was unusual with advanced disease when first seen.

38   The history of nephrolithiasis and peptic ulcers are common. Thirst and polyuria are secondary to the high serum calcium. Other manifestations include pancreatitis, muscle weakness, and hypertension.

39   A generalized osteopenia is seen secondary to the increased bone resorption. Cortical bone is resorbed at a faster rate than cancellous bone; this is manifest as subperiosteal resorption in the phalanges and distal clavicle. The skull may show a "salt and pepper" appearance, and cystic changes (brown tumor) will occur late in the disease process.

QUESTIONS

40 What are the two major mechanisms that cause the hypercalcemia that is seen in malignancy?

41 The physical medicine chronic pain service asks you to see a 33-year-old man with diffuse skeletal pain and muscle weakness of many months duration. He has no history of fractures, but his bone density is low. Laboratory data is:

Serum calcium	9.4	(8.5-10.6)
Serum phosphorus	2.0	(2.5-4.5)
Alkaline phosphatase	414	(20-135)
Parathyroid hormone	normal	
25 OH vitamin D	19	(9-50)
1,25 OH vitamin D	<5	(15-60)

Tetracycline-labeled bone biopsy was consistent with severe osteomalacia. Into which general category of metabolic bone disease does this patient fit?

42 The patient had a small soft tissue mass removed from his thigh several years earlier. It was diagnosed as an hemangiopericytoma. What is the likely diagnosis of the patient's metabolic bone disease?

43 Discuss the pathophysiology.

44 Which tumors are associated with this disease?

45 Following resection of the tumor, what treatment regime is indicated for the metabolic bone abnormalities?

46 A 10-year-old patient has presenting symptoms that include somewhat short stature and pain in the regions of her major joints. The x-ray film is shown (*Figure 3-8*). What are the likely causes of her problem?

Fig 3-8

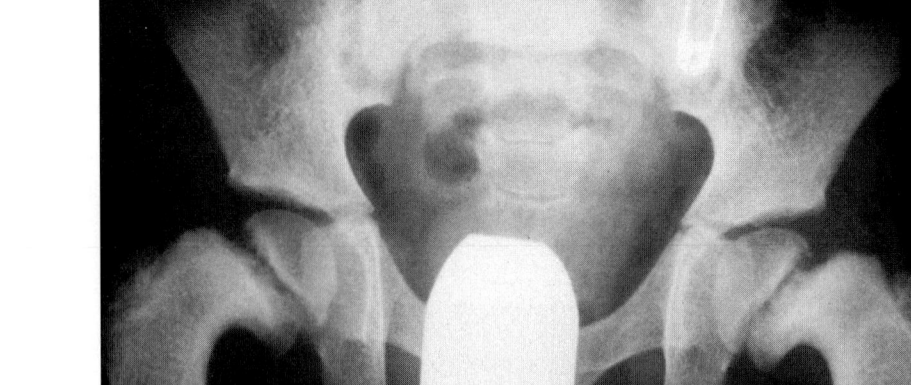

ANSWERS

40 Humeral hypercalcemia results from production of calcemic factor by the tumor. One specific factor, PTH-related protein, is believed to be the responsible factor in a large number of cases. Local or generalized bone destruction by the tumor tissue can be seen in myeloma, breast cancer, prostate cancer, and lymphomas.

41 Hypophosphatemic rickets and osteomalacia.

42 This represents tumor-associated or oncogenic osteomalacia. Although the tumors are often small and difficult to detect, the laboratory finding of hypophosphatemia, increased urine phosphate, a normal 25 vitamin D, and a low 1,25 vitamin D are classic for this syndrome.

43 The exact mechanism remains unclear, but it is believed that the tumor produces a factor that affects the function of the renal tubule blocking phosphate reabsorption, as well as produces a conversion of 25 vitamin D to 1,25 vitamin D.

44 Usually the tumor is benign and of mesenchymal origin. Vascular tumors seem to be the predominate type, but giant cell tumors and chondrosarcoma have been reported. Other tumors less frequently involved include breast, prostate, and oat cell carcinomas, multiple myeloma, and nonossifying fibroma.

45 Once the tumor tissue is removed, the metabolic abnormalities correct and usually require no further treatment.

46 The findings are those of active rickets, which may be caused by nutritional deficiency of vitamin D and calcium or renal disease.

QUESTIONS

47 Which regions of the physeal plate do you expect to show microscopic change?

48 The patient described in Q46 has rickets secondary to renal failure. What physiologic changes account for skeletal abnormalities?

49 List the major skeletal changes seen in childhood renal osteodystrophy.

50 A 42-year-old man has presenting symptoms that include spontaneous fractures of several ribs and his fourth lumbar vertebrae. A bone mineral density measurement is two standard deviations below his age-matched normal value. In the laboratory workup, which particular test should you order?

51 A 42-year-old female renal transplant patient was referred to the orthopedic clinic for increasing pain in both hips. Physical examination showed a positive Trendelenburg gait bilaterally and a painful decrease in the range of motion of both hips. X-ray film taken 3 years posttransplant are shown (*Figure 3-9*). What is the most likely cause of her symptoms?

Fig 3-9

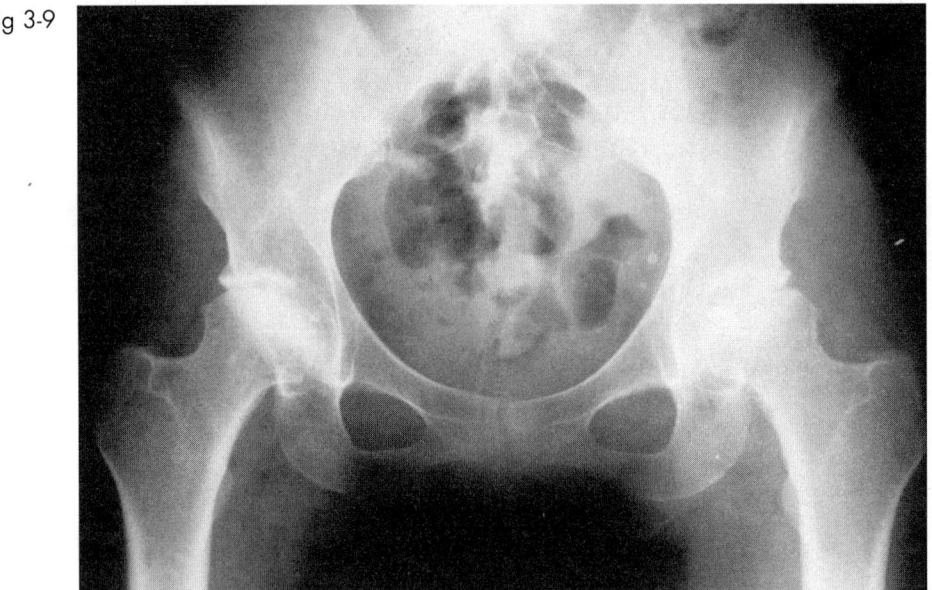

52 Which other skeletal areas are likely to be involved with this process?

53 Name the most common etiologic factors associated with avascular necrosis of the femoral head.

ANSWERS

47 The hypertrophic zone and the zone of provisional calcification. The hypertrophic zone becomes markedly widened, and provisional calcification does not occur. The reserve and proliferative zones remain normal.

48 The kidneys are responsible for the α-L-hydroxylation of vitamin D making the active form, 1,25 (OH) 2 D3, and for control of calcium and phosphate excretion. With renal failure, serum phosphate increases and vitamin D function is impaired, resulting in altered calcium availability. PTH is secondarily increased. Mineralization at the growth plate is impaired, and the skeleton becomes osteopenic. When aluminum-containing medication is used to bind the excess phosphate in the GI tract, a secondary aluminum-induced osteomalacia may occur.

49 Bowing of the long bones, enlargement of the wrists and ankles, frontal bossing of the skull, kyphosis, scoliosis, slipped epiphyses, and short stature.

50 The serum testosterone level. Although all of the risk factors are important, including alcohol intake, the most common cause of osteopenia in young men is hypogonadism.

51 The patient has bilateral avascular necrosis, which is likely caused by the high steroid dosage prescribed following her renal transplant. She was treated at a time before cyclosporine therapy was commonly used and, consequently, was treated with high-dosage steroids and Imuran.

52 The most common areas involved with steroid-induced avascular necrosis include the proximal humerus, the talus, the distal femoral condyles, and the femoral heads.

53 High-dose steroids, Caisson's disease, sickle cell disease, excessive alcohol intake, lupus, fractures of the femoral neck, hip dislocations, and radiation exposure.

QUESTIONS

54 Which of the currently available imaging modalities will detect femoral head avascular necrosis the earliest?

55 The treatment options for femoral head avascular necrosis include:

56 The same patient described in Q52 began to develop a clicking sensation in her right hip 8 years following her total hip replacements. She had no pain with normal walking. Her x-ray film is shown (*Figure 3-10*). What is your differential diagnosis of this lesion?

Fig 3-10

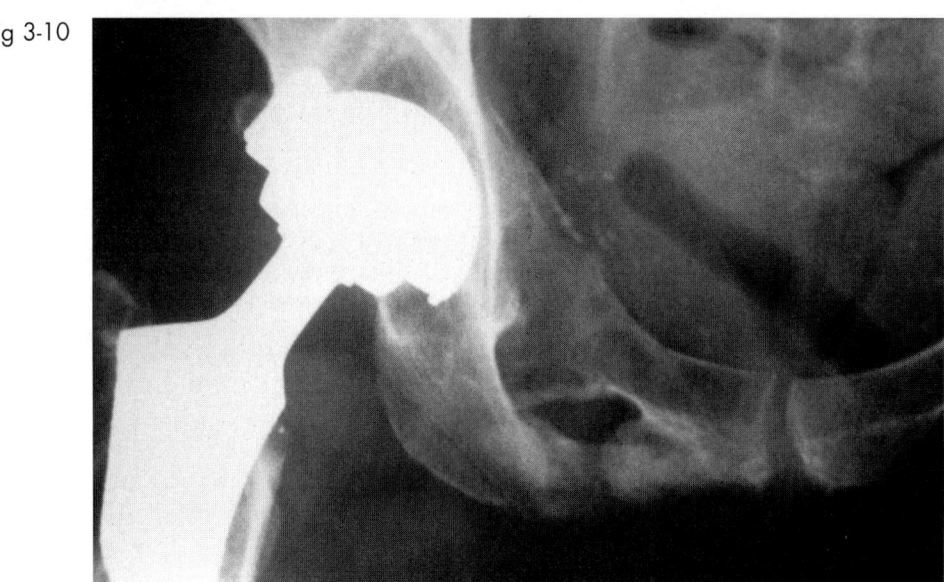

ANSWERS

54 MRI will detect the earliest changes in the femoral head. The technetium 99m bone scan will detect osteonecrosis before routine x-ray film studies.

55 (1) Protective weight bearing. This treatment is occasionally successful in preventing collapse of the femoral head, but often the disease progresses despite conservative care.
(2) Core decompression with or without bone graft. The literature is conflicting as to the results of this form of treatment. Success depends on the stage at which treatment is instituted, but the failure rate remains high.
(3) Joint arthroplasty. Although rotational osteotomy has been used, total joint arthroplasty remains the procedure of choice following femoral head collapse and the onset degenerative arthritis.

56 Infection, benign neoplasm, polyethylene wear debris were considered in the patient's differential diagnosis. She proved to have bone lysis, secondary to reaction to the polyethylene wear debris from the cup liner. Microscopically this tissue appears as small birefringent shards with a surrounding inflammatory reaction.

QUESTIONS

57 A 28-year-old woman developed gradual increasing pain in her left groin and hip region during the last trimester of pregnancy. The pain continued, and she presents to your office 1 month postpartum. Her pelvis film is shown (*Figure 3-11*). Laboratory data show normal white blood cell (WBC) count, erythrocyte sedimentation rate (ESR), alkaline phosphatase, calcium, and phosphorus. How can you confirm your diagnosis?

Fig 3-11

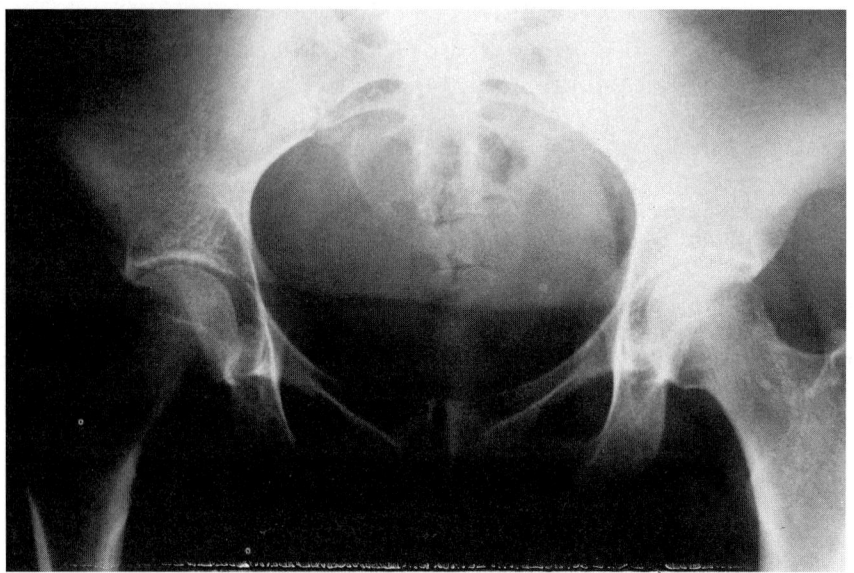

58 Which other areas of the skeleton might be involved with this syndrome?

59 How should this patient be treated?

ANSWERS

57 The patient's most likely diagnosis is transient regional osteoporosis of pregnancy. Laboratory data and synovial fluid analysis are usually within normal limits, but a bone scan may be positive in the area of involvement.

58 Transient regional osteoporosis of pregnancy usually involves the hip region. A similar syndrome seen in both men and women is not associated with pregnancy and has a similar presentation and course. It is commonly seen in the hip, knee, foot, ankle, and shoulder regions.

59 This is usually a self-limited condition and will resolve after delivery. Treatment in both groups mentioned in A58 should be symptomatic and consist of nonsteroidal antiinflammatory agents to control the discomfort and protective weight bearing to avoid injury to the osteopenic bone. Resolution should occur over a several month period.

QUESTIONS

60 A 24-year-old woman develops pain in her left arm after bumping into a door frame while riding in her wheelchair. An x-ray film of her left upper extremity is shown (*Figure 3-12*). What is her most likely metabolic defect?

Fig 3-12

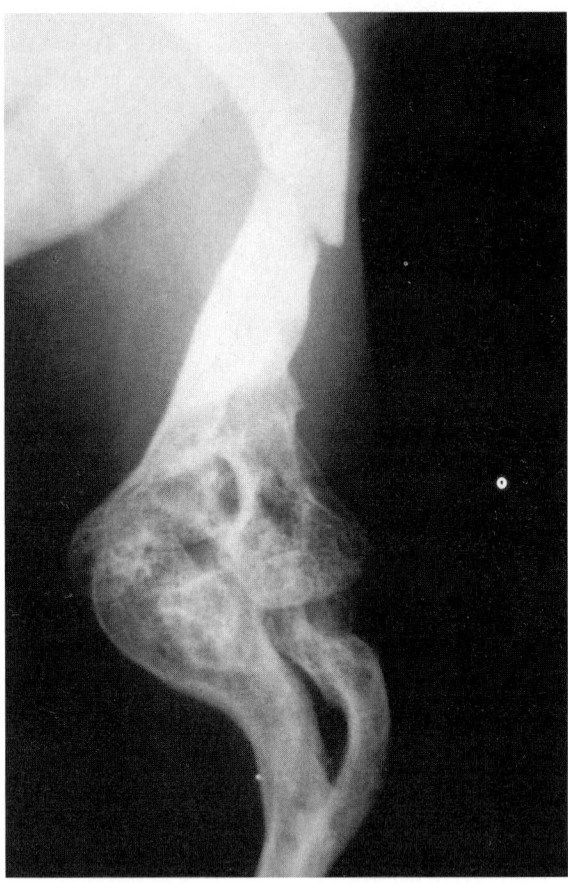

61 How can you use the laboratory to confirm your clinical diagnosis?

62 List the differential diagnoses of serial fractures in children.

63 Describe the genetics of osteogenesis imperfecta.

64 List the clinical classification system for osteogenesis imperfecta.

65 What are the major complications of Type III osteogenesis imperfecta?

66 A 22-year-old man is seen in the emergency room with a closed fracture of his left femur secondary to an automobile accident. He has no other significant abnormalities noted; he is taken to the operating room for closed intramedullary rod placement of his fractured femur. Shortly after induction of the anesthesia, the anesthesiologist notes that the patient has become tachycardiac, his carbon dioxide tension has increased, and his temperature is 38.8° C. Should you proceed with the surgical treatment of this patient? What is your working diagnosis?

ANSWERS

60   The patient's diagnosis is osteogenesis imperfecta, and the x-ray film shows the typical findings of a patient with a severe form of this disease. The metabolic defect responsible for this condition is an abnormality of structure or synthesis of Type I collagen.

61   The laboratory findings are usually normal and of little help in confirming the diagnosis. At times, nonspecific elevation of serum alkaline phosphatase and urinary calcium and hydroxyproline are present. Skin biopsy using special staining techniques may be more helpful in establishing the diagnosis in the milder forms of the disease.

62   Child abuse, congenital insensitivity to pain, and osteogenesis imperfecta.

63   Inheritance is thought to be predominantly autosomal dominant with some cases of autosomal recessive inheritance occurring in Types II and III. Most cases seem to be point mutations involving the pro alpha 1 and pro alpha 2 chains of the Type I collagen. These mutations occur at a variety of locations. A consistent defect is rarely found between affected lineages.

64   There are four clinical types defined at present.
Type I—Type I patients have little deformity, are normal in stature, and have infrequent fractures. Fifty percent of these individuals have hearing loss.
Type II—This form is fatal in infancy.
Type III—Patients with this form of the disease have short stature, multiple fractures, and usually some deformities present at birth. The teeth and hearing are commonly affected.
Type IV—This form of osteogenesis imperfecta is mild to moderate with some bone deformity and possibly short stature. Teeth involvement is common, but hearing loss occurs less often than in Type III.

65   Multiple recurrent fractures, long bone deformities, kyphoscoliosis, dentinogenesis imperfecta, ligamentous laxity, and hearing loss.

66   The most likely diagnosis is malignant hyperthermia, which can occur in healthy individuals with no known family history of the disorder. The safest course is to discontinue the surgical procedure and immediately institute treatment for malignant hyperthermia.

QUESTIONS

67 What is the treatment of choice for this syndrome?

68 What are the commonly involved agents that trigger malignant hyperthermia?

69 A 32-year-old man complains of pain in several skeletal sites including his right humerus and both femurs. He has had problems with his humerus since age 16 when he was diagnosed as having fibrous dysplasia. The x-ray film of his femur is shown (*Figure 3-13*). Current laboratory data show normal calcium and phosphorus levels, an alkaline phosphatase of 369 (normal = 117), and a normal urinary examination for calcium and phosphorus. Are these laboratory results compatible with fibrous dysplasia?

Fig 3-13

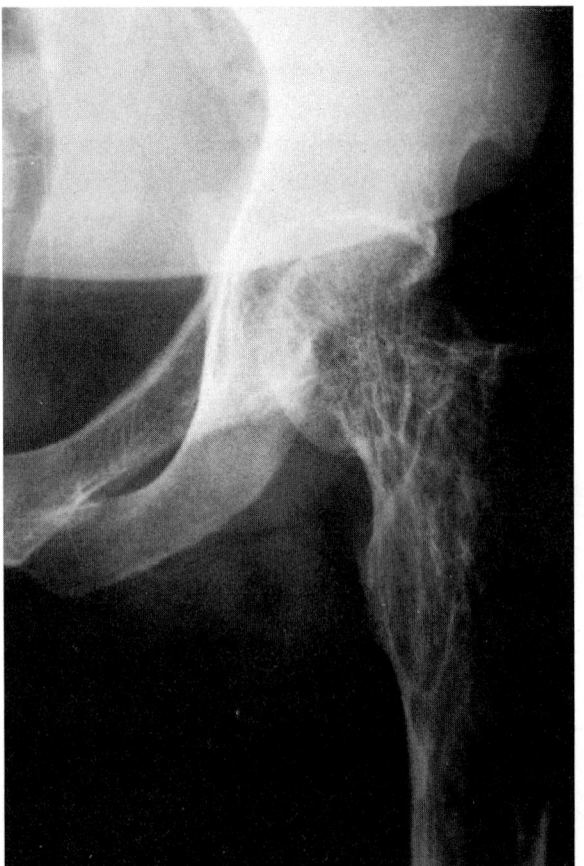

70 The patient also demonstrates several large irregular café au lait spots on his chest wall. What is your diagnosis now?

71 Name the common endocrine abnormalities seen in the Albright-McCune-Sternberg syndrome.

72 Is there medical treatment available for the bone lesions seen in fibrous dysplasia?

ANSWERS

67 Treatment of the acute crisis should include terminating the administration of anesthetic agents, administering dantrolene intravenously at a dose of 2 to 3 mg/kg, cooling the patient, and treating any electrolyte or cardiac disturbances.

68 Inhalation anesthetics, muscle relaxants (particularly succinyl choline), and possibly the intake of alcohol and cocaine.

69 Yes. The laboratory results are usually normal in the patient with fibrous dysplasia, but the results may also show an elevated alkaline phosphatase. Rarely phosphorus wasting is seen in the urine. This occurs in the Albright-McCune-Sternberg variety of fibrous dysplasia.

70 The three types of fibrous dysplasia include the monostotic variety, usually seen in the second and third decade; a polyostotic variety seen in children less than 10 years; and the Albright-McCune-Sternberg syndrome, a polyostotic variety with café au lait spots and multiple endocrine changes.

71 Thyrotoxicosis, Cushing's syndrome, acromegaly, hyperprolactinemia, hyperparathyroidism, and precocious puberty.

72 No, except in a rare phosphate wasting syndrome. In the patient with this variant, phosphorus and vitamin D supplementation may help to correct the generalized bone disease.

QUESTIONS

73 When should surgery be considered in this disease?

74 A 60-year-old woman is seen in your office questioning the value of a bone mineral density study. She asks if bone mineral density measurement is predictive of her chances of having a hip fracture in the future. What advise would you give?

75 How does the fracture risk increase with a decreasing bone mass?

76 Which of the current methods for measuring bone mineral density are associated with the lowest dosage of radiation?

77 List the major indications for performing bone mineral density measurements.

78 A 42-year-old woman with severe asthma has been on and off corticosteroids for many years. Her current dosage is 60 mg of prednisone per day, but she assures you that it is being tapered; and she should be off the drug soon. What would you expect her bone mineral density to show?

79 What are the effects of prednisone on bone to account for this change?

80 The patient's laboratory data showed the following serum values: Alkaline phosphatase 137, osteocalcin 1.8, calcium 9.2, phosphorus 3.1. What is the significance of the low osteocalcin value?

81 Name some of the disorders in which osteocalcin might be increased.

82 What influences serum alkaline phosphatase levels in this patient?

83 Describe the major biochemical markers of bone resorption.

ANSWERS

73 The bone lesions should not be treated surgically unless the disease is associated with significant or progressive deformity, pain, or multiple fractures. At times, biopsy is useful for making the diagnosis.

74 Studies indicate that hip fracture risk is proportional to femoral bone mineral density and to the age of the patient. Bone mineral density measurement is useful in assessing the overall fracture risk but will not give a definitive individual prognosis. The other major risk factor for fractured hips in the elderly is the propensity to fall.

ANSWERS

75 The risk increases 1.5 to 2.0 for each standard deviation decrease in the bone mineral measurement.

76 Dual energy x-ray film absorptiometry. The highest dosage is from quantitative computer tomography (CT) followed by single photon absorptiometry. The latter involves less than 15 mrem of radiation per examination. Dual photon and energy absorptiometry are associated with the lowest radiation dosages. The dual energy x-ray film absorptiometry is the most common method in use at this time.

77 1. Estrogen deficiency, if used as an assessment for the need of estrogen replacement therapy
2. X-ray film evidence of decreased bone mineral density, especially that seen on spinal x-ray films
3. Initiation of glucocorticoid therapy
4. Patients with proven primary hyperparathyroidism, if treatment decisions need to be evaluated

78 A marked decrease for her age.

79 Corticosteroids cause an increase in the urinary calcium loss, a decrease in intestinal absorption of calcium, decreased osteoblast function, and increase in the bone resorption rate. All of these adversely effect the bone's ability to maintain its normal architecture and mineral content.

80 Osteocalcin is synthesized by the osteoblasts. Although most is incorporated into the matrix, some is released and measurable in the serum. The function of osteocalcin is not entirely known; however, it is a marker of the bone formation rate. It is increased in certain high turnover states and is decreased when the formation rate is decreased. In this case the decrease is secondary to the glucocorticoid effect on the osteoblasts.

81 Paget's disease, hyperthyroidism, hyperparathyroidism, and acromegaly.

82 Alkaline phosphatase may be increased by bone formation and by bone resorption. It is a mark of bone turnover in diseases such as Paget's disease, but levels in corticosteroid-treated patients may not be helpful because both formation and resorption may be effected.

83 Several markers found in the urine are elevated in association with increased bone resorption. These include urinary calcium, hydroxyproline, and pyridinoline. The latter two are both collagen degradation products. In addition the bone biopsy specimens often show an increase in the osteoclast numbers in the patient with active bone resorption.

QUESTIONS

84   You are asked to see a 12-year-old boy with short stature secondary to truncal shortening, genu valgus, kyphosis, and coroneal clouding. He also has short phalanges. The elbow and wrist joints appear lax to your examination. You were told that the admitting physician is considering a diagnosis of mucopolysaccharidosis. If this is so, what type do you suspect, and how can you confirm your diagnosis?

85   You are asked by the family if this disease is inherited and if prenatal diagnosis would be possible if they consider having another child. How do you respond?

86   The surgeons are considering an abdominal operation on the patient with Morquio's syndrome, requiring a general anesthetic. They ask if you know of any precautions they should take.

87   You are now the local expert in managing patients with mucopolysaccharidosis; you are asked to see another patient with median nerve dysfunction and normal intelligence. His laboratory data show increased urinary chondroitin and dermatan sulfate, and he has an abnormality of α-L-iduronidase deficiency. You immediately recognize which type of mucopolysaccharidosis?

88   In spontaneous or natural fracture healing, what is the apparent role of transforming growth factor-β (tgf-β)?

89   What is the probable function of tgf-β during the enchondral stage of fracture repair?

90   Name some other noncollagenous proteins believed to be important in fracture repair.

91   A 41-year-old marathon runner complains of pain in her left hip area of 2 months duration. Her routine x-ray films are in normal limits. What advice would you give?

ANSWERS

84 Skeletally, several varieties of mucopolysaccharidosis are similar to this patient, but the only type with lax joints is type IV, Morquio's syndrome. This diagnosis can be confirmed by a urinary examination showing increased keratin sulfate. A more definitive method is to perform enzyme assays on cultured fibroblasts, leukocytes, or serum.

85 All of the types of mucopolysaccharidosis are autosomal recessive in inheritance except for type II, Hunter's syndrome, which has sex-linked recessive inheritance. It is possible to perform diagnostic enzyme assays on amniotic fluid.

86 The patient with Morquio's syndrome presents a major anesthetic risk because of C1-2 instability. Patients with mucopolysaccharidosis types I, II, and VI have a less incidence of C1-2 instability, but they still have a significant risk.

87 Scheie's syndrome, type I-S, is characterized by the symptoms described in Q87 plus stiff joints and a propensity to develop carpal tunnel syndrome. The enzyme changes in Scheie's syndrome are the same as seen in Hunter-Hurler syndrome, but the latter is associated with mental retardation.

88 Having been deposited from an outside source, TGF-β is present in the fracture callus, initially localized in the hematoma. Subsequently it is synthetized by the cells active in the healing process. It probably has a regulatory function throughout the healing cascade, effecting cell proliferation, differentiation, and matrix synthesis.

89 It seems to promote the transition from cartilage production to bone production by decreasing the synthesis of type II collagen and increasing the synthesis of type I collagen during this phase.

90 Plate derived growth factor (PDGF), insulin-like growth factor (IGP-II), epidermal growth factor (EGF), and fibroblasts growth factor (FGP), have been shown to be involved. Many other factors currently being investigated are also important for the fracture healing mechanism.

91 The patient needs further evaluation, including basic laboratory data and a bone scan. Throughout the evaluation, she should limit her activity to protected weight bearing on the right lower extremity.

QUESTIONS

92 The bone scan was completed (*Figure 3-14*). What is your probable diagnosis and management?

Fig 3-14

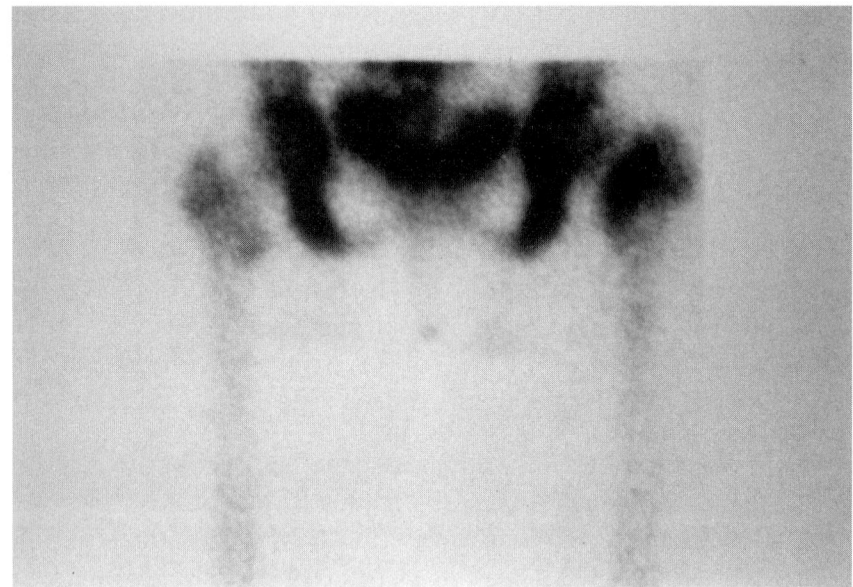

93 Describe some possible risk factors associated with the symptoms of the stress fracture described in Q92.

ANSWERS

92 The history and bone scan are compatible with a stress fracture to this area. She definitely should limit weight bearing activities and is probably a candidate to have internal fixation of her femoral neck because she is at risk of sustaining a displaced fracture. The differential diagnosis might include metastatic disease and possibly osteoid disease.

93 Estrogen deficiency, osteoporosis, and osteomalacia. In addition to her running activities, which put a high mechanical stress on the bone, her estrogen status should be investigated since it is often deficient in high-performance female athletes. A general metabolic bone work-up would be helpful to confirm that there are no other underlying metabolic diseases. A general decrease in bone mineral density has been demonstrated in young people with stress fractures.

QUESTIONS

94 A 55-year-old woman with Type I diabetes complains of pain in her right hip area of 2 months duration. Routine x-ray films of her pelvis and hips are normal. She has had no trauma, but she thinks the pain began while using a lower-extremity, low-resistance exercise machine. The delayed image of her bone scan is shown (*Figure 3-15*). What is your diagnosis, and how would you manage the patient.

Fig 3-15

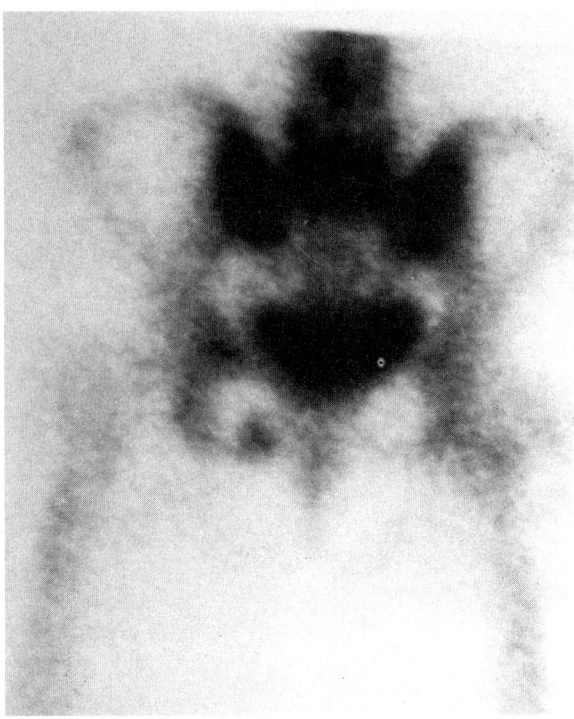

95 One year later repeat films, showed definitive changes of healing stress fracture. What are her major risk factors for developing this fracture?

ANSWERS

94   The most probable diagnosis is a stress and insufficiency fracture of her inferior and superior pubic rami. Initial management should be to reduce her activity level and decrease weight bearing across her right hemipelvis.

95   Diabetes causes a decrease in collagen production and a decrease in osteoblast function, both of which lead to diffuse osteopenia and delayed fracture healing. Associated vasculitis and neuropathy may also play a role.

QUESTIONS

96 A colleague shows you the x-ray film shown (*Figure 3-16*). He says that the patient has had some hip discomfort for several years. She has had no trauma, but reports a history of longstanding gastro-intestinal disease. What is your presumptive diagnosis?

Fig 3-16

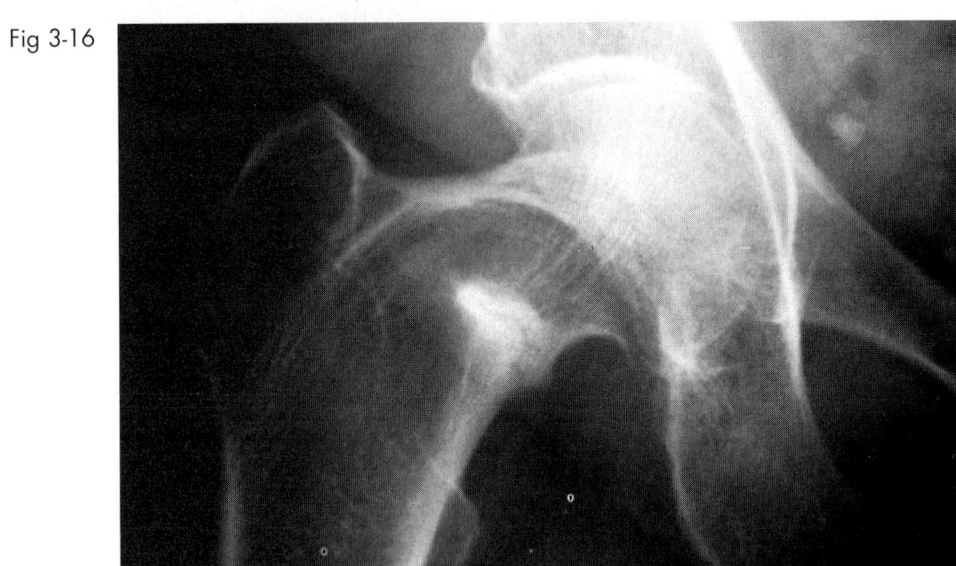

97 A patient with known hyperthyroidism has severe osteopenia. What parameters from a tetracycline-labeled bone biopsy would you expect to reflect her condition?

98 List the major indications for performing a tetracycline-labeled bone biopsy.

99 What are the typical findings in a tetracycline-labeled biopsy from a patient with osteomalacia?

ANSWERS

96   Such stress fractures or looser zones are characteristic of osteomalacia. Other common locations for stress fractures in osteomalacic patients include the ischial and pubic rami, the axillary border of the scapula, and the ribs. A laboratory work-up that includes serum levels of calcium, phosphorus, alkaline phosphatase, and PTH and possibly the vitamin D metabolites should be confirmatory. If not, a bone biopsy may be indicated.

97   Hyperthyroidism shows a classic example of an increased bone turnover and will show increase in both osteoblast and osteoclast numbers, thinning of the trabecular seams and possibly cortical porosity, a normal or accelerated mineralization rate, and a normal to slightly increased osteoid surface area. The osteoid seam thickness will be slightly narrowed.

98   Although biopsy is indicated for individuals with bone disease of an undetermined etiology, it is especially useful in suspected osteomalacia, in the management of patients with renal osteodystrophy, in young patients with osteopenia, and in the evaluation of patients who are not responding to conventional treatment programs.

99   The biopsy reflects the stages of the disease. In an early mild form the changes seen are similar to that in secondary hyperparathyroidism. This includes an increased turnover state similar to hyperthyroidism but will have associated marrow fibrosis. The intermediate stage of osteomalacia is associated with increased osteoid thickness with continuing signs of increased resorption. The fully developed osteomalacia pattern on bone biopsy shows a low turnover state with little resorption, wide osteoid seams (> 15 mm) and a decreased mineralization rate (mineralization lag time > 100 days).

CHAPTER 4

Hand and Wrist

Timothy S. Loth

QUESTIONS

1   The chief of general surgery at your hospital asks you to look at his right dominant long finger, which he just jammed into a stretcher while transferring a patient. From the time of the accident he has been unable to actively extend the distal interphalangeal (DIP) joint. Profundus function is intact, and the skin is intact. There is tenderness over the dorsal aspect of the DIP joint, and he has a 50° extension lag. Radiographic films of the finger demonstrate no bony injury. What is the diagnosis, and how would you manage this aggressive surgeon who wishes to continue operating?

2   A 35-year-old symphony conductor injured her right long finger approximately 2 months earlier, but she does not recall the mechanism of injury. She complains of DIP joint pain and an inability to extend the distal phalanx. On physical examination she has a characteristic mallet finger deformity with no bony changes noted on radiographic films. How should this problem be treated?

3   The conductor from Q2 underwent a period of splinting for 12 weeks and subsequently underwent a therapy program to wean from the splint and to commence range-of-motion exercises. She returns to your office with a 45° extension lag at the DIP joint with an associated swan-neck deformity of the finger. Passive range of motion is normal and free of pain. She asks you to do something about the deformity of her finger. What are your recommendations?

4   A 56-year-old man came to the emergency room with marked swelling and pain in his hand, complaining of an inability to sleep 18 hours after sustaining several cat bites to the dorsum of his hand. The hand is diffusely swollen with purulent material exuding from the puncture wounds. There are several tender epitrochlear nodes. Axillary nodes are nontender. Lymphangitic streaking is present to the elbow. Describe your management of this patient.

ANSWERS

1 The patient has a mallet finger. A mallet finger is a result from either an avulsion of bone from the base of the distal phalanx with the attached terminal extensor tendon, or it is a rupture of the terminal extensor. Treatment of a tendinous mallet finger is full-time splinting of the DIP joint in full to slight hyperextension for 6 to 8 weeks with a period of weaning from the splint. The splinting must be continuous; otherwise, the tendon will heal in a lengthened position resulting in a residual extension lag. To allow the patient to continue operating, we fabricated extra splints that could be gas sterilized and applied with sterile tape or Velcro following surgical scrub. Another option for treatment would be pinning the DIP joint in full extension with a transarticular Kirschner wire (K-wire) for 6 weeks. The latter treatment risks damage to the articular surface by the K-wire, as well as increases the potential for infection and nail deformity.

2 This patient has a chronic mallet finger. Even as late as 3 months, patients have been treated with extension splinting over a period of 8 to 12 weeks with correction of the mallet deformity. The finger should be splinted in full extension to slight hyperextension as described in the Q1 except that the duration should be extended 2 to 6 weeks.

3 There are several methods of reconstructing a mallet finger with associated swan-neck deformity. One of the better techniques is a release of the central slip over the proximal interphalangeal (PIP) joint, which rebalances the extensor mechanism. The patient is allowed active range of motion shortly after the operation with intermittent splinting of the PIP and DIP joints in an extension gutter over a 3-week period to prevent extensor lag at the PIP joint. This treatment has proved effective in correcting the swan-neck and mallet deformities. Other corrective techniques include surgically shortening the terminal extensor tendon or spiral oblique ligament reconstruction.

4 After obtaining wound cultures, it is advisable to start the patient on a penicillinase-resistant medication (to treat staphylococci) and penicillin (to treat Pasteurella and anaerobes.) Pasteurella multocida is a particularly aggressive organism that can develop abscesses within 24 hours of cat bites. The infected wounds should be debrided, drained, and left open until resolution of the infection has occurred. Other antibiotics, such as Augmentin, have recently been advocated for treatment of Pasteurella. Intervenous (IV) therapy is continued until there has been a substantial wound response, namely, an absence of purulent drainage, a resolution of erythema, and a marked diminution in pain. Usually 3 to 7 days after drainage the patient can be placed on oral antibiotics tailored to the culture sensitivities.

QUESTIONS

5 What are the options for treatment for a 58-year-old woman with deformity and pain from idiopathic osteoarthritis of the DIP joint?

6 Describe the treatment of a coronal dorsal hamate fracture.

7 What is the most common problem following a malunion of an unreduced, displaced, coronal dorsal hamate fracture?

8 Describe a salvage procedure for severe posttraumatic, small finger CMC arthrosis.

9 Describe the treatment of an Adriamycin chemotherapeutic agent extravasation that occurred 10 hours earlier to the dorsum of the hand of a 65-year-old woman. The dorsal hand is indurated, swollen, and exquisitely tender to a level approximately 3 cm proximal to the wrist. Reddish pigmentation is noted in an area 3 cm by 3 cm in diameter at the site of extravasation.

ANSWERS

5 Conservative measures include intermittent splinting, nonsteroidal antiinflammatory medications, and local corticosteroid injections. Surgical options include DIP joint replacement arthroplasty versus DIP joint arthrodesis. Arthrodesis is favored because it is longlasting and has fewer complications than joint replacements.

6 Although coronal dorsal hamate fractures can frequently be reduced, it is difficult to maintain the reduction. Because this is an intraarticular fracture and subluxation (dislocation), large displaced fragments should be anatomically reduced and internally fixed. Smaller hamate fragments may be excised, sutured to their site of origin, or ignored after reduction. Pinning of the carpometacarpal (CMC) joint is advisable if the injury is unstable after reduction. Pins are removed in 4 to 6 weeks.

7 Arthrosis of the small finger CMC joint with associated weakness in grip strength.

8 Interposition arthroplasty and CMC arthrodesis have been advocated for this problem. The latter is preferred because of durability, reliability, and maintenance of excellent hand function.

9 The approach to acute extravasations of chemotherapeutic agents is controversial. These agents are generally grouped, based on their toxicity, as either *vesicants* (agents that are highly toxic to tissues) or *irritants* (agents that frequently produce inflammatory reactions but rarely produce extensive necrosis). Adriamycin is a potent vesicant and, depending on the volume involved, is likely to produce a necrotic ulcer unless rapidly débrided and thoroughly irrigated. Delayed primary closure of the wound is recommended in 2 to 3 days. The débridement should remove tissues with the pigmentation of Adriamycin (i.e., the reddish pigment) and any grossly necrotic tissue. It is generally recommended that these extravasations be surgically drained as soon as possible, ideally within 72 hours. Beyond 72 hours, experimental studies have shown that extensive necrosis has frequently occurred and that at this point the débridement is too late to prevent necrosis. Débridement is limited to excising dead tissue and residual vesicant.
Others prefer to take an expectant approach, because not all vesicant extravasations go on to necrosis. In this therapeutic approach the hand is placed in a bulky dressing and ice or warm compresses are applied, and the injury is evaluated intermittently. If necrosis develops, the ulcer is débrided and skin coverage obtained. Injectable antidotes are of questionable benefit.

QUESTIONS

10 The patient from Q9 was treated with elevation, warm compresses, and observation of the extravasation. The figure shown (*Figure 4-1*) shows her hand 2 weeks following her injury. What are the options for treatment at this point?

Fig 4-1

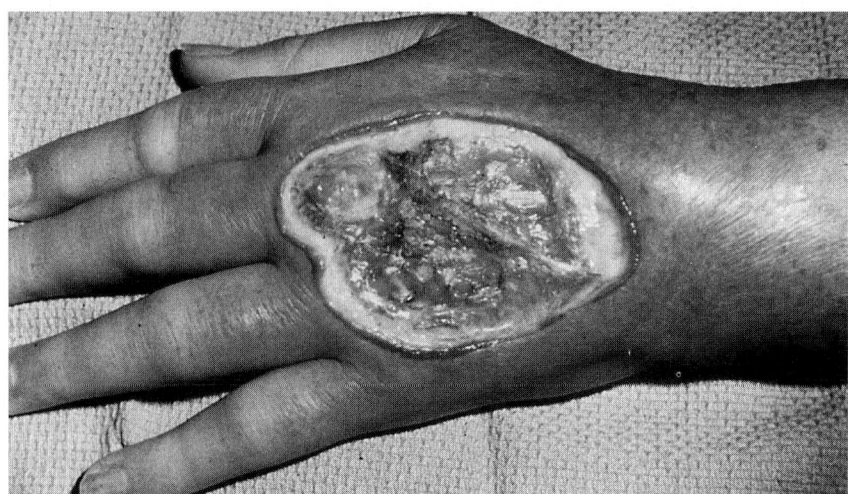

11 This 58-year-old man has noted progressive loss of motion in his ring and small fingers associated with thick cords in the palm. What is his diagnosis, and what are your recommendations regarding his treatment? (*Figure 4-2*)

Fig 4-2

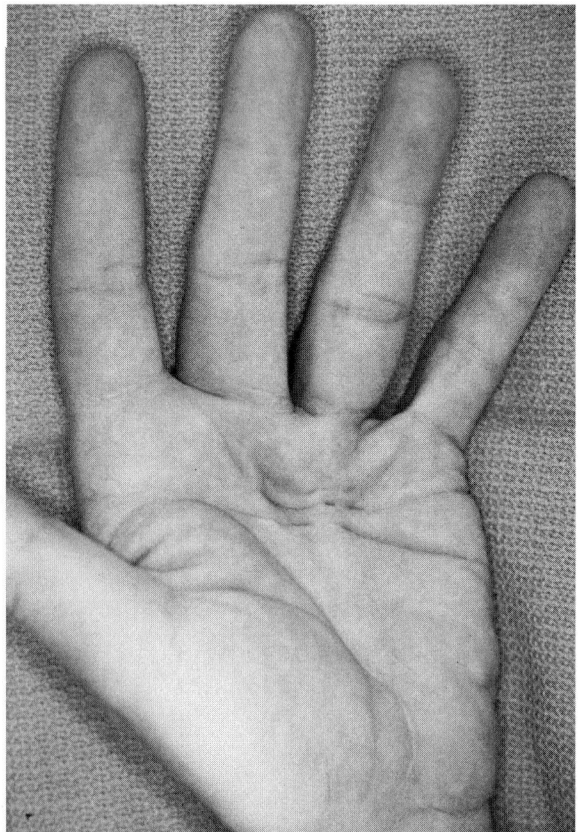

ANSWERS

10   Unfortunately, once an extravasation has reached a point of full thickness ulceration in the hand, permanent joint stiffness develops regardless of the subsequent treatment. This is one of the major arguments favoring early intervention to prevent extensive necrosis from occurring. At this point, extensive débridement of the ulcer is necessary to eliminate residual chemotherapeutic agent. Retained vesicant in the ulcer bed can cause skin graft necrosis several months after the extravasation. Once a clean bed has been established, an ulcer of this size requires flap coverage. An ipsilateral radial forearm flap is ideal for coverage of this wound. It provides stable full thickness coverage to the defect with acceptable donor site morbidity and without the necessity for microvascular transfer. Other options include posterior interosseous flap or abdominal pedicle graft.

11   The patient has Dupuytren's contractures of the ring and small fingers. Surgery is recommended for 20° to 30° contractures of the metacarpophalangeal (MCP) joint and any contracture of the PIP joint.

QUESTIONS

12   A 58-year-old woman who complains of a painful nodule located over the proximal flexion crease of the hand in the axis of the ring finger. The firm, tender mass is 5 mm by 5 mm in the fascial layer. It does not transilluminate and does not move with the flexor tendon. There is no family history of palmar masses, although she states that her father and uncle have had problems with bands in the palm, which had caused contractures of the fingers. What is the differential diagnosis for the mass, and how would you treat it?

13   A 65-year-old man with recurrent Dupuytren's contracture comes to the office complaining that his small finger is again bent at the PIP joint. He has had two previous surgeries that have failed to produce long lasting correction of the PIP contracture. The small finger is held at 90° of flexion at the PIP joint and he has no active extension and only 10° of active flexion. Radiographic films of the digit demonstrate mild joint space narrowing at the PIP joint. The finger is always getting in his way and interferes with his golf game. He requests that the finger be amputated. Discuss the options for treatment.

14   A 52-year-old right-hand dominant waste management worker lacerated his left thumb on a windshield wiper 5 days earlier. Over the past 3 days he has noted increasing pain and swelling in the thumb with intermittent purulent drainage and an inability to sleep because of throbbing pain. On physical examination there is fusiform swelling of the thumb. It is tender volarly from the tip into the palm. Active motion was minimal because of pain. The interphalangeal (IP) joint is held in mild flexion, and passive extension of the thumb IP joint caused severe pain. There is a 1.5 cm oblique laceration over the flexion crease of the thumb IP joint with purulent material draining from it. What is the patient's diagnosis, and how should he be treated?

15   What is the treatment of choice for an open tendinous mallet finger at the DIP joint?

ANSWERS

12 Because the nodule is located slightly proximal to the typical location of a volar retinacular ganglion cyst and because it does not transilluminate, one would consider additional differential diagnostic possibilities including solid tumors such as lipoma, neurilemmoma, or giant cell tumor of the tendon sheath. Based on the family history of cords in the palm, the most likely diagnosis is a Dupuytren's nodule. The acute tenderness of the nodule is usually temporary, but it can be decreased through steroid injection directly into the nodule. The presence of plantar fibromatosis (Lederhosen's disease) would help confirm the diagnosis.

13 In a patient who has had two failed attempts at eradicating Dupuytren's contracture of the PIP joint of the small finger (assuming that these surgeries were adequately performed), the patient's request for an amputation is not unreasonable. A disarticulation at the PIP joint may serve him well and would obviate the need for extensive postoperative rehabilitation. Another option is PIP joint arthrodesis in a better position. This procedure would maintain finger length and avoid the potential problem of painful neuromas following amputation, but there is a risk of nonunion at the arthrodesis site. The last option would be to perform a third excisional surgery, possibly skin grafting the site and releasing the joint contracture. In a patient with two failed operations on severe PIP joint Dupuytren's contracture, embarking on a third excision of the diseased tissue is rarely rewarding for the patient.

14 The patient has flexor pollicis longus septic tenosynovitis. With infection present at least 3 days, he will require incision and drainage with resection of the flexor tendon sheath between the flexor pulleys. The purulent material should be cultured and gram stained, and the patient should be started on IV antibiotics including coverage for gram-negative organisms because of his occupation. The wound should be left open and allowed to close secondarily or with a delayed primary closure once the infection has adequately resolved.

15 Under metacarpal block anesthesia with a digital tourniquet after wound irrigation and débridement, the tendon should be repaired with a nonabsorbable suture after pinning the DIP joint in extension with a K-wire. The postoperative therapy is the same as for a closed tendinous mallet finger, except that the pin should be removed 4 to 6 weeks after surgery. With open joint injuries it is advisable to administer an IV antibiotic to reduce the risk of infection.

QUESTIONS

16 A 26-year-old right-hand dominant man comes to the emergency room 1 hour after a severe crush injury to the right hand after being trapped in a printing press. The hand is covered with green ink and markedly swollen with lacerations at the level of the distal flexion creases of all of the fingers. There are linear lacerations running along the axis of the long finger from the PIP joint to the base of the palm, which then runs ulnarward at the wrist flexion crease. Another 270° laceration runs across the base of the thumb leaving a 2 cm skin bridge dorsally, 1 cm proximal to the MCP joint. All of the fingers have two point discrimination greater than 15 mm, but sharp and dull discrimination was intact. Intrinsic muscle function was absent. Extrinsic muscle function was intact although extremely limited because of pain and swelling. Radiographic films demonstrate a dislocation of the trapezial-metacarpal joint. Once the ink was cleaned from the tips of the fingers, capillary refill was noted to be less than 5 seconds. Describe your approach to this injury.

17 At the delayed primary closure it is noted that the patient's fingers are extremely stiff and have assumed a position of metocarpophangeal (MCP) extension and IP flexion. What can you do intraoperatively to help improve finger motion and correct this abnormal hand posture?

18 During the delayed closure surgery, you are unsuccessful in maintaining the hand in a "safe position;" the fingers spring back into a claw position. It is further evident that the well-fitted dressing with splints are not going to be able to maintain the "safe position." What else can be done to maintain adequate position of the fingers?

ANSWERS

16 The major concerns in this case are as follows:

(1) *Compartment syndrome of the intrinsic muscles.* With severe crushing injury, there must be a high index of suspicion for compartment syndrome. In the hand the intrinsic muscles are divided into multiple compartments, each of which would require decompression in this type of injury. The diagnosis of compartment syndrome can be confirmed through intracompartmental pressure determination. In this case the dorsal and palmar interossei, the thenar, hypothenar, and adductor compartments required release. The thenar musculature was completely destroyed requiring extensive débridement.

(2) *Contaminated, open, crushing injury.* Although neurapraxia can account for the sensory deficit, assuming that all of the deficit is produced by the crush injury can give a false sense of security, and one might miss a lacerated nerve. Simultaneous with the complete débridement of devitalized and heavily contaminated tissue, one should explore lacerations to rule out reparable nerve injuries. For this type of injury it would be appropriate to release the carpal and ulnar tunnels to decompress the nerves at these potential sites of compression.

(3) *Skeletal injury.* The thumb trapezial-metacarpal joint was found to be completely unstable. The thenar musculature was largely destroyed, and the thumb metacarpal was dislocated. A repair was carried out of the volar-oblique ligament and the joint capsule, and the trapezial-metacarpal joint was pinned in a reduced position with a .062 K-wire for 6 weeks.

(4) *Rehabilitation.* To facilitate rehabilitation of the hand, the digits were placed in a "safe position;" 70° to 80° of MCP joint flexion with the IP joints in nearly full extension. The skin was left open because of the significant swelling, and the patient was returned to the operating room 5 days postoperatively for delayed primary closure.

17 Manipulation of the digits under anesthesia can often dramatically increase range of motion of the fingers and help facilitate better positioning. Placing the hand in a well-fitted compression dressing that maintains a safe position with strict postoperative elevation should help.

18 Temporary K-wire fixation of the MCP joints in 70° to 90° of flexion is a useful technique for maintaining the "safe position" in the face of marked swelling from crush injury or severe burns to the hand.

QUESTIONS

19 Despite a conscientious program of postoperative therapy with edema control and splinting in excellent position, the patient develops a flexion contracture of the long finger. This appears to be related to a linear scar, which was the result of one of the palmar lacerations he sustained in the original accident described in Q16. He lacks 30° of PIP and 45° of DIP extension. How should this problem be corrected?

20 A 26-year-old woman complains that fingers in both of her hands feel cold, numb, and tingly, which is aggravated by exposure to cold. She has noticed hand color changes consisting of white, followed by painful red digits. At times the fingers have remained white for over an hour, and this condition has caused her a great deal of pain. On physical examination her fingers are pink but cool to the touch. Allen's test demonstrates good flow both from the radial and ulnar arteries. What is her most likely diagnosis:

21 How should this patient be initially worked up?

22 The patient's noninvasive vascular studies confirmed vasospastic disease without obstructive lesions. Based on these findings, what are your treatment recommendations?

23 The same patient has done fairly well for approximately 2 years following institution of your recommendations; however, this winter she noted nearly constant severe pain in the fingers. When she comes to your office she has ischemia of the ring and long fingers with a 5 mm ulcer at the radial border of the ring finger. The patient states that she has faithfully followed your recommendations but continues to have problems. What are your options at this point?

ANSWERS

19 Flexion contractures of the digits can result from a number of causes. Linear scar crossing a joint palmar to the axis of rotation of the finger can produce limitation of flexion. Flexor tendon shortening or adhesions can produce limited extension. At the PIP joint, thickening of the check rein ligaments can produce flexion contracture at this joint, as can capsular contractures as a result of significant joint injuries. The initial approach to this problem is an aggressive program of therapy including dynamic and static splinting in attempt to achieve full extension. If this is not effective, Z-plasty of the scar with sequential release of any other sites of limitation is necessary. This may require tenolysis, check rein ligament release, and possibly collateral ligament release and skin grafting.

ANSWERS

20   Raynaud's disease.

21   History and serologic testing should be directed toward ruling out connective tissue disease. Rheumatoid factor (RF), antinuclear antibodies (ANA), complete blood count (CBC), and erythrocyte sedimentation rate (ESR) are helpful initial screening tests. Noninvasive vascular studies are also helpful to confirm vasospastic disease through cold immersion stress testing of the digits. Doppler studies may suggest fixed arterial lesions.

22   The patient is instructed to keep her hands warm at all times. Mittens are more effective in keeping the digits warm than gloves because mittens prevent cold air from surrounding each digit. Chemical hand warmers are also an effective supplement to keep the fingers from getting cold. If these measures are ineffective, pharmacologic treatment consisting of calcium channel blockers, such as nifedipine, have been effective in managing the patient with vasospastic disease. The patient is instructed to cease smoking and caffeine intake.

23   Because Raynaud's syndrome frequently precedes the development of full-blown connective tissue disorders, it would be worthwhile to reassess the patient for connective tissue disease. The development of an ulcer at the tip of the finger is usually indicative of fixed arterial lesions. Repeating noninvasive vascular studies may be helpful; however, an arteriogram would be diagnostic for occlusive disease. Before sending her for vascular studies, one should consider performing a peripheral nerve block of the median and ulnar nerves at the wrist to see if this reverses the ischemia. If the peripheral nerve block reverses the ischemia, there is a vasospastic component to her disease, which, if controlled, would benefit digital circulation and may allow healing of the ulcer and prevent further necrosis. Maximal pharmacologic management should be pursued before considering surgical intervention. Digital sympathectomy may be indicated if severe, uncontrolled pain or unhealing ulcers persists after an adequate trial of calcium channel blockers and vasodilators.

QUESTIONS

24 What is a digital sympathectomy?

25 A 28-year-old construction worker complained of ulnar wrist pain and numbness and tingling in the ulnar two digits following an episode 3 weeks earlier in which he was pounding his snow plow onto the front of his truck using the heel of hand as a hammer. Since that time the ulnar two digits have felt cool and tingly. Describe the differential diagnosis.

26 What would confirm the diagnosis of hypothenar hammer syndrome or ulnar artery thrombosis?

27 How is Allen's test performed?

28 A 43-year-old secretary complains of gradual onset of progressive difficulty in writing. She denies any previous history of trauma or any neurologic conditions in her family history. She is otherwise healthy and takes no medications. She denies any paresthesias or muscular weakness. Her physical examination demonstrates normal motor and sensory function in the extremity. Her deep tendon reflexes are 2+ and bilaterally equal. When asked to write, she is noted to grasp the pen awkwardly and write in an extremely slow and labored manner. After 45 seconds she is unable to write further because of an inability to effectively hold the pen. What is this patient's most likely diagnosis, and how can it be confirmed?

29 What are the characteristic EMG findings in the patient with focal dystonia?

30 What are your treatment recommendations for the patient with writer's cramp (focal dystonia)?

ANSWERS

24 A digital sympathectomy is adventitial stripping of sympathetic fibers over a segment of digital artery in the palm and fingers. In patients with vasospastic component of their ischemic disease, digital sympathectomy interrupts the sympathetic outflow that causes constriction of the digital vessels.

25 Hypothenar hammer syndrome is associated with alterations in sensation and circulation of the ulnar digits. It is caused by using the ulnar base of the hand as a hammer, resulting in thrombosis of the ulnar artery, which is traumatized over the hook of the hamate. The arterial injury produces vasospasm and ischemia with intermittent emboli from the thrombus in the ulnar artery. Other conditions that

ANSWERS

may be responsible for his symptoms would be direct trauma to the ulnar nerve in Guyon's canal or ulnar tunnel syndrome. A hamate fracture can also produce paresthesias in the ulnar two digits. Other diagnostic considerations would be cubital tunnel syndrome and vasospastic and occlusive vascular diseases.

26 Absence of blood flow from the ulnar artery on Allen's testing would be highly suggestive of a thrombosis of the ulnar artery. This could be confirmed through color-flow Doppler evaluation or arteriogram.

27 The patient is asked to make a tight fist and straighten the fingers completely three consecutive times while the physician occludes the radial and ulnar arteries just proximal to the wrist. After the third fist, the patient is asked to relax the hand. The investigator then releases the ulnar artery, maintaining compression over the radial artery. If there is a complete superficial palmar arch, all of the fingers will pink up with release of the ulnar artery within 5 seconds. The test is then repeated, this time maintaining compression over the ulnar artery and releasing pressure over the radial artery to check its patency.

28 The patient most likely has writer's cramp, also known as focal dystonia. The diagnosis can be confirmed through electromyogram (EMG) studies.

29 There is excessive cocontraction of the antagonist and agonist muscles consisting of abnormally prolonged bursts of electrical activity.

30 The treatment of this condition has generally been frustrating. An initial approach consists of changing the hand posture during writing and adjusting the writing implement using different types of pen diameters and other types of writing devices. The patient is analyzed by occupational therapists with attention to body posturing and proper writing techniques. Medical management with oral or IV beta blockers and anticholinergics have had limited success. A new promising technique involves the injection of botulinum toxin into the most active dystonic muscles (identified by EMG while the patient is writing). These injections have facilitated temporary weakening of the muscles injected, resulting in a temporary functional improvement through selective weakening of the overactive muscles. A significant drawback is the need for maintenance injections on a monthly to bimonthly frequency.

QUESTIONS

31   An 18-year-old polevaulter missed the landing pit, falling on his extended right wrist. He had immediate pain and swelling and came to the emergency room where radiographic films were obtained. What do these films show (*Figures 4-3A and 4-3B*)?

Fig 4-3 **A**

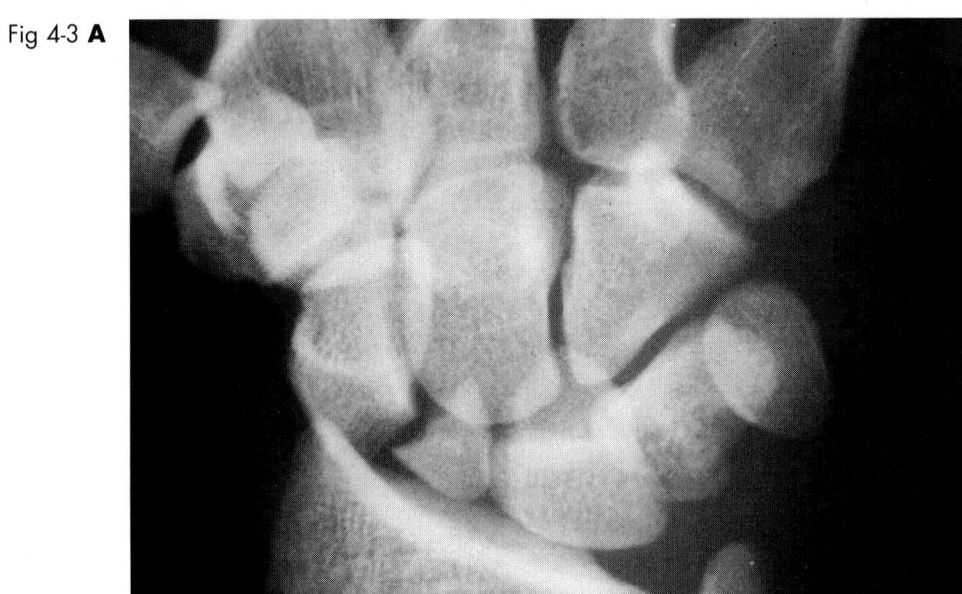

Fig 4-3 **B**

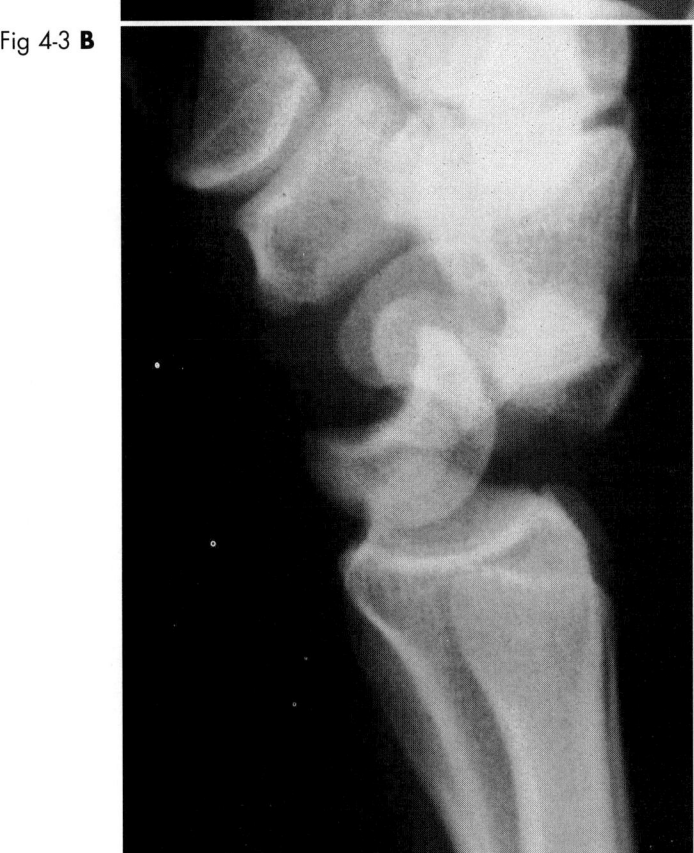

32   What is the recommended treatment for this injury?

ANSWERS

31   The anteroposterior (AP) and lateral radiographic films of the right wrist show a dorsal trans-scaphoid perilunate dislocation.

32   A closed reduction under anesthesia can be obtained by placing the hand in traction with approximately 10 pounds of weight applied to the arm. The reduction maneuver is performed with the lunate supported by the surgeon's thumb over the palmar wrist so that it is not pushed volarly out of the lunate fossa as the midcarpal joint is reduced. It is recommended that the scaphoid be anatomically reduced and fixed with K-wires or screws. The luno-triquetral joint is also exposed, reduced, and pinned. Palmar exposure is sometimes indicated in patients who have had median nerve compromise to release the carpal tunnel. (*Figure 4-4*)

Fig 4-4

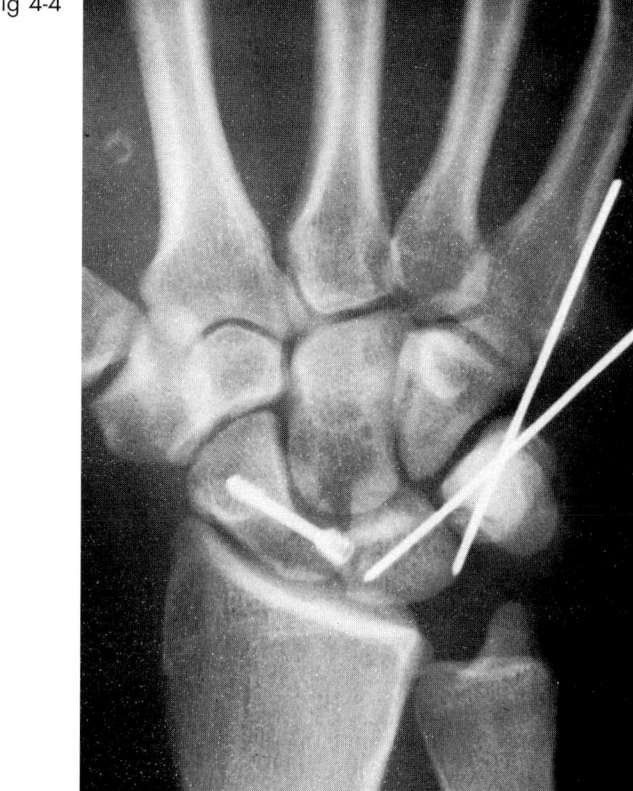

QUESTION

33 A 25-year-old, right-hand dominant man fell while skateboarding, sustaining an injury to his right thumb. His radiographic film (*Figure 4-5*) demonstrates an intraarticular fracture of the base of the thumb metacarpal. Describe your management of this patient.

Fig 4-5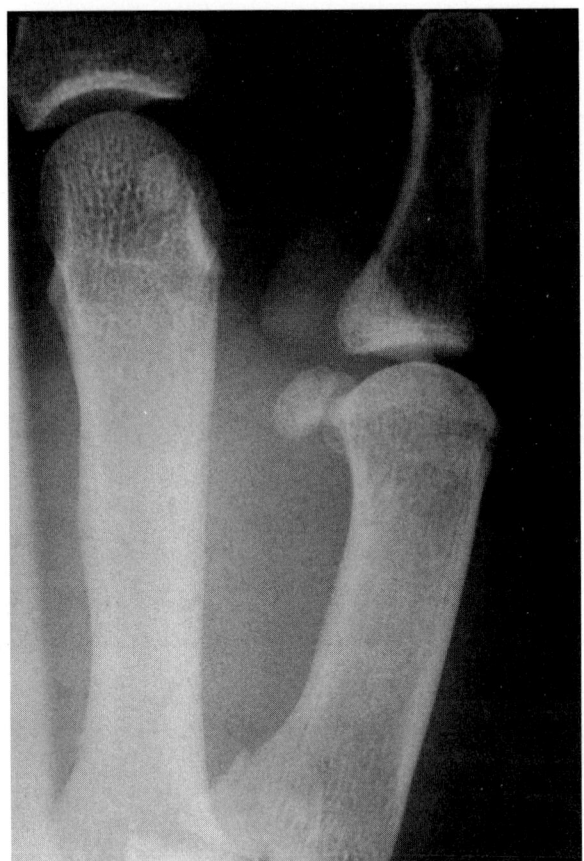

ANSWER

33 This intraarticular fracture of the base of the metacarpal is displaced approximately 1 mm. In assessing whether a patient would benefit from surgical intervention, one considers whether sufficient clinical improvement can be obtained through surgery. An attempt at closed treatment should be strongly considered. Tomograms obtained in a thumb spica cast demonstrated minimal displacement. If additional displacement were noted on thumb tomograms, surgery would be indicated.

QUESTIONS

34 This 48-year-old woman sustained a gunshot wound to the right hand with a 3 mm entry wound between the long and ring fingers at the proximal palmar crease and a ragged 1.5 cm exit wound over the dorsal midshaft of the metacarpal. Radiographic films are shown (*Figures 4-6A and 4-6B*). Describe management of this patient.

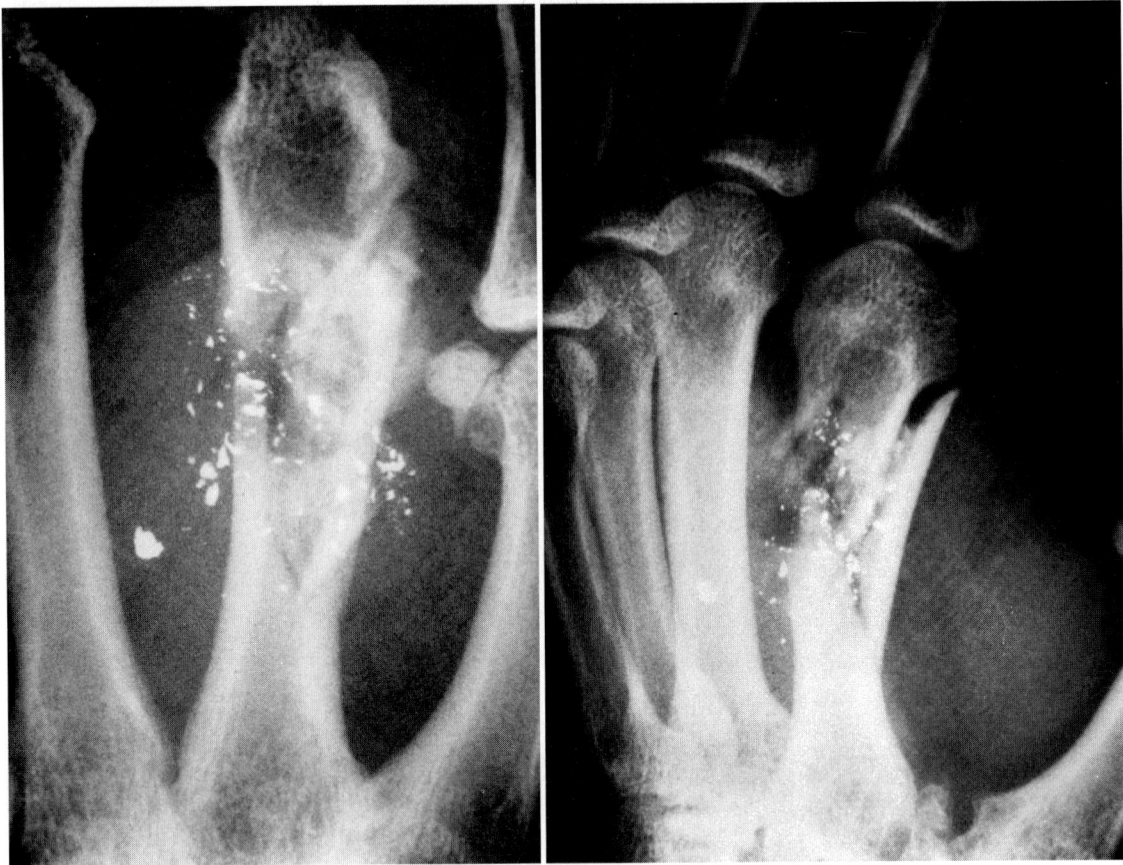

Fig 4-6 **A**   Fig 4-6 **B**

35 A 25-year-old laborer inadvertently caught his long finger in a router at work, sustaining complex nail bed injury involving complete avulsion of the nail with a laceration extending in a stellate manner from the midportion of the sterile matrix proximally through the germinal matrix. There is a comminuted fracture of the distal phalanx at its midportion with an associated tuft fracture. How should this fracture and nail bed injury be managed?

36 The patient in Q35 returns to your office 6 months following the repair with a split nail. What causes this problem?

ANSWERS

34   Following assessment of tendon function and neurovascular status, the patient should be taken to the operating room for débridement of the wound. Attention should be directed toward an elimination of gross contamination thorough irrigation of the fracture and wound débridement and an assessment of tendon, nerve, and blood vessel integrity. If possible the wounds should be loosely closed. It is controversial whether extensive internal fixation is desirable in low velocity gunshot wounds. Because of minimal shortening and no angular or rotational malalignment, this particular patient was treated with IV antibiotics for 24 hours and splinted. No bone grafting was required, and the patient had an excellent functional result with a healed fracture. For high velocity gunshot wounds resulting in significant soft tissue disruption, external or internal fixation may be desirable.

35   Acutely, the best management consists of judicial débridement of the wounds, removal of any residual nail to fully expose the nail bed, and meticulous repair of the nail bed using fine absorbable sutures such as 6-0 or 7-0 Vicryl. The fracture should be reduced and, if necessary, stabilized with K-wires. Even if rigid bony fixation is not achieved, the K-wires can impart additional soft tissue stability, which aids wound healing. If the fingernail is intact following cleansing, it can be replaced to prevent scar formation between the germinal matrix and the nail fold. Alternatives to keep the nail fold open include Xeroform gauze and Silastic nail splints, left in place for 2 weeks. The digit is then splinted, and range of motion of the free joints is pursued in 3 to 5 days.

36   Split nail is produced by a scar in the germinal or sterile matrix. This scar causes an area where there is a deficiency in the production of nail cells, which results in the split.

QUESTIONS

37   A 35-year-old laborer smashed his distal phalanx between a forklift and a box at work, sustaining a comminuted tuft fracture with an associated soft tissue injury. He had been treated with repair of the soft tissues, irrigation of the fracture site, and wound closure. After 2 months, he has noted a marked decrease in tenderness of the finger-tip and has good range of motion of the digit. However, the patient has also noted a transverse ridge in the proximal fingernail. He is concerned that he may have a permanent fingernail deformity and wonders what can be done. What is your response to this patient's inquiries?

38   A 50-year-old woman complains that the fingernail of her index finger has been painful and intermittently draining purulent material at its base over the past 6 months. The nail is nonadherent at the tip. There is erythema around the base, but it is not particularly tender. No purulent material is noted. There is diffuse swelling at the base. There is a blue-green discoloration of the nail plate. What is the most likely diagnosis?

39   What are the indications for surgery for a Bennett's fracture?

40   Describe the Wagner approach to the trapezial-metacarpal joint.

ANSWERS

37 Minor transverse nail ridges frequently occur following application of tourniquets to the upper extremity or following episodes of hypoxia. These ridges tend to resolve spontaneously as the nail grows out; they usually do not produce any permanent nail deformity. On the other hand, if his distal phalanx fracture has produced irregularity of the phalanx following healing of the fracture, it is possible that nail growth can be disturbed by phalangeal malunion. A radiographic film of the distal phalanx would be appropriate to ensure that this is not the case.

38 The patient most likely has onycholysis, a condition in which the nail is no longer adherent to the nail bed. In the early stages the condition is relatively painless. It is frequently seen in women who keep their nails long. This condition may occur in one or several nails; usually only one part of the nail is separated from the nail base. The nail is susceptible to repeated minor trauma that may extend the involved area, producing associated pain. The nail bed becomes contaminated by bacteria or yeast leading to purulent drainage. Blue, green, or blackish discoloration of the nail plate typically represents *Pseudomonas aeruginosa* contamination. If the condition is not corrected fairly early, the exposed nail bed becomes keratinized, and it is almost impossible to reattach the nail.

39 There is some controversy regarding the indications for surgery with advocates of both closed reduction and open reduction with internal fixation. It is recommended that displacement greater than l mm should be treated with closed reduction and percutaneous pinning. If this technique is unsuccessful, open reduction and internal fixation is recommended.

40 The incision runs along the radial axis of the thumb metacarpal in the interval between the abductor pollicis longus and the thenar muscles. The incision then extends proximally along the radial border of the flexor carpi radialis tendon. Subperiosteal elevation of the thenar muscles exposes the trapezial-metacarpal joint and the metacarpal base.

QUESTION

41   An 18-year-old high school student jammed his thumb playing bas-
      ketball. Because this continued to hurt despite pulling on it, he came
      to the office where radiographic films were obtained (*Figure 4-7*).
      What is the treatment of choice for this injury?

Fig 4-7

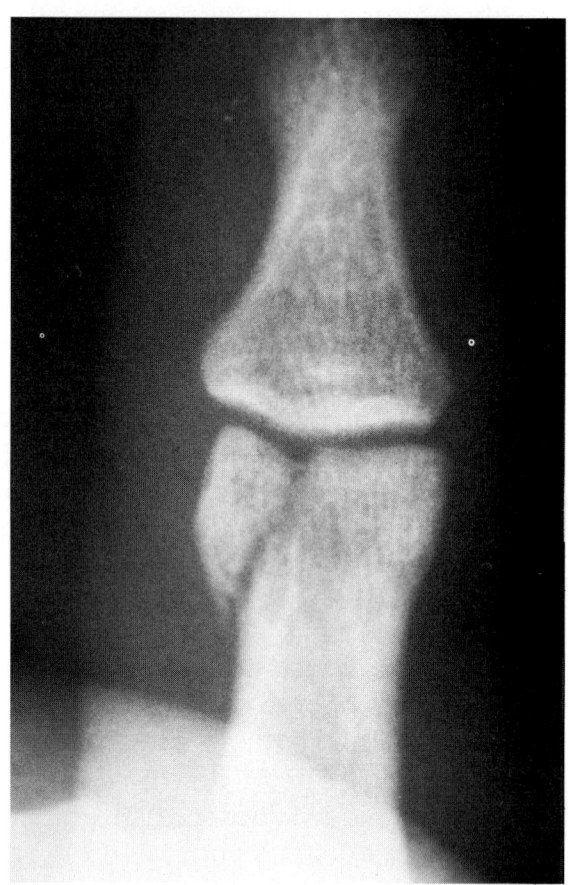

ANSWER

41 Because of the rotation of the fragment with intraarticular step off, the treatment of choice is to perform reduction of the fragment with internal fixation. Closed reduction can be attempted under C-arm image intensification using finger traction with manipulation or a reduction clamp, such as a Blaylock clamp, to facilitate reduction. The fracture can then be percutaneously pinned. Another option is to perform open reduction and internal fixation with K-wires or a small lag screw. The advantages of the latter are that one can visually assure that the reduction is anatomic and, if the fixation is deemed rigid, an early motion program can be started.

QUESTION

42   Three weeks following an injury to the index finger, a 16-year-old football player is brought to your office because he has persistent pain over the ulnar base of the index finger. He has limited range of motion of his finger and is tender over the ulnar base of the proximal phalanx. There is moderate swelling in this area. A radiographic film (*Figure 4-8*) demonstrates an avulsion fracture of the base of the proximal phalanx. He wishes to continue playing football because his hand is no longer bothering him much. What is your treatment?

Fig 4-8

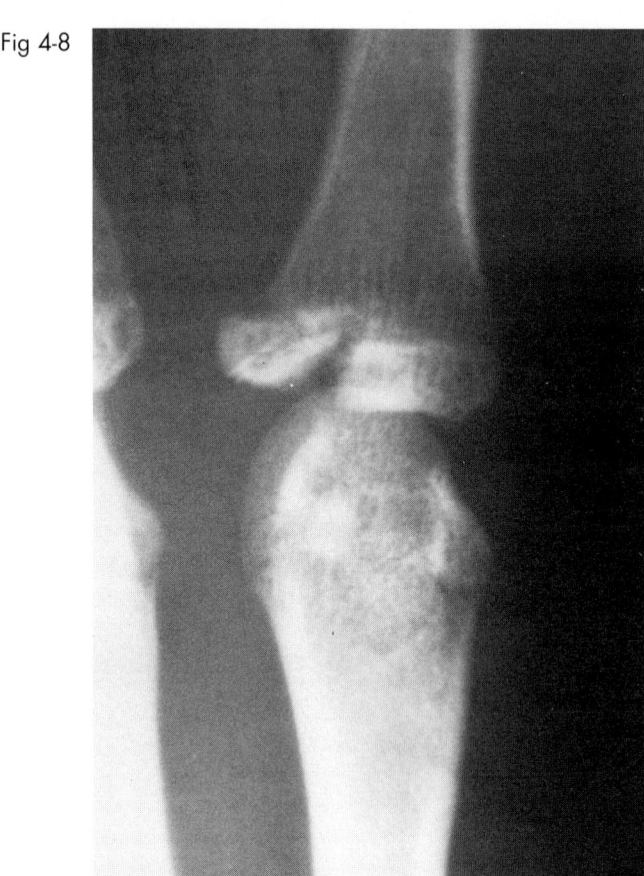

ANSWER

42 This intraarticular avulsion of the ulnar base of the proximal phalanx is in an unacceptable position that would result in posttraumatic arthrosis. An open reduction with take-down of the partially united fracture was in order. Fixation with a lag screw was performed. With stable fixation, early range of motion can be started.

QUESTION

43   This 12-year-old boy fell from a skateboard, injuring his ring and small fingers. On evaluation he has swelling and tenderness at the bases of the proximal phalanges and has rotational deformity of the ring finger (*Figures 4-9A, 4-9 B, and 4-9 C*). What is the nature of the injury, and how should he be treated?

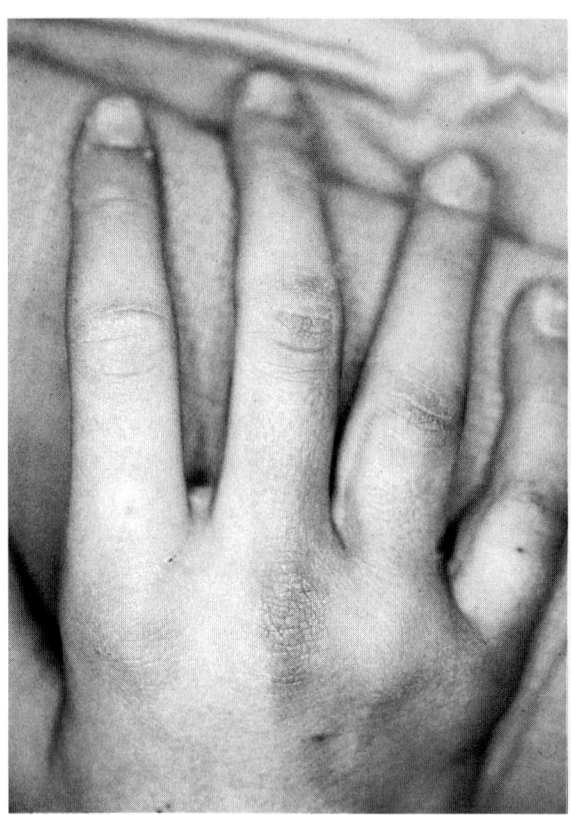

Fig 4-9 **A**

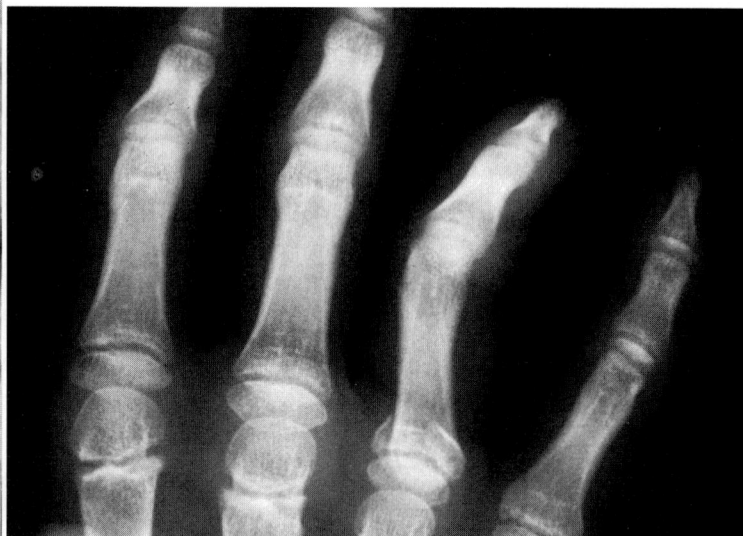

Fig 4-9 **B**

Fig 4-9 **C**

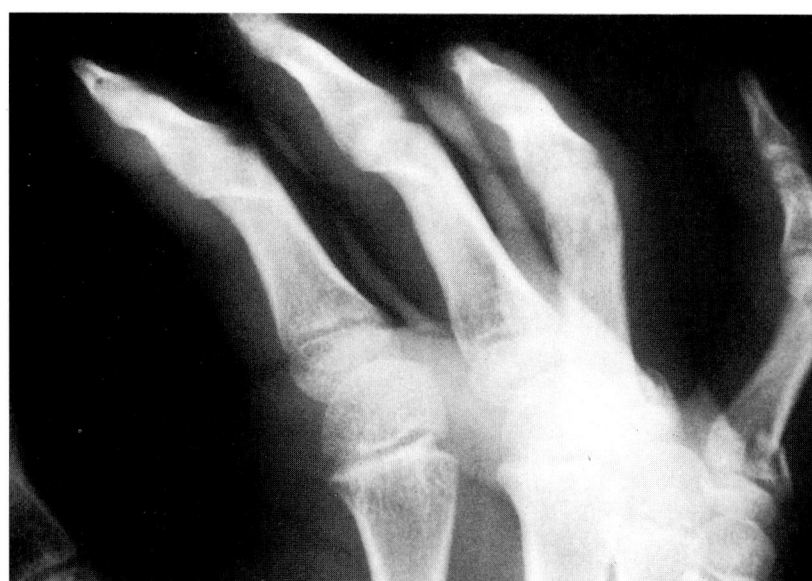

ANSWER

43 These are Salter-Harris type II fractures of the bases of the ring and small finger proximal phalanges with associated rotational and angular deformities. Closed reduction under hematoma block anesthesia is usually effective in facilitating a stable reduction. It is rare that operative intervention is required in this type of injury. The fractures typically go on to union in 3 to 6 weeks.

QUESTION

44 A 28-year-old soccer goalie was kicked in the hand while attempting a save. Physical examination demonstrates ulnar deviation and radial rotation of the small finger. This digit is swollen and tender with limited motion because of pain. A radiographic film (*Figures 4-10A, 4-10B, and 4-10C*) of the hand demonstrates fracture of the proximal phalanx. Describe the treatment of this injury.

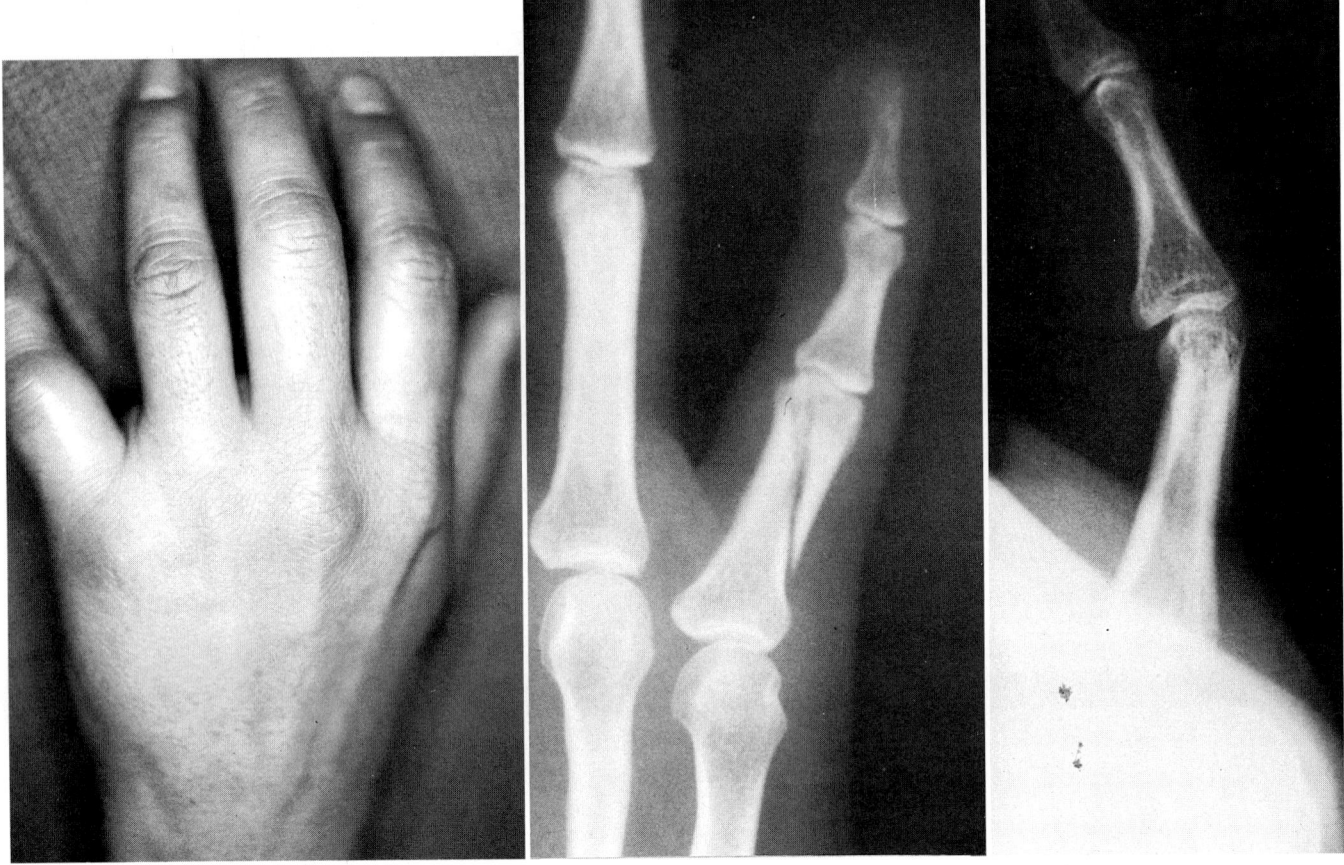

Fig 4-10 **A**   Fig 4-10 **B**   Fig 4-10 **C**

ANSWER

44 Closed reduction should be performed following adequate anesthesia (ulnar nerve block and hematoma or metacarpal block). If reduction can be held with buddy taping and splinting, closed treatment should be continued. This particular fracture proved unstable requiring closed pinning (*Figure 4-11*). If after pinning the fracture no motion is detected under fluoroscopy, early active range of motion with protective splinting between exercises can be initiated.

Fig 4-11

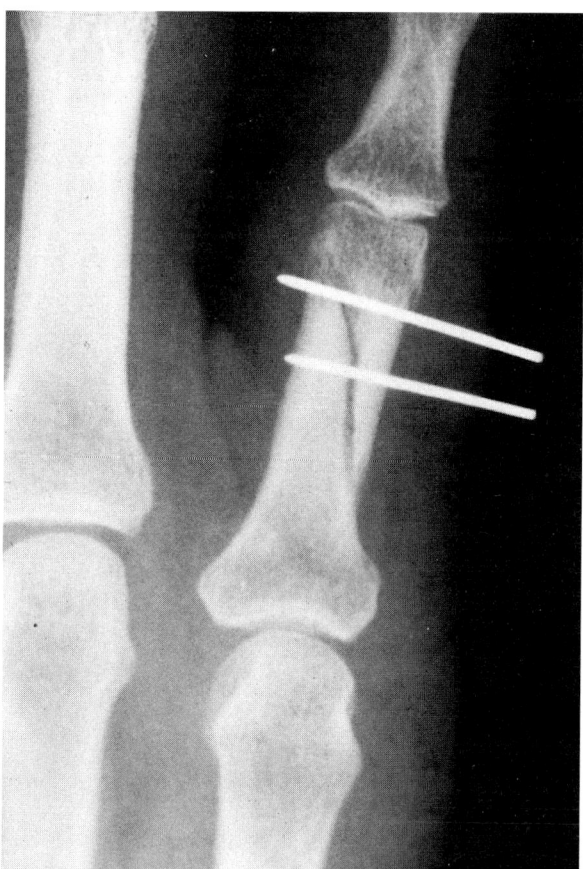

QUESTIONS

45 A 32-year-old mechanic injured his thumb while playing football. The thumb was caught in another player's face guard and jerked radially. The thumb was swollen and markedly tender over the ulnar aspect. He demonstrated no end point of his ulnar collateral ligament (UCL) MCP joint to stress testing. The radiographic film is demonstrated below (*Figure 4-12*). What is the diagnosis, and what should the treatment involve?

Fig 4-12

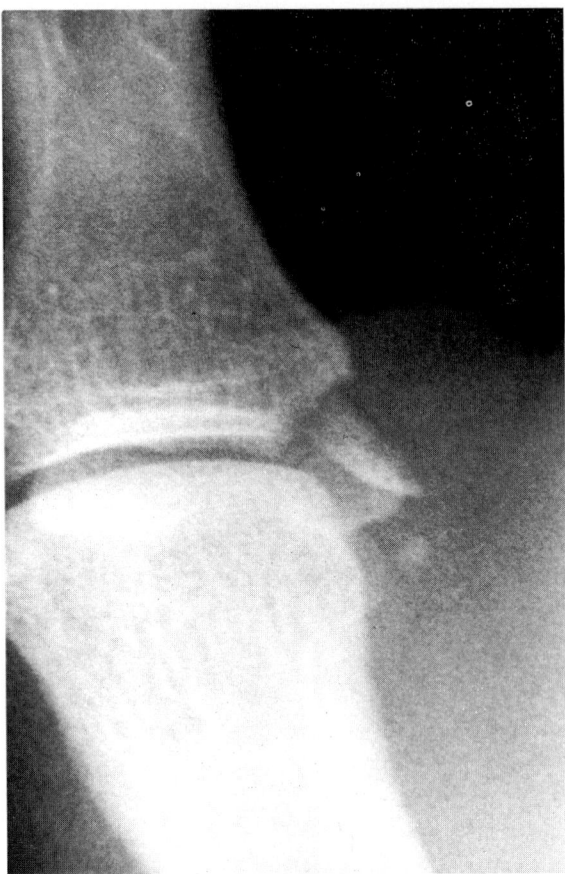

46 What is a Stener lesion?

47 What are clinical indications for repair of the ulnar collateral ligament of the thumb?

ANSWERS

45 The patient has an avulsion injury of the ulnar base of the proximal phalanx of the thumb. Treatment of a fragment displaced to this degree would require open reduction and internal fixation (*Figure 4-13*).

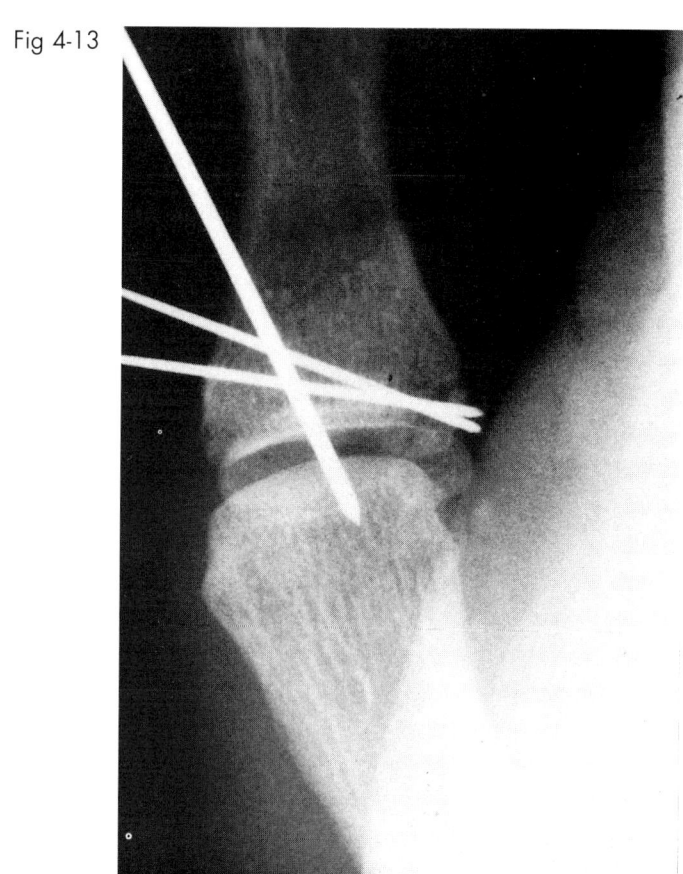

Fig 4-13

46 The Stener lesion was described by Bertil Stener following exploration of 39 cases of complete rupture of the UCL of the thumb MCP joint. In 25 cases he found interposition of the adductor aponeurosis between the base of the proximal phalanx (where the collateral ligament had been avulsed) and the retracted stump of the collateral ligament. The adductor apparently becomes interposed between the torn ligament end, and the base of the phalanx as the thumb is widely abducted during the injury. With the adductor interposed between the ligament and its site of attachment, prognosis for a stable thumb is poor if left to "heal" in this position.

47 Clinical stress testing can be helpful in distinguishing partial from complete ruptures. In the acute injuries it is often helpful to block the area with an anesthetic agent, performing either a digital block or a pericapsular block. The MP joint should be stressed in positions of 0° and 30° of flexion. If no end point is identified with stress testing, it is clear that the collateral ligament is completely ruptured and should be repaired.

QUESTIONS

48 What are some of the radiographic techniques used to determine the need for repair of the UCL of the thumb MCP joint?

49 A 28-year-old nurse fell injuring her right small finger around the MCP joint. Her skin is intact, and she is neurovascularly intact. Describe your treatment of this intraarticular fracture (*Figures 4-14A and 4-14B*).

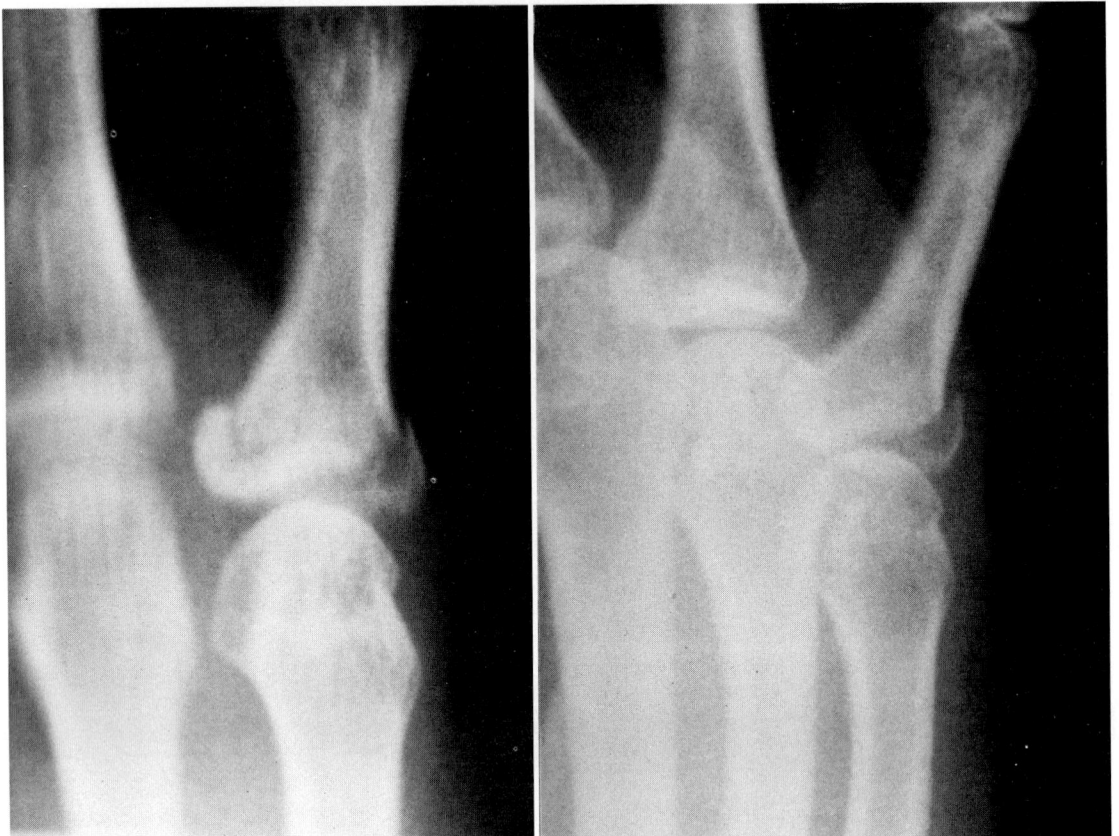

Fig 4-14 **A**   Fig 4-14 **B**

50 How is treatment of radial collateral ligament (RCL) injury of the thumb MCP joint different from treatment of the UCL?

51 A patient with a bony gamekeeper's thumb returns to the office 6 weeks after operative repair. K-wires have been removed 4 weeks postoperatively. On examination the patient is still swollen and tender over the UCL. The MP joint is stiff. The radiographic films demonstrate an absence of bony healing between the fragment and the base of the proximal phalanx. What should be done about this bony "nonunion?"

52 The patient returns 3 weeks after initiation of the rehabilitation program and after stress testing of the UCL demonstrates moderate pain and persistent instability. What are the treatment options at this point?

ANSWERS

48   Some of the radiographic techniques include the following:
(1) Plain radiographic films may demonstrate displaced and rotated fragment of the base.
(2) Stress radiographic films of the MCP joint will indicate that surgery is recommended if there is greater than 10° to 15° of instability noted compared with the opposite uninjured side or if there is greater than 30° stressed abduction arc.
(3) Thumb MCP joint arthrogram as described by Bowers, can demonstrate a displaced or trapped UCL tear.
(4) Magnetic resonance imaging (MRI) is another promising, though expensive, imaging technique. Most complete tears can be identified clinically.

49   The comminuted intraarticular fracture of the base is a formidable problem. Fragments of this size are often difficult to manipulate and stabilize. The risk of stiffness with open reduction and internal fixation is substantial particularly because rigid fixation is not always possible. Closed reduction is unlikely to remain stable. Percutaneous pin fixation alone is another option that has limited expectations for success because of the large compressive force across the joint. Combinations of internal or percutaneous fixation and external fixation are promising options. In this particular case, external fixation was elected. An anatomic reduction was achieved through ligamentotaxis, which was maintained by the distraction afforded by the fixator.

50   There is little difference between the two. For complete ruptures, operative repair is recommended. For partial tears of the RCL, 4 weeks of immobilization is recommended.

51   Not all avulsion fractures of the base of the proximal phalanx of the thumb MCP joint go on to bony union, but they can develop an asymptomatic fibrous union. A stress test of the UCL should be performed. If the joint is stable, one should proceed with a gradual rehabilitation program. After 2 to 3 weeks the patient is reevaluated. Because of joint stiffness from recent immobilization, one can be misled into believing that the collateral ligament is stable. Once postimmobilization stiffness is worked out, the collateral ligament stability should be reassessed.

52   The presence of significant instability at this point indicates a treatment failure. Additional cast immobilization will not be effective in "tightening up" the repair. The repair should be explored and a repeat repair performed. If the tissue is inadequate for simple open reduction and internal fixation (ORIF), the bony fragment may be excised and the ligament advanced into the base of the proximal phalanx, or a ligament reconstruction may be performed similar to those used in chronic UCL injuries.

QUESTIONS

53   Describe some of the options available for reconstructing chronic UCL ruptures.

54   How can the PIP joint be stabilized in dorsal fracture and dislocation in which greater than 50% of the articular surface is involved?

55   An 18-year-old football player caught his small finger in another player's shoulder pads, snapping the finger. Tendon function appeared to be intact except for an inability to adduct the finger. There was swelling around the MCP joint, and tenderness localized primarily over its radial aspect. Radiographic films were normal. What is the differential diagnosis for this injury?

56   How can the diagnosis of torn RCL of the MCP joint be made?

57   How should this ligament tear be treated?

58   What is the salvage procedure for several failed reconstructions of the UCL of the thumb MCP joint?

59   True or False. The reestablishment of adequate blood flow in and out of an amputated extremity is the key to successful replant surgery.

60   True or False. Because reestablishment of circulation is the number one priority in successful replant surgery, following débridement and preparation of the injured structures for replantation, reestablishment of arterial and venous circulation become the next step in the reattachment process.

ANSWERS

53   If the old ligament can be identified, it can be reinserted into the base of the proximal phalanx similar to a primary repair using pull-out suture or bone anchor. Scarred remnants of capsule can also be used to fashion a collateral ligament and can be either sutured to the base of the phalanx or imbricated over itself. The adductor pollicis insertion into the ulnar sesamoid can be transferred to the base of the proximal phalanx for a dynamic reconstruction. Free and pedicled tendon grafts have been used as well, consisting of palmaris longus, plantaris, or extensor pollicis brevis.

54   The PIP joint can be stabilized through a volar plate arthroplasty with bone grafting or through open reduction and internal fixation if there is a large bony fragment. It is necessary to obtain good fixation if one elects to perform open reduction and internal fixation because of the significant forces that work against the fracture fixation. If volar plate

ANSWERS

arthroplasty is performed, it is often advisable to bone graft the sulcus distal to the volar plate to fill in this area and give support to the volar plate or use a sublimis slip to fill this interval to prevent dislocation. Traction is another option that appears promising with the use of either an external fixator or a traction device.

55 Pain around the radial aspect of the MCP joint with associated swelling and an inability to adduct the finger are highly suggestive of an injury to the RCL of the MCP joint. Capsular tear, chondral fracture of the metacarpal head, and ruptured interosseous muscle are other diagnostic considerations.

56 Although there are a number of sophisticated diagnostic tests available, including MRI, the simplest and least expensive is a stress test of the RCL. This is performed by placing the MCP joint in a position of 90° of flexion and applying an abduction stress to the joint. This must be compared with the opposite, unaffected hand to take into account idiosyncratic ligamentous laxity. If there is significant difference in laxity, the diagnosis is made.

57 Incomplete ligament tears can usually be treated with splint or cast immobilization with MP joint at about 45° of flexion for 3 to 4 weeks. Once acute tenderness subsides, buddy taping the digits for an additional 3 to 4 weeks is recommended.
The acute management of complete RCL tears of the MCP joints is controversial. Nonoperative treatment can be successful; however, the percentage of failures is much lower using direct surgical repair. The nonoperative treatment for complete tears is similar to the treatment for incomplete tears with immobilization in a cast or splint for 4 to 6 weeks and with subsequent buddy taping. Index finger RCL repair is mandatory because of the need for MCP radial stability for pinch.

58 Although an additional graft to reconstruct the ligament may be attempted, the most reliable procedure for failed reconstruction of the UCL would be a thumb MCP joint arthrodesis.

59 True. Without reestablishment of adequate circulation to the amputated part, the surgery is a waste.

60 False. Although reestablishment of circulation to the severed part is the number one priority, bony stability and tendon repair must precede vascular reconstruction so as not to disrupt the delicate microsurgical anastomoses when performing those gross motor tasks. In proximal extremity amputations, temporary arterial shunting before bone and tendon repair can maintain extremity viability and allow subsequent microvascular repairs.

QUESTIONS

61 A patient sustained an Urbaniak type I ring avulsion injury. The wound is débrided and nicely closed to avoid postoperative scarring, and a bulky dressing is applied. The patient returned to the hospital several hours later stating that his finger had become pale. What errors in the initial management may have led to this circulatory compromise?

62 In the absence of any arthritic changes in the wrist, what is the best approach to the treatment of ulnar impaction syndrome?

63 In what position should the wrist be radiographed to document ulnar variance?

64 Although ulnar positive variance is associated with ulnar impaction syndrome, ulnar negative variance is associated with what wrist condition?

65 What is Kienböck disease?

66 What is the etiology of Kienböck disease?

67 What is the most popular treatment for Lichtman's stage II and III Kienböck disease with ulnar neutral or ulnar minus variance?

68 A 65-year-old woman complains of catching at the PIP joint of her ring finger. She describes the PIP joint becoming locked into flexion and is able to demonstrate it in your office. She says it is much worse in the morning; she frequently awakes with the digit held in a locked position. What is the diagnosis and how should she be treated?

69 What physical findings would one expect with a trigger digit?

ANSWERS

61 There are several potential pitfalls in dealing with ring avulsion injuries in which circulation is intact. There is a temptation to perform a cosmetic closure on these wounds, which is a major mistake. The wounds should be closed loosely because of swelling, which develops from the significant avulsive component of this injury. Swelling may lead to circulatory compromise in a tightly closed wound. The dressing should be loosely applied so that it does not become a source of compression. In addition, the patient should be instructed in arm elevation for the next 48 hours. If the patient appears unreliable, admission to the hospital for observation and enforced elevation is advisable.

ANSWERS

62 An ulnar shortening procedure is a good solution for painful wrist caused by ulnar impaction with documented neutral or ulnar plus variance.

63 Because extremes of pronation and supination alter the ulnar variance, this determination should be made with the forearm in a neutral position.

64 Ulnar negative variance is most frequently associated with Kienböck disease.

65 Kienböck disease is an avascular necrosis of the lunate.

66 Although controversial, most experts believe that the avascular necrosis is the result of a posttraumatic insult to a susceptible wrist (i.e., negative ulnar variance and single vessel perfusing the lunate). Occult lunate fractures have been identified in early Kienböck disease and are felt to represent a traumatic sequelae.

67 Distal radius shortening or ulnar lengthening. The rationale for either of these treatments is to achieve a better distribution of force at the level of the radioulnar interface with the lunate. Of the two procedures proposed, the radial shortening is technically less demanding.

68 This most likely is a trigger finger. Treatment would consist of an injection of the flexor tendon sheath with a mixture of steroid and anesthetic, which is frequently curative. Alternative treatments include splinting programs to maintain the MP joint in extension. The last option is surgical release of the A-1 pulley, which is reserved for cases in which conservative treatment was not successful.

69 The best finding is having the patient demonstrate the triggering. This can usually be elicited by asking the patient to make a tight fist and then to extend the digits. The affected finger will be maintained in flexion at the PIP joint and then suddenly snap into extension as the thickened part of the flexor tendon passes under the A-1 pulley. Sometimes the patient has to manually straighten the finger to overcome the locking. Typically, the patient will have marked tenderness overlying the A-1 pulley and nodular enlargement of the flexor tendon in this area.

QUESTIONS

70 A 52-year-old rheumatoid woman complains of spontaneous long finger catching. She recalls no injury. On physical examination she has full flexion of the digits; however, when she attempts to extend the fingers, she is unable to obtain full extension of the long finger MCP joint. There is dorsal swelling and tenderness around this area. She lacks 30° active extension at the MCP joint. In addition, the digit deviates 20° ulnarly at the MP joint with attempted digital extension. With passive assistance, however, the digit can be brought into full extension and held in this position. Radiographic films were unremarkable for revealing a pathologic condition at this joint. Likewise, the wrist is minimally involved with the rheumatoid disease. What is the diagnosis, and how should she be treated?

71 A 35-year-old cook is referred by his company doctor for "locking" of the long finger MCP joint. There is no history of trauma, and on physical examination there is no swelling noted. The digital range of motion demonstrates near normal flexion, but there is a 40° lack of active and passive extension at the MP joint. His extensor tendon feels intact, and his neurosensory examination is intact. Apart from slight enlargement of the radial condyle of the metacarpal head, there are no radiographic abnormalities. What is this patient's diagnosis and treatment?

72 A 39-year-old laborer at an industrial plant complains of lateral proximal forearm pain that developed spontaneously without specific injury approximately 2 months earlier. He complains of weakness in the extremity with heavy use of the hand but denies numbness, tingling, or paresthesias. He is not tender over the lateral epicondyle but has moderate tenderness at a point 6 cm distal to the lateral epicondyle and pain with resisted long finger extension. There is no motor weakness. Resisted wrist extension produces minimal pain, but resisted supination is extremely painful at the aforementioned site of tenderness. Radiographic films of the elbow were normal. What is the patient's differential diagnosis?

73 How is this diagnosis confirmed?

74 How is radial tunnel syndrome treated?

ANSWERS

70 Trigger finger in a patient with rheumatoid disease may be caused by a number of problems ranging from the classical triggering at the A-1 pulley to other entities, such as nodular involvement of the flexor tendons at various levels. In this particular case the patient is experiencing locking because of subluxation of the extensor mechanism over the long finger MCP joint as a result of attritional rupture of the radial sagittal band. Although nonoperative treatment can be successful through a program of splinting, a more reliable treatment is operative repair or reconstruction of the sagittal band.

71 Locking MCP joint is usually associated with a metacarpal head osteophyte or prominence, which catches on the collateral ligament or volar plate producing limitation of full extension. Although gentle manipulation can be attempted, forceful attempts at unlocking the joint should not be made. Given time, the joint will sometimes unlock spontatneously. I have injected the joint with a mixture of steroid and anesthetic to facilitate reduction of inflammation, which may be responsible for the previously well-tolerated bony metacarpal head prominence, causing impingement on an edematous volar plate or collateral ligament. If after several weeks the joint is not unlocked, then operative intervention is warranted with exploration of the joint with removal of the impinging source. Some patients will experience unlocking of the joints with an interval of symptom-free motion followed by a relocking of the joint. In this event, early operative intervention is recommended.

72 Differential diagnosis for nontraumatic lateral proximal forearm pain includes lateral epicondylitis (tennis elbow), osteochondritis dissecans, radial tunnel syndrome, and cervical radiculitis. Of these, the most likely diagnosis is radial tunnel because of the localized pain distal to the lateral epicondyle, pain with resisted middle finger extension, and forearm supination.

73 Radial tunnel syndrome is principally a clinical diagnosis. Abnormalities in the sensory distribution of the radial nerve are rare because the compression in radial tunnel is usually distal to the branching of the superficial branch of the radial nerve. Detectable muscle weakness is uncommon. Radiographic films and electrodiagnostic tests are normal in the vast majority of radial tunnel syndrome patients. Frequently, anesthetic injection in the area of maximal tenderness will temporarily alleviate the pain and help confirm the diagnosis.

74 Nonoperative treatment consists of rest and wrist splinting in a dorsiflexed position for a period of 4 to 6 weeks. Surgical release of the radial tunnel is indicated when conservative care fails to alleviate the symptoms.

QUESTIONS

75 What structures are implicated as sites of entrapment in radial tunnel syndrome?

76 A 32-year-old banker complains of a mass at the base of the thumb, which has worsened over the past few weeks. He notices intermittent tingling in the thumb, which is aggravated by bowling. Physical examination demonstrates a firm 10 mm by 2 mm mass palpable on the ulnar aspect of the thumb at the level of the MP joint. Rolling and percussion of the mass produces paresthesias in the thumb tip. What is this patient's diagnosis?

77 Describe treatment of "bowler's thumb."

78 This 3-year-old boy smashed his index finger in a door jam at home, sustaining an injury seen in the radiographic film shown (*Figure 4-15*). There was a 1 cm laceration overlying volar distal flexion crease. Tendon function, sensation, and circulation were intact. Describe your management of this patient.

Fig 4-15

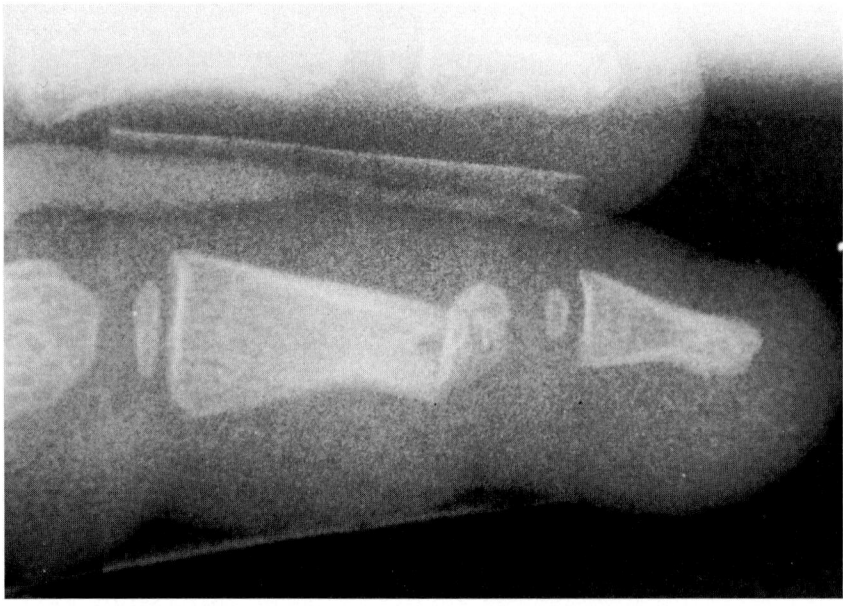

ANSWERS

75 Sites include the arcade of Frohse, tendinous edge of extensor carpi radialis brevis, radial recurrent vessels, and fibrous bands anterior to the radial head.

76 This patient has "bowler's thumb," which is perineural fibrosis of the ulnar digital nerve of the thumb caused by repeated pressure of the bowling ball against the nerve. This condition is usually seen in fairly avid bowlers, and, upon further questioning the patient admits that he was a tournament-level player. Varying degrees of this condition can occur ranging from intermittent pain and numbness to constant sensory changes along the ulnar aspect of the thumb.

77 Although surgical decompression with neurolysis and aponeurectomy may be performed, the best results have come from early recognition and conservative treatment. If recognized early, the elimination of the repeated trauma through cessation of bowling, adjustment of the bowling ball grip through redrilling the thumb hole, or application of accommodative padding have been helpful. A shield or splint can sometimes be a helpful adjunct for those patients who are severely addicted.

78 This displaced angulated middle phalanx neck fracture requires open reduction with K-wire fixation. The laceration site should be irrigated and débrided.

QUESTION

79 Describe treatment of a 42-year-old laborer who sustained injury seen in the radiographic films shown (*Figures 4-16A and 4-16B*). Physical examination demonstrates a tear in the skin volar to the IP joint. She has poor flexion of the digit and minimal extension at the IP joint of the thumb.

Fig 4-16 **A**

Fig 4-16 **B**

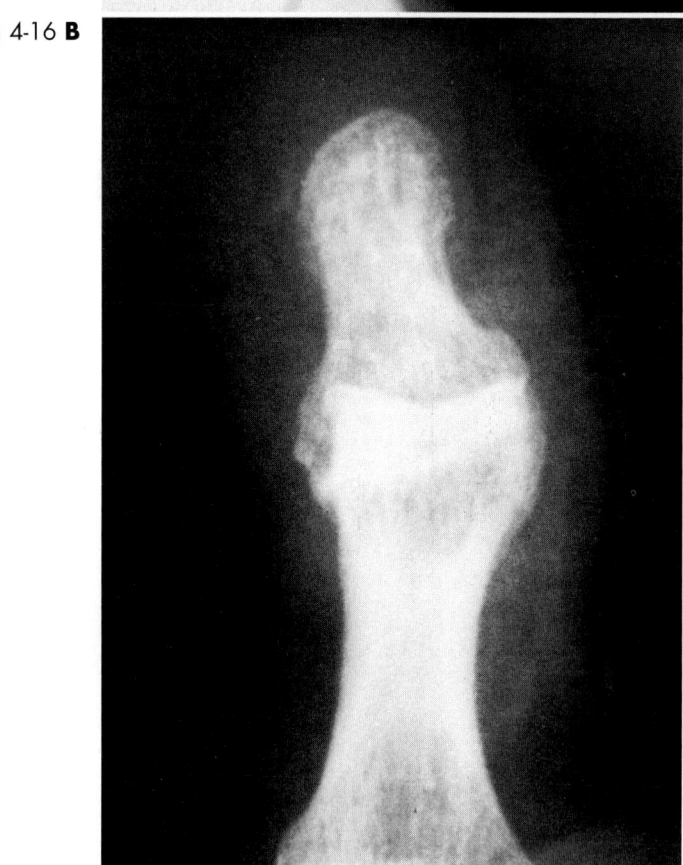

ANSWER

79   This dorsal dislocation of the IP joint of the thumb should be treated with cleansing and débridement of the open laceration with reduction of the dislocation. Stability should be assessed after reduction through stressing the collateral ligaments. Active flexion and extension should also be tested to rule out tendon injury.

QUESTIONS

80 The patient in Q79 had a reduction performed and was then referred to your office 1 month later with persistent pain in the thumb and limited range of motion. Radiographic films were obtained(*Figure 4-17*). What is your approach to this problem?

Fig 4-17

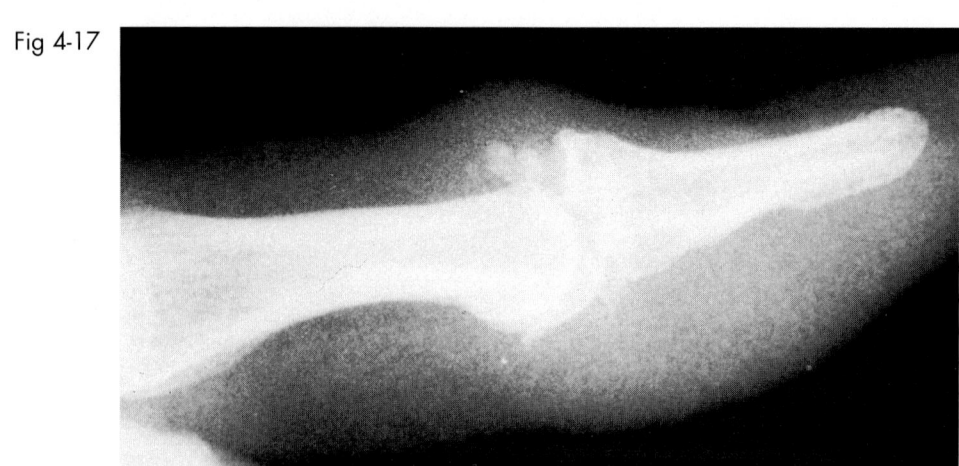

81 A 35-year-old man comes to the office with an angular deformity of his small finger. He says that it was injured when he was 10 years old and has never been treated (*Figure 4-18*). He has pain-free motion, which is 70% normal. What is your recommendation regarding treatment?

Fig 4-18

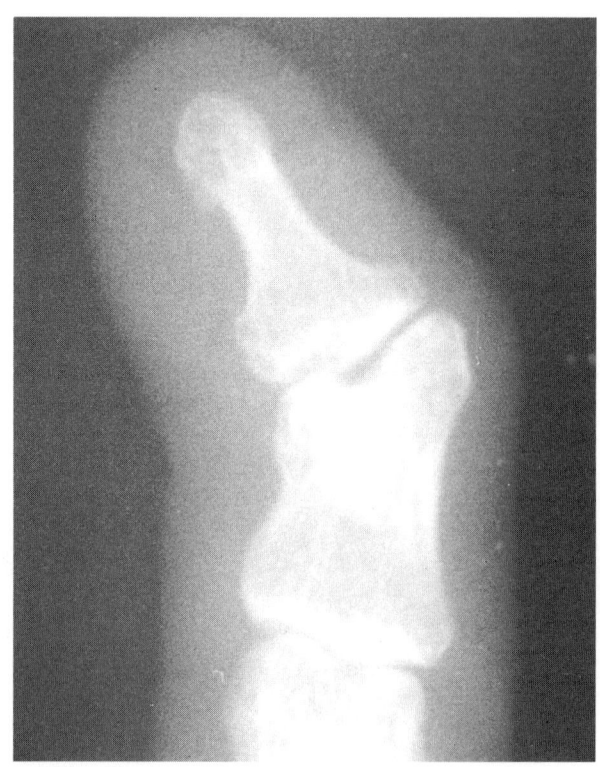

ANSWERS

80 The patient has an unstable dorsal dislocation that redislocated. Treatment is open reduction with a volar plate arthroplasty versus DIP joint arthrodesis.

81 The radiographic film demonstrates severe irregularity of the DIP joint referable to collapse of the ulnar condyle. The patient probably had an intraarticular ulnar condyle fracture that healed in this malunited position. Owing to the remodeling capacity of childhood, his digit has taken on this appearance with relatively good function. Treatment options range from accepting the deformity to performing an opening wedge osteotomy to realign the digit. If there were loss of motion with articular deterioration, consideration would be given for a DIP joint arthroplasty or arthrodesis.

QUESTIONS

82 This 35-year-old nurse slammed her long finger in a car door on the way to work. She comes to your office with a subungual hematoma involving 50% of the nail, throbbing pain, and the radiographic film shown below (*Figure 4-19*). Tendon function and the skin are intact. How should this be treated?

Fig 4-19
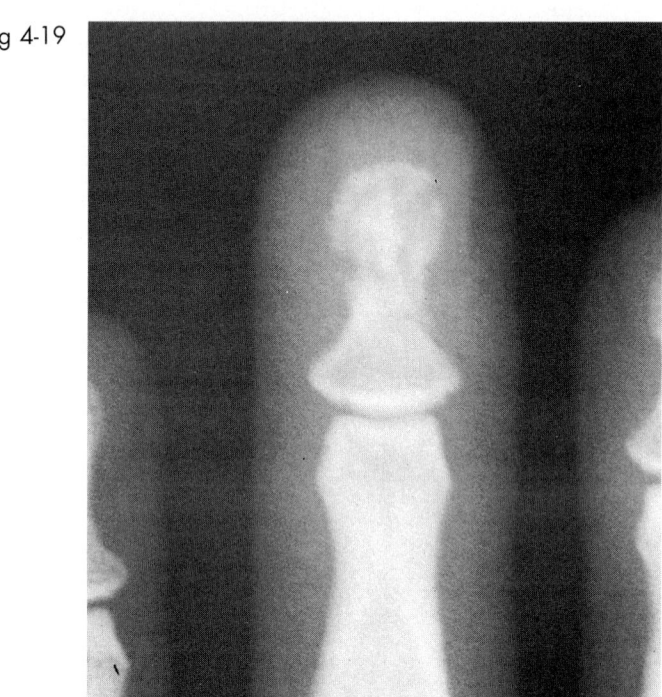

83 This 35-year-old laborer sustained a distal phalanx tuft fracture 3 months earlier and underwent a period of splint treatment. He comes to your office because of persistent pain and deformity of the finger. A radiograph film is shown (*Figure 4-20*). On physical examination there is gross motion at the tip of the finger at the level of his fracture site with obvious dorsal angulation of the tip of the finger. How would you approach this problem?

Fig 4-20
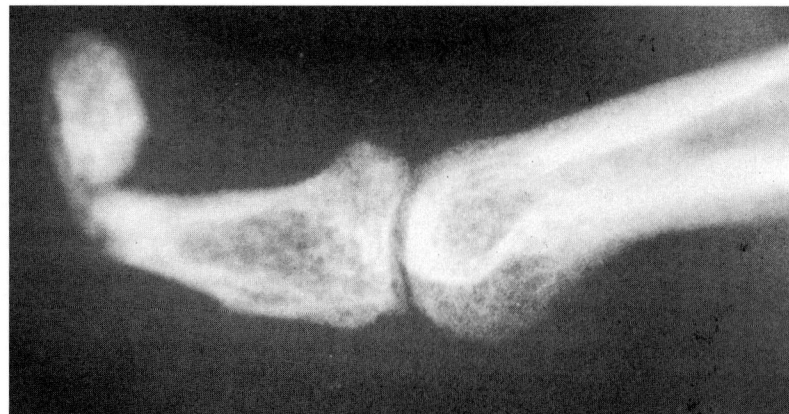

ANSWERS

82 Assuming there is no angular deformity on lateral radiographic films, this comminuted tuft fracture should be treated in a closed manner with splinting for a period of 3 to 6 weeks until the digit is comfortable. The subungual hematoma can be relieved through making one or two small holes in the nail to allow it to drain. It is controversial whether the nail should be elevated to inspect for nail bed injury and potential repair.

83 This large tuft fracture should have been stabilized acutely with K-wire fixation or with adequate splinting to avoid this deformity. At this point our treatment is excision of the tuft fragment versus bone grafting and fixation. To provide stability for the fingertip and avoid hook nail deformity, one would favor correction of the deformity with grafting and fixation with K-wires.

QUESTION

84 This 10-year-old girl sustained a Salter-Harris type II fracture of the small finger, proximal phalanx 6 months ago. She was treated with splinting of the digit only. The patient was concerned because her small finger abducted excessively relative to the opposite finger. She complains of this cosmetic deformity. Her AP radiographic films taken at the time of injury and taken in your office today are shown (*Figures 4-21A, 4-21B and 4-21C*). Her digital range of motion is completely normal with no rotational abnormality and no overlap of the digits. The patient wants your recommendation regarding how difficult it would be to correct this abnormality and asks whether this injury was poorly treated.

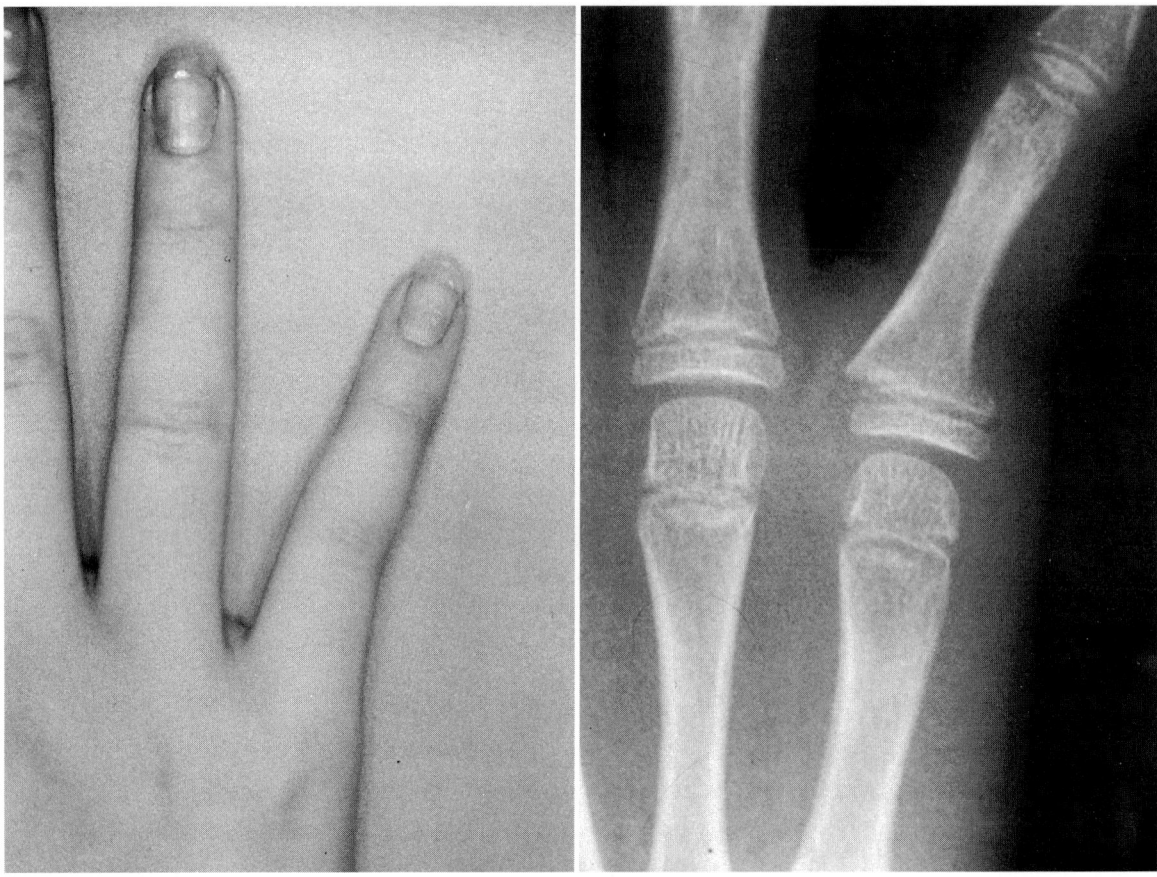

Fig 4-21 **A**   Fig 4-21 **B**

ANSWER

84   The patient's Salter-Harris type II fracture obviously was angulated and should have undergone a closed reduction at the time of her injury. These fractures are usually stable after reduction, can be treated with buddy taping and splinting, and usually heal with minimal problems. At this point there is mild angular deformity noted without functional impairment; the deformity would require an osteotomy of the proximal phalanx for correction. Recommendation would be to accept this relatively mild deformity. There may be continued minor correction with additional growth; however, conventionally one does not see significant improvement with radioulnar angulation in phalangeal fractures.

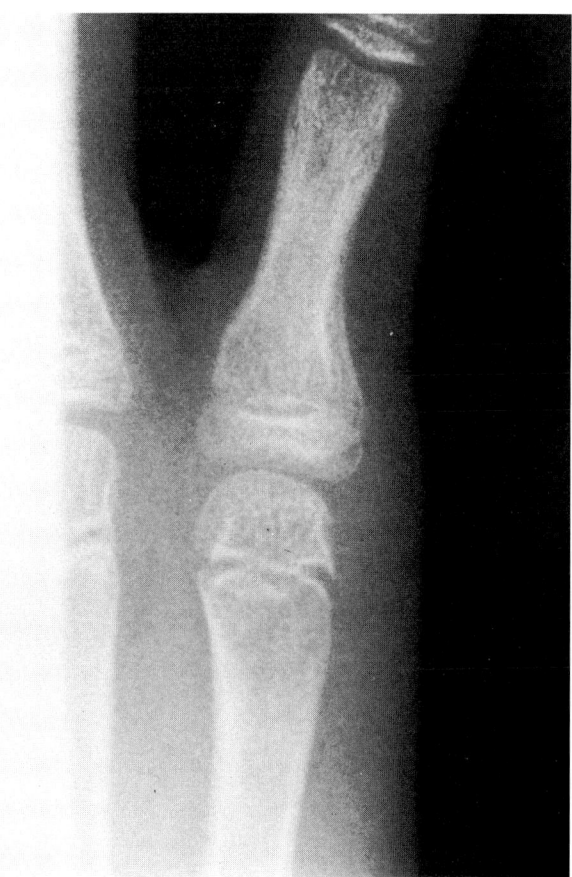

Fig 4-21 **C**

QUESTION

85 This 4-year-old boy smashed his finger in a car door sustaining injury around the PIP joint of the small finger. A radiographic film is shown (*Figure 4-22*). How should this fracture be treated?

Fig 4-22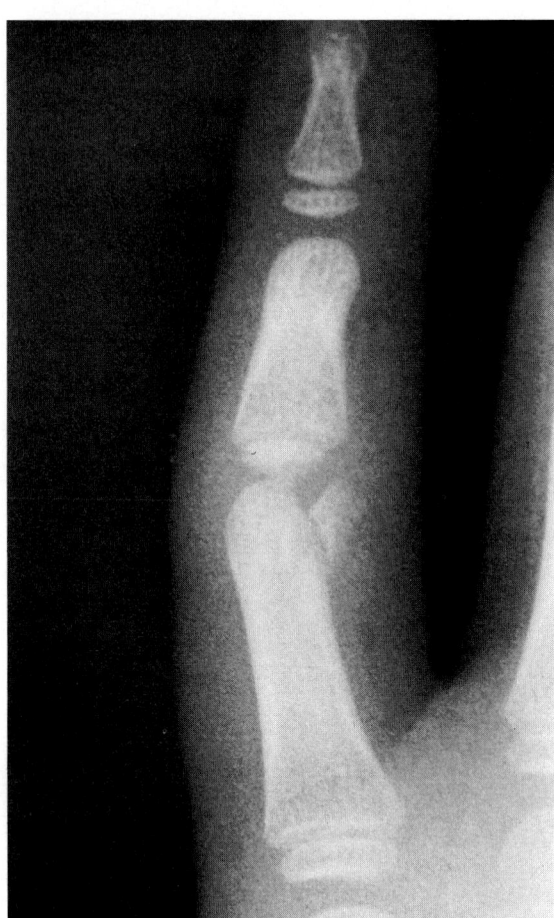

ANSWER

85   In general, displaced, intraarticular fractures should be treated with open reduction and internal fixation. This is particularly true in pediatric fractures wherein the seemingly small fracture fragments are covered with cartilage and can be extremely large and often constitute significant portions of the articular surface. This fracture will require open reduction and internal fixation of a large volar radial condylar fracture (*Figure 4-23*).

Fig 4-23

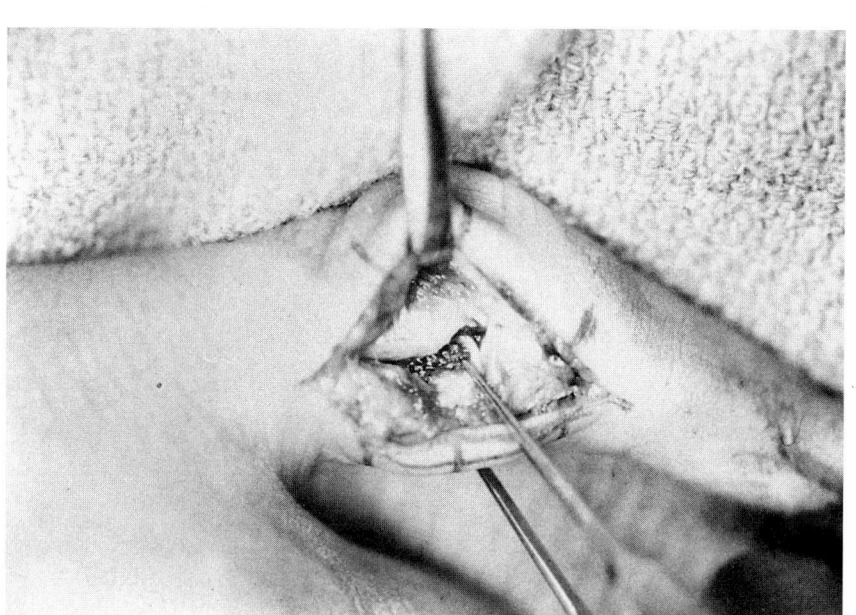

QUESTION

86 This 25-year-old, fourth year medical student fell off his bike sustaining a fracture to the PIP joint of his index finger. Radiographic films (*Figures 4-24A and 4-24B*) are shown below. Describe the management of this fracture.

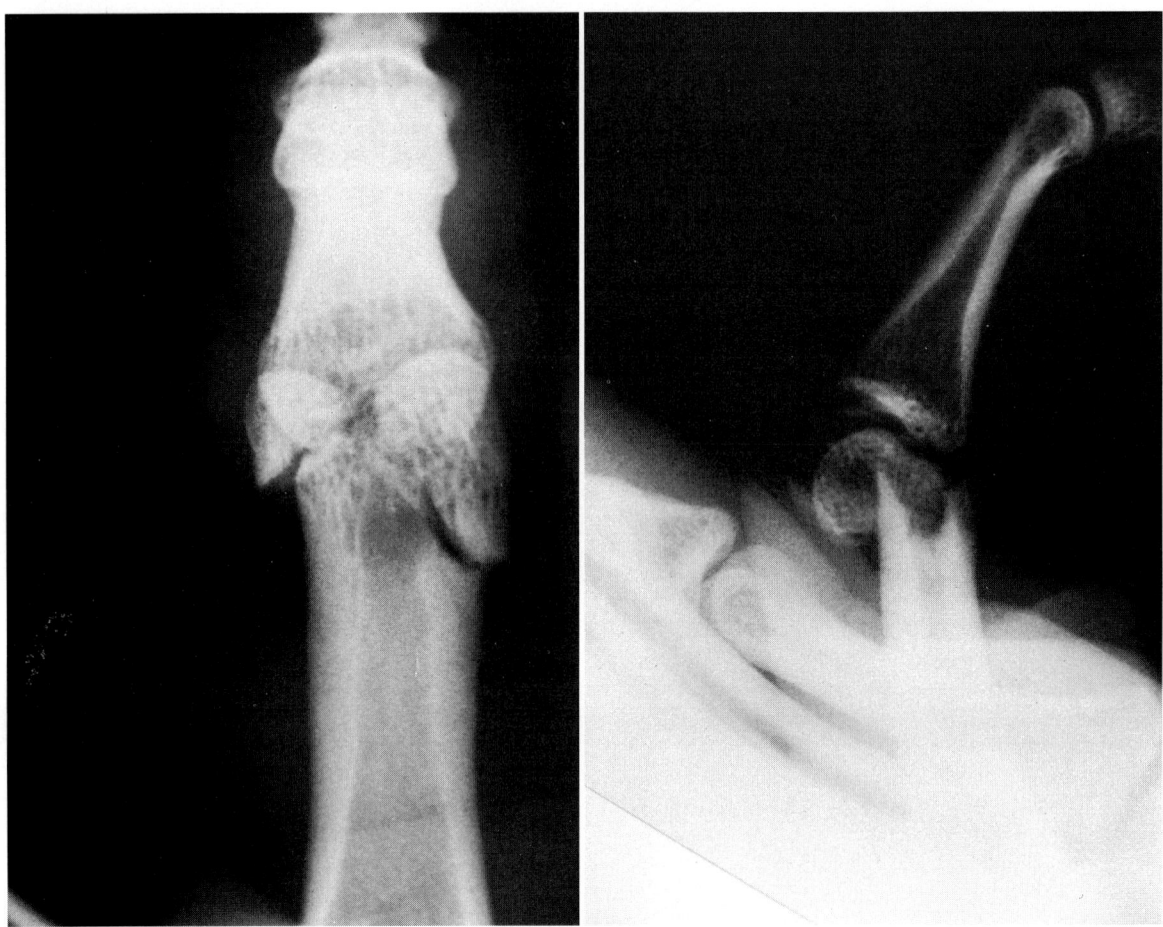

Fig 4-24 **A**   Fig 4-24 **B**

ANSWER

86   This Y-intercondylar fracture is unstable and requires some form of fixation after reduction. Closed reduction with percutaneous pinning and application of traction, an external fixator to maintain alignment through ligamentotaxis, or open reduction and internal fixation are accepted approaches to this difficult fracture.

QUESTION

87 This 56-year-old woman underwent an osteotomy for a slowly progressive rotational deformity of the right long finger. A radiographic film taken 2 weeks postoperatively is shown (*Figure 4-25A*). The radiographic film at the bottom of the page (*Figure 4-25B*) was taken 3 months after surgery when she came to your office for the first time. Physical examination demonstrates gross motion at the osteotomy site, and there is little active or passive motion at the PIP joint. How should this problem be approached?

Fig 4-25 **A**

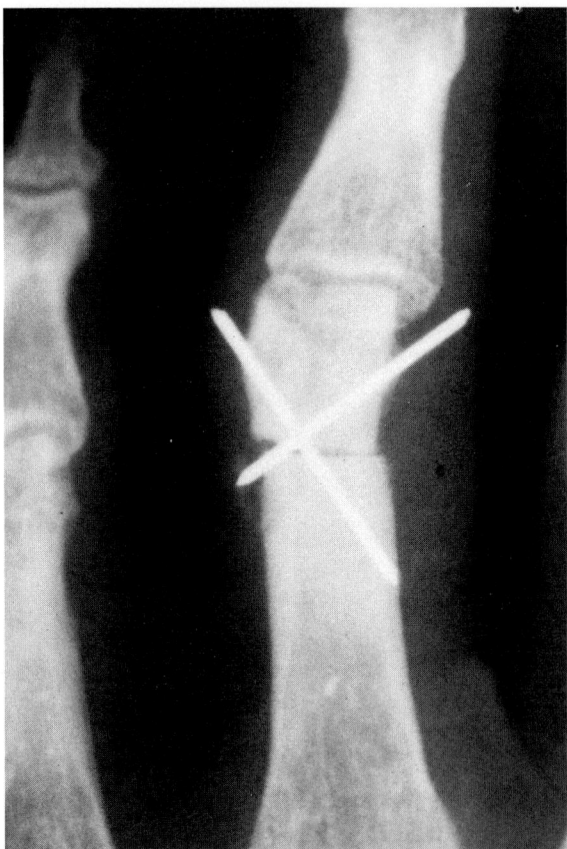

Fig 4-25 **B**

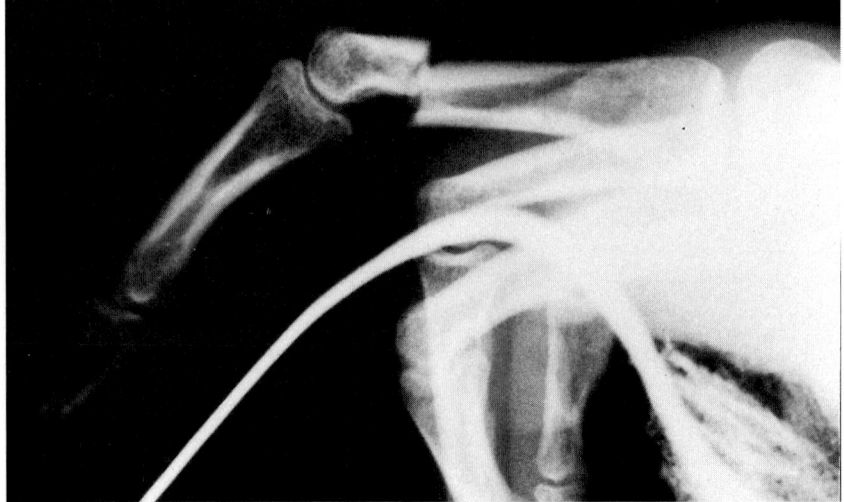

ANSWER

87   This nonunion of the proximal phalanx neck should be repaired through open reduction and rigid internal fixation using K-wires, interosseous wires, or miniplate and screws. The osteotomy site should be bone grafted and compressed. Strong consideration should be made for PIP joint capsulotomy with institution of early postoperative range of motion.

QUESTIONS

88 Describe the indications for surgery of index and long finger metacarpal shaft fractures.

89 What are the indications for surgery for ring finger metacarpal shaft fractures?

90 What are your indications for operative treatment of small finger metacarpal shaft fractures with regard to angulation and shortening?

91 List seven general indications for surgery in metacarpal and phalangeal fractures.

92 What are the indications for operative intervention in metacarpal head fractures?

ANSWERS

88 The general indications for open reduction and internal fixation of any fracture of the hand include open fractures, multiple fractures, unstable fractures, and fractures with rotational or angular deformities not corrected by manipulation. Specifically with regard to the index and long fingers, if after manipulation there is greater than 10° of angular deformity in the AP plane, a shortening greater than 3 mm to 4 mm, more than 5° radioulnar angulation, any residual malrotation, or segmental bone loss, one should consider operative intervention. Bear in mind that these are guidelines that must be applied selectively for each patient.

89 Because of the increased mobility of the ring finger ray through the CMC joint, increased angulation can be accepted in shaft fractures of the ring finger metacarpal. If after closed reduction it is determined there is greater than 20° of dorsal or palmar angulation, greater than 5° radioulnar angulation, greater than 3 mm to 4 mm of shortening, any residual malrotation, or segmental bone loss, surgery should be considered.

90 After closed reduction, more than 30° of AP angular deformity, more than 5° radioulnar angulation, greater than 3 mm to 4 mm of shortening, or any residual malrotation are indications for surgery in small finger metacarpal shaft fractures.

91 (1) Open fractures
(2) Displaced intraarticular fractures
(3) Malrotation, seen most often in spiral and short oblique fracture patterns
(4) Displaced phalangeal neck fractures
(5) Fractures with bone loss
(6) Multiple hand and wrist fractures associated with significant soft tissue injury
(7) Multitrauma with associated hand fractures

92 Displaced fractures with ligament avulsion and osteochondral fractures usually require surgical intervention. Coronal, sagittal, and oblique fractures with displacement should be operatively treated. Comminuted intraarticular fractures sometimes may benefit from surgical intervention providing adequate bone stock remains for fixation. Occasionally, external fixation is helpful in realigning comminuted, intraarticular fragments.

QUESTIONS

93 What are the indications for surgery on index and long finger metacarpal neck fractures?

94 What are the indications for surgery for ring finger metacarpal neck fractures?

95 What are the indications for surgery on small finger metacarpal neck fractures?

96 This 1-year-old infant is brought to your office with a congenital abnormality of the thumb seen in the photographs shown (*Figures 4-26A and 4-26B*). What is the Wassel classification of this thumb deformity?

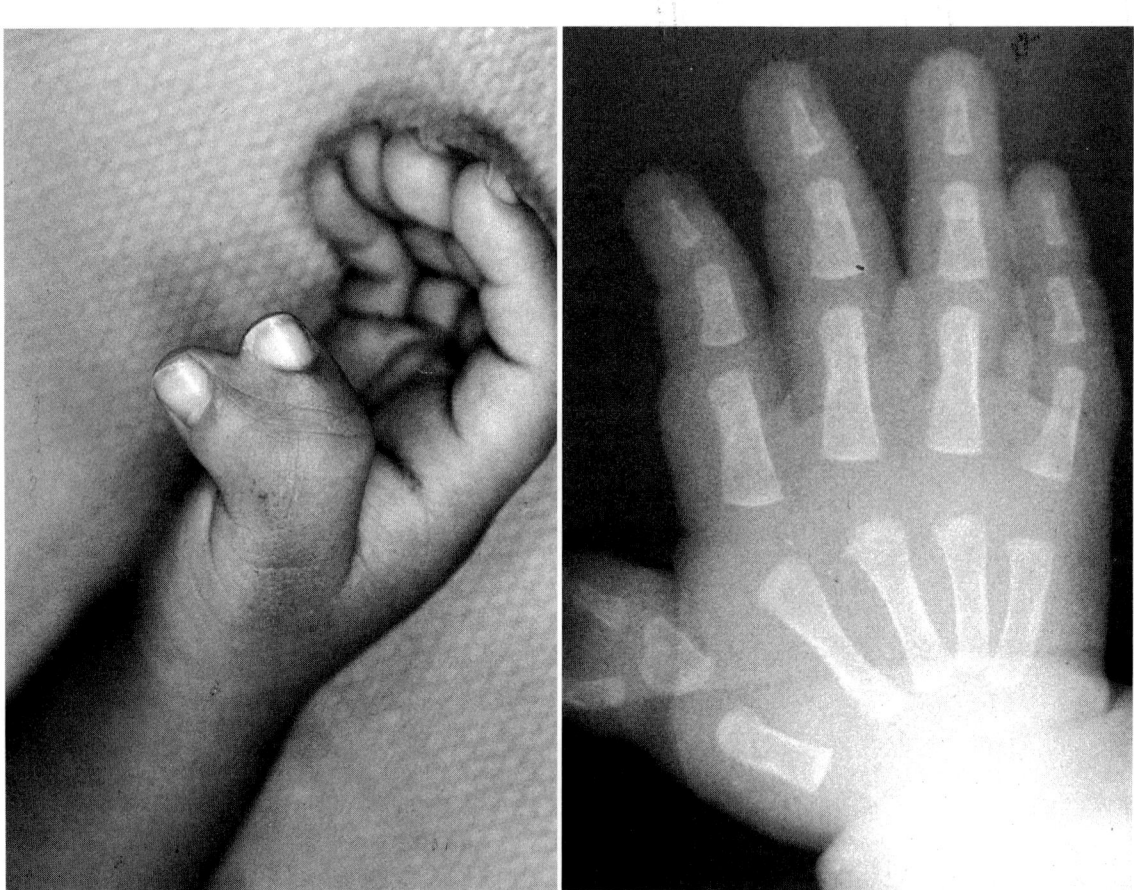

Fig 4-26 **A**   Fig 4-26 **B**

ANSWERS

93 Fractures that displace more than 50% of the cortical contact area with greater than 5° to 10° angulation or greater than 10° rotational abnormality should have open reduction and internal or external fixation.

94 Although this is somewhat controversial, authors have quoted ranges from 20° to 40° of angulation as the upper limits of acceptable reduction for ring finger metacarpal neck fractures.

95 Again, this is controversial in that there is a wide range of acceptable limits described by a number of authors. These numbers range from 30° to 70° of angulation as long as there is no loss of PIP extension and no more than a 10° rotational abnormality.

96 This Wassel type III has characteristic partial duplication of the proximal phalanx with a complete duplication of the distal phalanx and DIP joint.

QUESTIONS

97   When should surgery be performed to correct the problem in Q96?

98   Which of the extra thumbs would be removed in the reconstructive procedure?

99   During reconstructive surgery, why is the radial element usually removed in congenital duplication of the thumb?

100   Describe the details for the surgical reconstruction for this thumb.

101   What is the Bilhaut-Cloquet procedure?

102   What medical conditions are associated with Wassel type II preaxial polydactyly?

ANSWERS

97 The optimal age is controversial. Surgery can be done any time from 3 months and older. At approximately 1 year of age, the structures are adequately developed so that reconstruction is not excessively tedious, and the anesthesia risk is minimal.

98 Usually the radial thumb is excised.

99 The radial thumb is usually smaller than the ulnar digit, and there is no interference with the ulnar neurovascular bundle, which accounts for sensibility on this important aspect of the thumb used in prehension and opposition. In addition, the UCL usually does not require reconstruction with the excision of the radial thumb. This is desirable because stability of the UCL is essential in thumb function.

100 Skin flaps are outlined over the radial aspect of the thumb with excision of the distal phalanx and osteotomy of the proximal phalanx. A periosteal flap should be preserved along the radial aspect of the thumb proximal phalanx for reconstruction of RCL of the IP joint. The joint may need to be temporarily stabilized with a transarticular pin to facilitate protection of the collateral ligament reconstruction. In this particular thumb the UCL required reconstruction because of laxity as well.

101 To join the remaining radial and ulnar segments and to facilitate creation of a single thumb, the Bilhaut-Cloquet procedure involves the resection of a central wedge of tissue and bone between the duplicated thumbs with repair of the nail and bony apposition.

102 Wassel types I through VI are *not* associated with medical syndromes. In contrast, triphalangeal thumb (Wassel type VII) preaxial polydactyly can have associated medical problems.

QUESTIONS

103 This 5-year-old boy was brought to your office by his parents for removal of the extra finger on the right hand (*Figures 4-27A and 4-27B*). How is this polydactyly treated surgically?

Fig 4-27 **A**

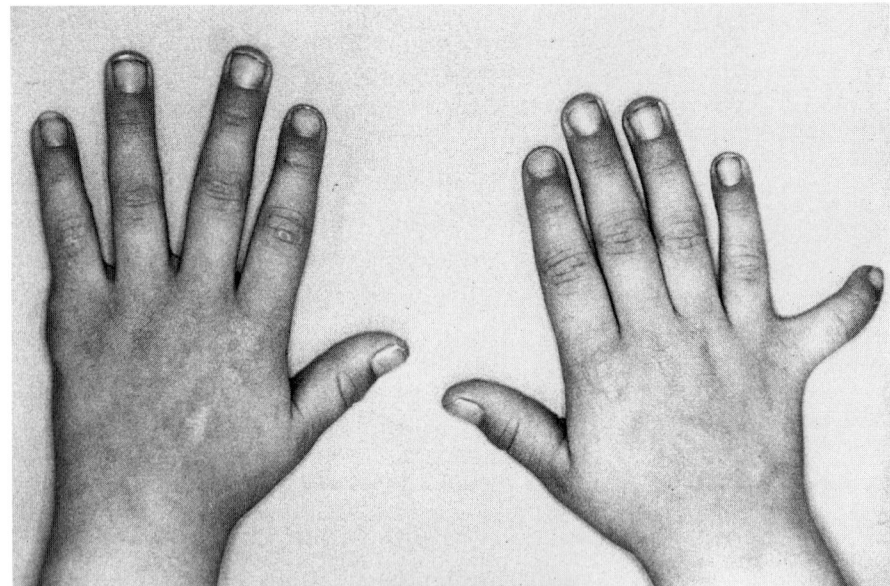

Fig 4-27 **B**

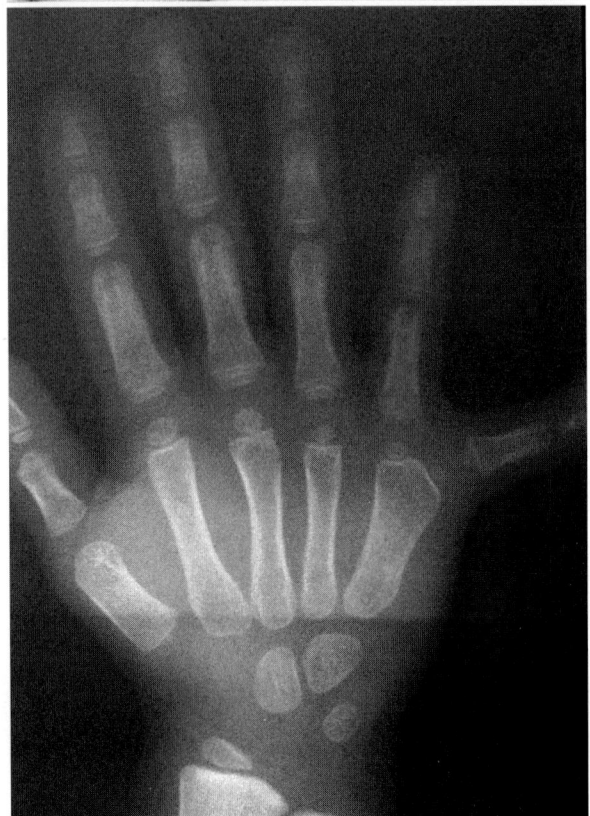

104 What medical conditions are associated with postaxial polydactyly?

ANSWERS

103 This patient requires excision of the accessory digit with osteotomy through the metacarpal head to remove the excess growth plate. Failure to trim the metacarpal head results in abnormal ulnar growth at the MCP joint, producing subsequent hand deformity. A periosteal flap should be elevated from the accessory digit to allow reconstruction of the UCL of the MCP joint.

104 In most black infants, postaxial polydactyly usually represents expression of an autosomal dominant trait, without associated medical problems. However, postaxial polydactyly in infants with no family history should be thoroughly evaluated for anomalies. These abnormalities include bladder obstruction, cataracts, eye defects, cleft lip, deafness, polycystic kidneys, chronic nephritis, hypogonadism, heart defects, hydrocephalus, mental deficiency, and imperforate anus.

QUESTIONS

105 A 35-year-old man who came to your office with elbow pain asked if you could also look at his small finger. Both small fingers radially deviate at the level of the DIP joint (*Figure 4-28*). He has full range of motion of the digits and no complaints of pain. He states that his small fingers have always deviated but not bothered him. What is the diagnosis and treatment?

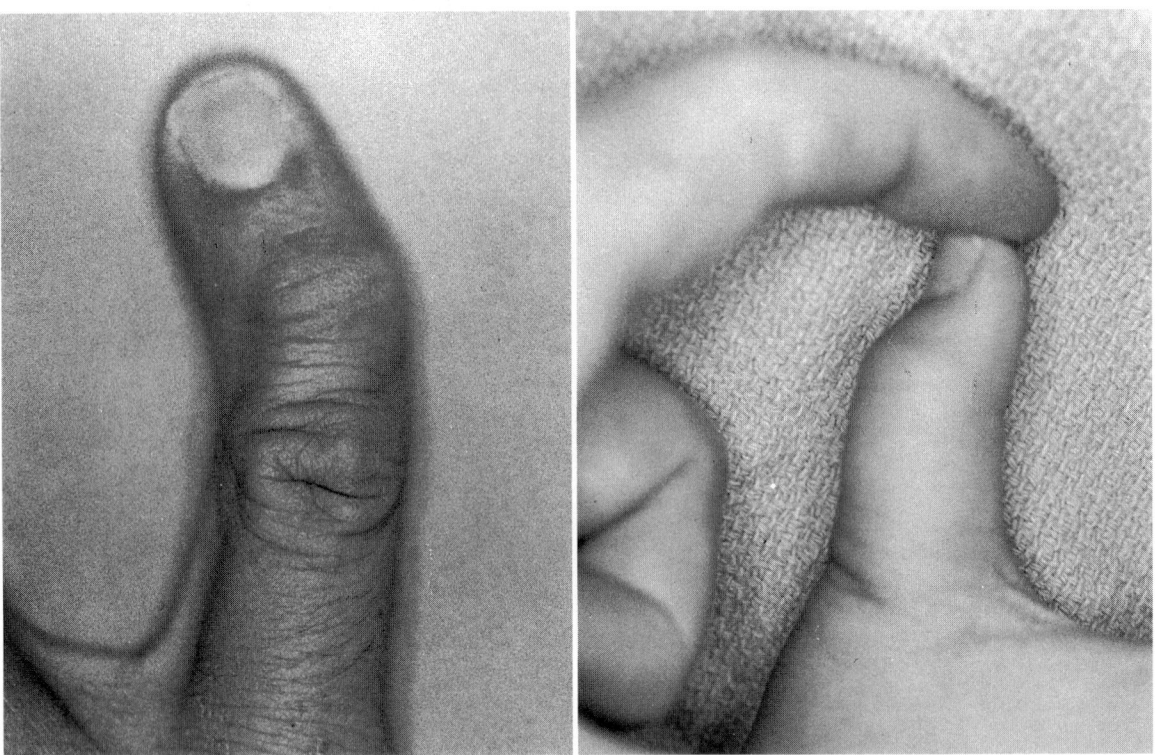

Fig 4-28   Fig 4-29

106 This 3-month-old boy was brought to your office because the parents noted that he is unable to fully extend his thumb. There is no history of congenital abnormalities in the family. Figure 4-29 demonstrates the extent of passive extension of the thumb. Actively, the thumb will extend no farther than 30° short of neutral. There is no other evidence of congenital problems. Apart from the loss of extension of the DIP joint, physical examination demonstrates good flexion of the thumb. The remaining digits are normal. He has a fullness in the flexor tendon overlying the volar MCP joint. What is the diagnosis?

107 How should this patient be treated?

ANSWERS

105   Diagnosis is clinodactyly, and this patient's condition requires no treatment. Clinodactyly is an angular deviation in the radioulnar plane usually caused by middle phalangeal asymmetric growth. Surgery is not recommended unless there is digital overlapping with fist making that interferes with function.

106   This condition most likely represents congenital trigger thumb, wherein there is enlargement of the flexor pollicis longus tendon at the level of the A-1 pulley in the thumb. Its incarceration would account for the lack of extension at the IP joint of the thumb.

107   There is controversy regarding treatment of congenital trigger thumb and trigger fingers. Some authors favor passive stretching by the parents and splinting, and others favor benign neglect with the expectation that some will spontaneously unlock their digits. Other orthopedists recommend surgical release upon diagnosis because of reports in the literature of a low percentage of spontaneous correction. A reasonable, middle-of-the-road approach is surgical release at 9 to 12 months of age if the digit has not spontaneously unlocked.

QUESTION

108　This 35-year-old man sustained a closed humeral fracture in a motor vehicle accident as pictured in Figure 4-30A. When he came to the emergency room, he was asked to extend his wrist and fingers as seen in Figure 4-30B. He had complete loss of MCP and wrist extension. What is his problem in reference to the hand, and how should it be managed?

Fig 4-30 **A**

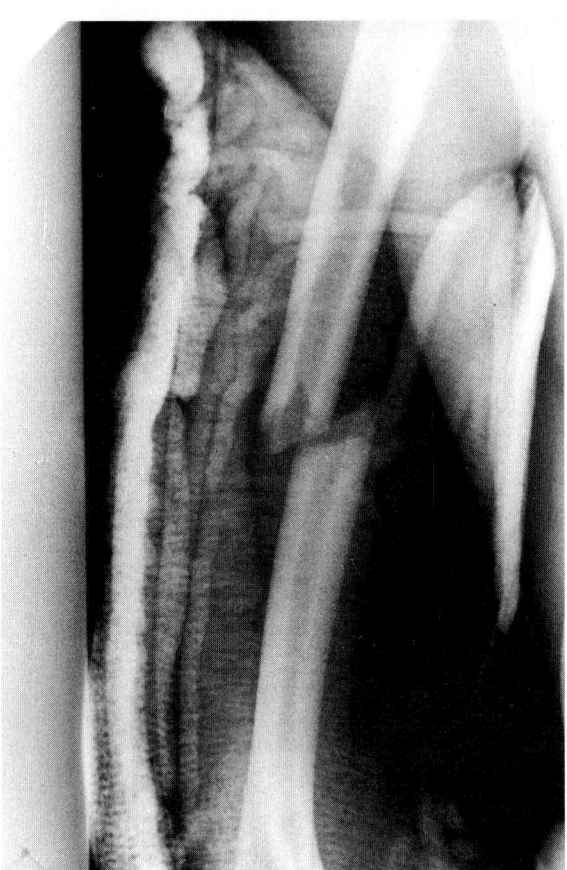

Fig 4-30 **B**

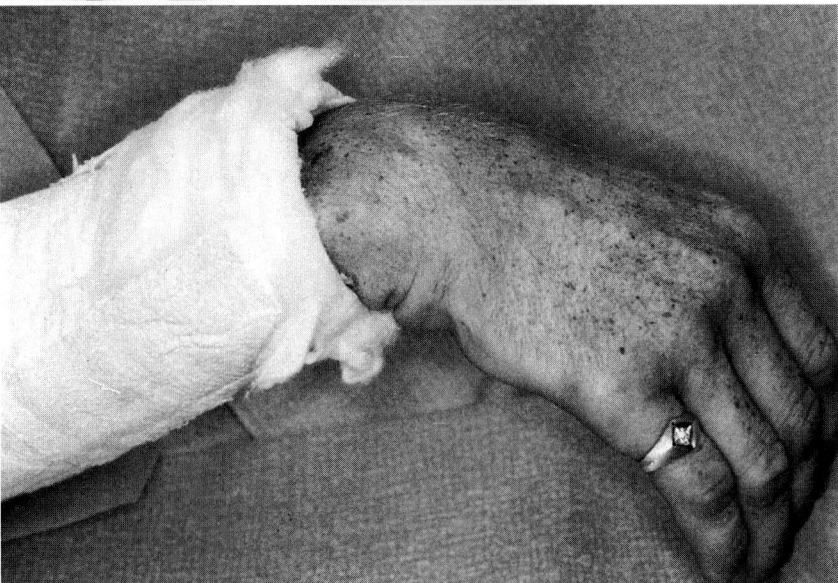

ANSWER

108 This humeral fracture is associated with a radial nerve palsy, which accounts for lack of MP extension of the digits and loss of wrist extension. Because he has a closed injury with the nerve palsy already in effect, one would expect a high likelihood of spontaneous nerve recovery without exploration; over 90% experience spontaneous recovery. Management would consist of splint, fracture brace, or cast for the humeral fracture and wrist splinting and physical therapy to maintain mobility of the digits.

QUESTIONS

109 Four months later the fracture has healed, but the patient in Q108 shows no clinical signs of recovery of his radial nerve function. What should be done now?

110 An 80-year-old woman fell at home sustaining a spiral fracture of the distal humerus. She is neurologically intact and has subsequently lost radial nerve function after application of a cast. Radiographic films demonstrate excellent alignment. How should she be managed?

111 A 38-year-old woman was unloading her horse from a trailer and sustained a midshaft, completely displaced transverse humerus fracture with 1 cm of overlap of the bone ends. A coaptation splint and collar and cuff were applied, and the patient noted dysesthesias in the sensory distribution of the radial nerve with subsequent loss of digital MCP and wrist extension. The coaptation splint was removed with return of nerve function within 5 minutes. A hanging cast was then applied, and there was a similar loss of radial nerve function within minutes with restoration of nerve function with removal of the cast. A plaster slab was then applied over the radial aspect of the arm, and she was placed in a sling. In this position there was no nerve dysfunction, although she continued to have significant pain without improvement in fracture position. What is your approach to this patient?

112 What are the two principal mechanisms of tendon healing in flexor zone 2?

ANSWERS

109 Repeat electrodiagnostic studies should be obtained and compared with those obtained earlier in the clinical course (3 to 4 weeks after injury). In the absence of any clinical or electrodiagnostic improvement, exploration is indicated after $3^1/_2$ to 4 months of observation in closed injuries.

110 Loss of the radial nerve function following manipulation or application of cast necessitates exploration of the nerve. In this particular case the nerve was intact, although it was tented over a spike of bone and located in the fracture site. The nerve was freed from incarceration, and the distal humerus was stabilized.

111 Because the nerve is in a vulnerable position and the fracture fragments are in marginal position, surgical exploration with ORIF of the fracture is recommended. Removal of the nerve between the humeral fragments and compression plating yielded an excellent result.

112 Tendon healing occurs through extrinsic healing, which is mediated through fibroblast ingrowth and is dependent upon adhesion formation between the tendon and surrounding tissue. The adhesions provide blood supply to the healing tendon; however, they may interfere with smooth gliding in the tendon sheath. The other process is intrinsic tendon healing, which, as the name implies, occurs through tenocyte mediated joining of opposed tendon ends. Theoretically, this type of healing produces fewer adhesions. Blood supply for the healing tendon is provided through intact vincular systems, and further nutrition is provided through synovial fluid bathing the healing site.

QUESTION

113   This 58-year-old woman slipped on the ice and sustained a right distal radius fracture, which was seen initially by a family-practice doctor who placed her in a short-arm cast. She is referred to you 1 week after the injury; these radiographic films (*Figures 4-31A and 4-31B*) were obtained in your office. Is this an adequate reduction?

Fig 4-31 **A**

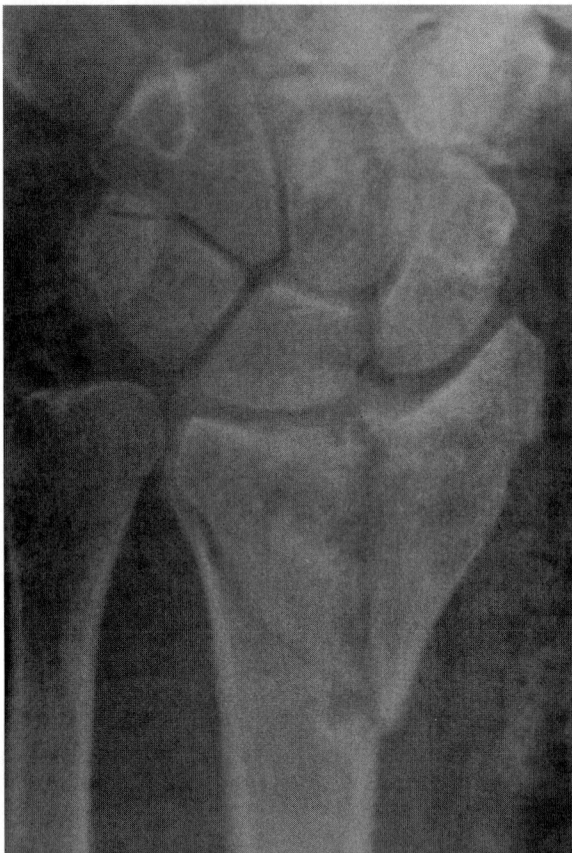

Fig 4-31 **B**

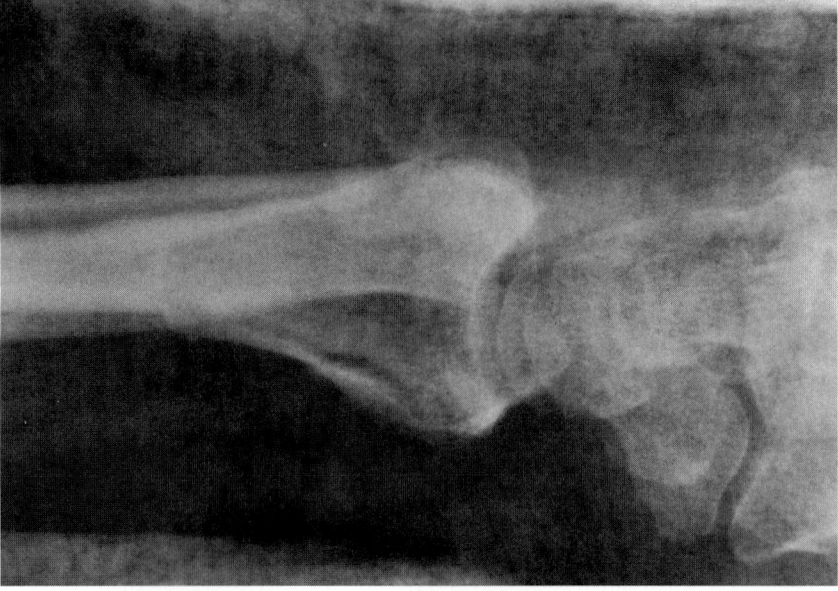

ANSWER

113   Although a lateral radiographic film looks fairly good, the AP is suggestive of a significant intraarticular step-off.

QUESTIONS

114 How would you further evaluate this fracture with regard to adequacy of reduction?

115 The radiographic film shown (*Figure 4-32*) is from the tomogram series from the patient described in Q113. What is your recommendation regarding treatment?

Fig 4-32

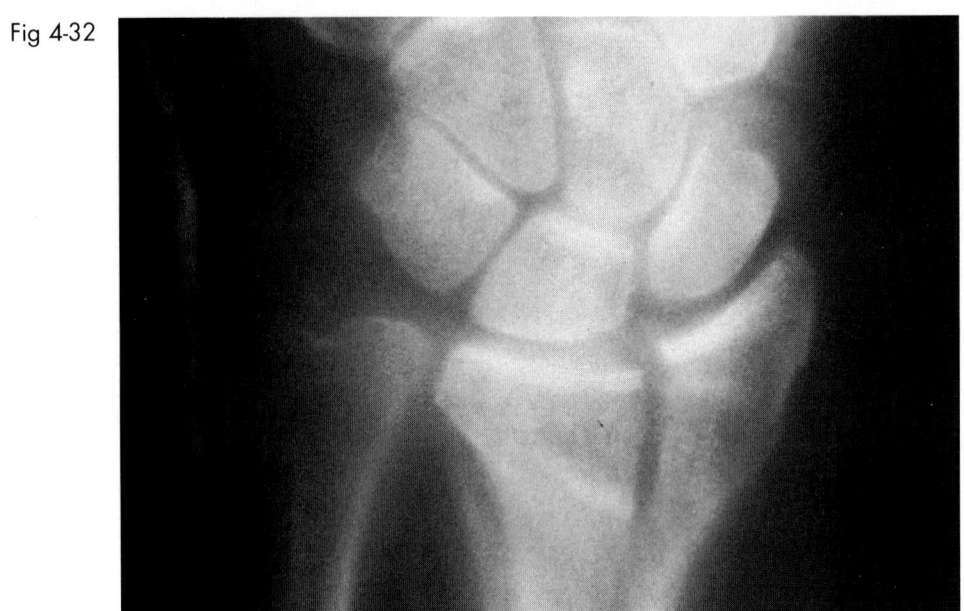

116 Describe the course of the radial nerve from its origin in the brachium through the arm.

117 A 51-year-old golfer complains of spontaneous onset of medial elbow pain 3 months earlier, which has progressively worsened. He is tender over the medial epicondyle and has pain with resisted pronation and wrist flexion. Radiographic films were normal. Describe your management of this patient.

ANSWERS

114   Tomograms or a computed tomography (CT) scan of the wrist.

115   Although somewhat controversial, there is general agreement that an intraarticular step-off greater than 1 mm to 2 mm should be corrected. Assuming that this patient is in reasonable health, surgical reconstruction should be considered. Percutaneous pinning with external fixation application or open reduction and internal fixation are appropriate.

116   The radial nerve is a branch of the posterior cord of the brachial plexus that runs posteriorly, leaving the axilla through the "triangular space." This "space" is bordered superiorly by the inferior part of the teres major, laterally by the humeral shaft, and medially by the long head of the triceps. The radial nerve is then accompanied by the profunda brachii as it passes obliquely across the posterior humerus between the lateral and medial heads of the triceps. It then travels in shallow groove, deep to the lateral head of the triceps. It penetrates the lateral intermuscular septum, running posteriorly to come into the anterior compartment of the arm. Here it is bordered medially by brachialis muscle and laterally by the brachioradialis proximally and the extensor carpi radialis longus (ECRL) distally. The radial nerve divides into the superficial branch and posterior interosseous nerve at approximately the level of the lateral epicondyle of the humerus.

117   Initial nonsurgical management of medial epicondylitis consists of rest and nonsteroidal antiinflammatory medication. Patients are instructed to avoid provocative activities. Corticosteroid injection and counterforce bracing are often beneficial. After symptoms have subsided, a rehabilitation program consisting of progressive stretching and isometric exercises can be initiated. Surgery is reserved for cases unresponsive to conservative care.

QUESTIONS

118   The illustration shown (*Figure 4-33*) is the lateral view of a 10-year-old child's wrist. The patient's mother noticed this lump with the wrist in a flexed posture. The mass is 1 cm by 1 cm in size, pain-free, and readily transilluminates. What are the treatment options?

Fig 4-33

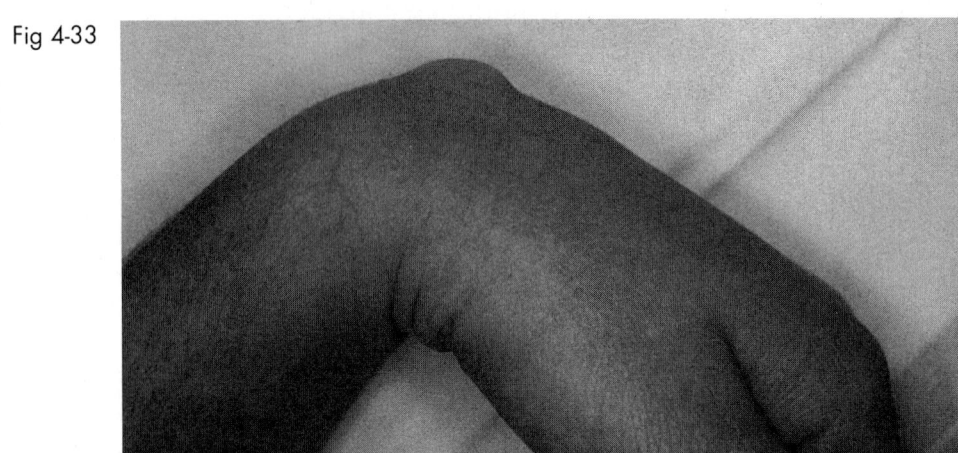

119   Describe the site of origin of most dorsal carpal ganglion cysts.

120   A 10-year-old girl has deformities of her left hand that have become progressively painful. A radiographic film is shown (*Figure 4-34*). What is the patient's diagnosis, and how should this problem be approached?

Fig 4-34

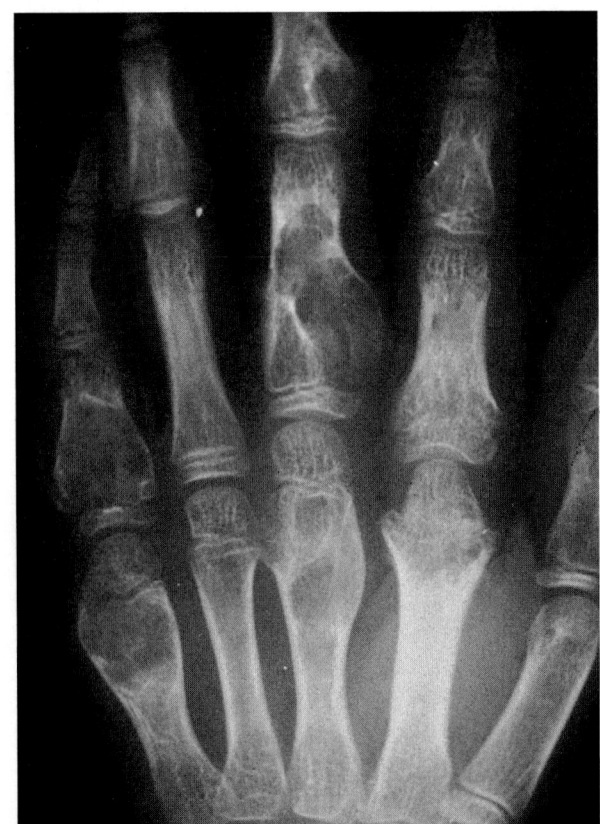

ANSWERS

118   A dorsal wrist mass in this area that is pain free and transilluminates is most likely a dorsal carpal ganglion cyst. Other diagnostic possibilities include giant cell tumor, extensor tenosynovitis, exostosis, or a soft tissue tumor. Because the wrist is a fairly characteristic location for a dorsal carpal ganglion cyst, treatment recommendations depend on the patient's degree of symptomatology. If the mass changes significantly in size or character, biopsy should be considered. An asymptomatic patient can be followed as needed. If the parent or the patient expresses symptoms with activities that do not respond to a period of splinting, surgical excision or mass aspiration may be considered.

119   The typical location of the base of the stalk of a dorsal carpal ganglion cyst is the dorsal scapholunate capsule and ligament.

120   The patient has multiple enchondromatosis. In a patient with symptomatic enchondromata with significant thinning of the cortex, one would consider excision.

QUESTIONS

121 A 50-year-old secretary slammed her finger in a cabinet drawer at work 1 week earlier and came to your office with swelling of her affected index finger. On physical examination there is lobulated nodular swelling dorsally and palmarly overlying the middle phalanx. The skin demonstrates no significant changes. Neurosensory examination is intact. Her digital range of motion is near normal. A radiograph is shown (*Figure 4-35*). She wants to know whether her proposed operation will be covered under workers' compensation. What is your response?

Fig 4-35

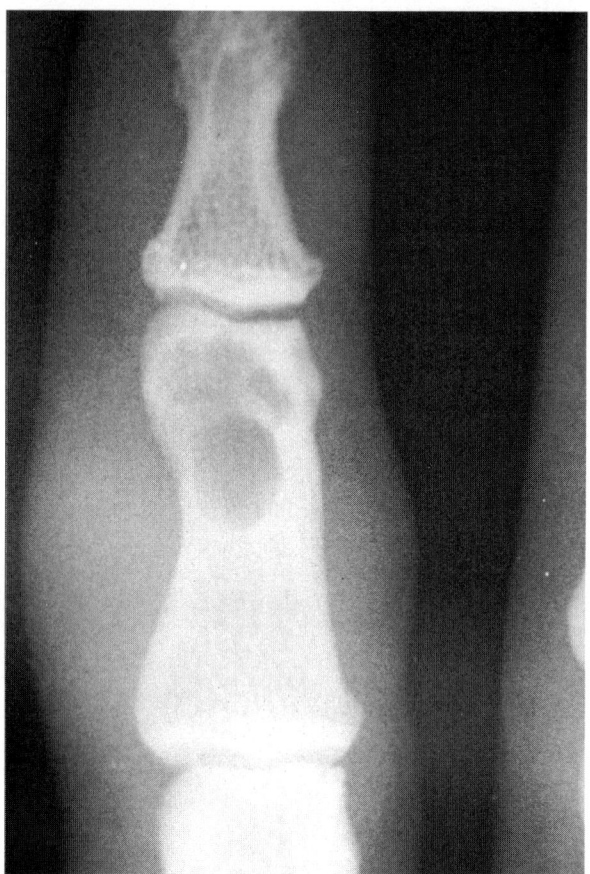

122 What is your diagnosis?

ANSWERS

121 The radiographic changes seen are consistent with a longstanding process of more than 1 week's duration. It is likely that slamming her finger in a cabinet had nothing to do with the process that has produced enlargement of the digit and erosion of the bone.

122 The most likely cause of gradual erosion of the middle phalanx (suggested by the rounded appearance and sclerotic margins of the defect) with associated soft tissue enlargement in several lobulated areas in the digit is a giant cell tumor of the tendon sheath.

QUESTION

123 A 4-year-old boy was brought to your office by his parents because of a painless radial enlargement of the index finger over the PIP joint. A radiographic film is shown (*Figure 4-36*). What is the diagnosis and recommended treatment?

Fig 4-36

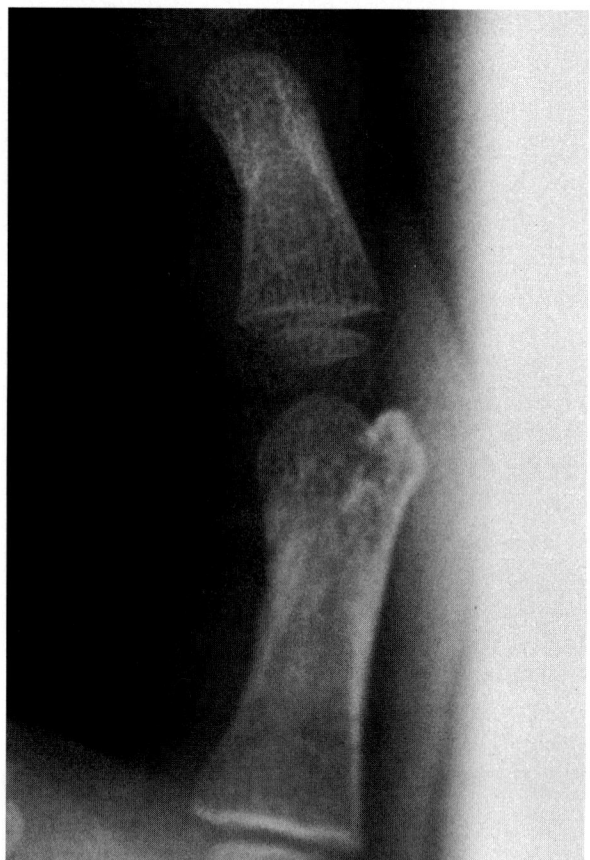

ANSWER

123   This enlargement has the characteristic appearance of an osteochondroma of the proximal phalanx. Treatment is excision of the osteochondroma with reattachment of the RCL.

QUESTION

124 The photograph shown (*Figure 4-37A*) demonstrates a recurrent mass in an 8-year-old boy. Six months ago he had excision of an osteochondroma from the forearm, and there has been gradual return of marked deformity of the forearm as noted in the radiographic film shown (*Figure 4-37B*). What is the differential diagnosis?

Fig 4-37 **A**

Fig 4-37 **B**

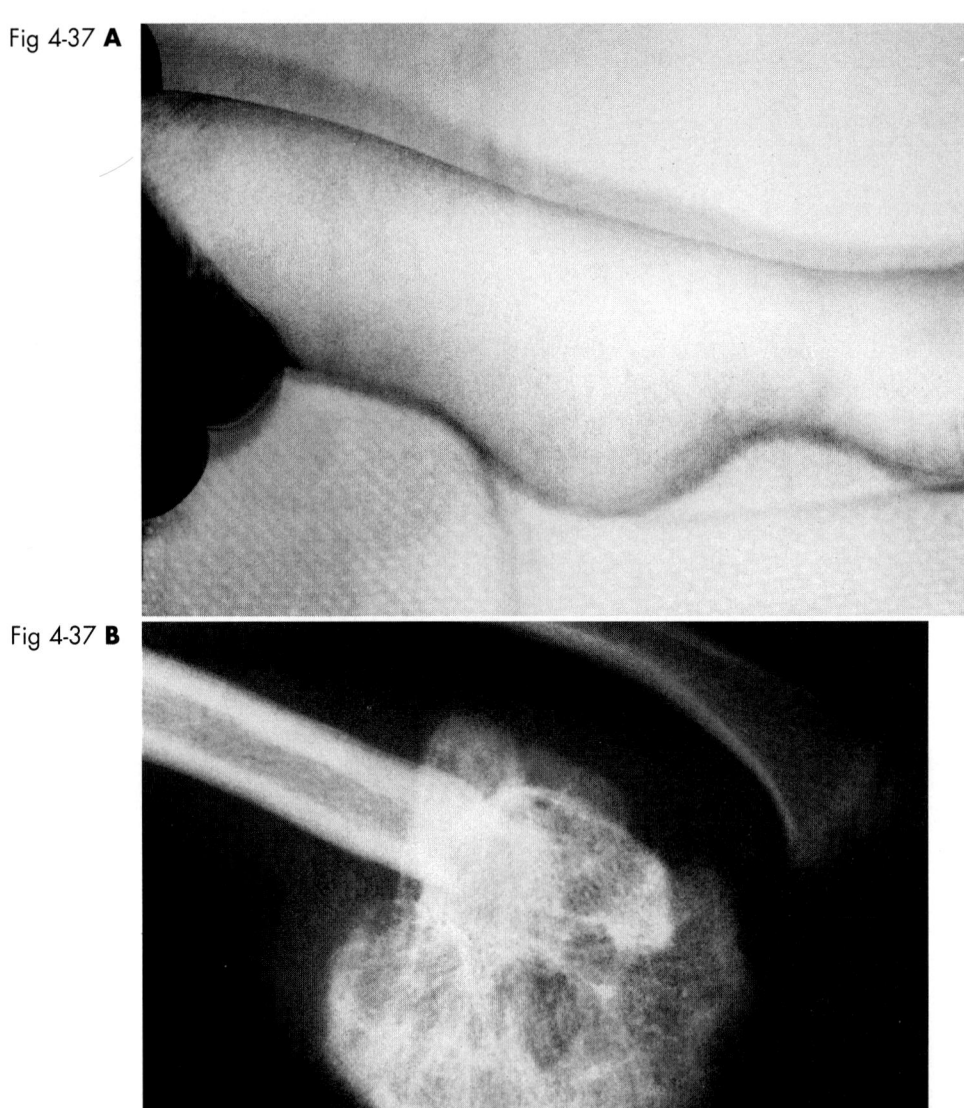

ANSWER

124 Recurrence of a mass following excision of an osteochondroma would suggest that there was an incomplete resection and that this is simply recurrence of the osteochondroma. The rate at which this mass has recurred is disturbing, suggesting a malignant process. One would have to consider osteosarcoma in the differential diagnosis. The radiographic film demonstrates fairly mature bone favoring a more benign process such as an osteochondroma. The pathologic specimen after the second resection demonstrated a recurrent osteochondroma.

QUESTIONS

125 A 14-year-old girl has complained of right wrist pain after a fall in gymnastics class. The wrist has remained symptomatic, and she complains of a dorsoulnar prominence with deformity. Careful questioning reveals that this deformity had been present before her injury. A radiographic film of the right wrist is shown (*Figure 4-38*). What is the diagnosis?

Fig 4-38

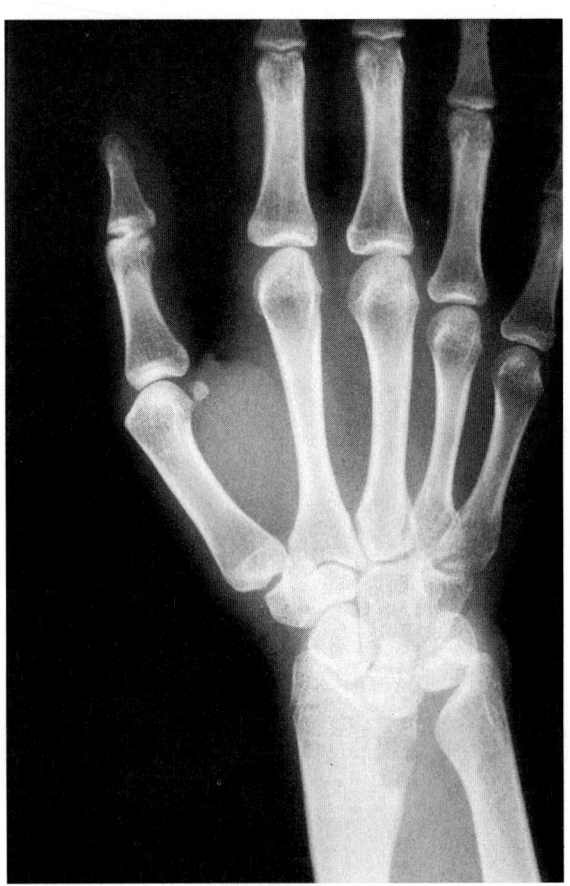

126 How would you confirm this diagnosis?

ANSWERS

125 Madelung's deformity.

126 Often radiographic films of the opposite wrist will demonstrate a similar deformity. A radiographic film of the left wrist is illustrated (*Figure 4-39*). Characteristic radiographic changes include decreased radial length with triangular shape, usually associated with early fusion of the ulnar half of the distal physis. There is often an area of lucency at the ulnar border of the distal radius, with ulnar and volar angulation of the distal radial articular surface. The ulna is shortened with enlargement of the ulnar head, associated with dorsal subluxation. The carpus tends to be wedge shaped with the apex located proximally.

Fig 4-39

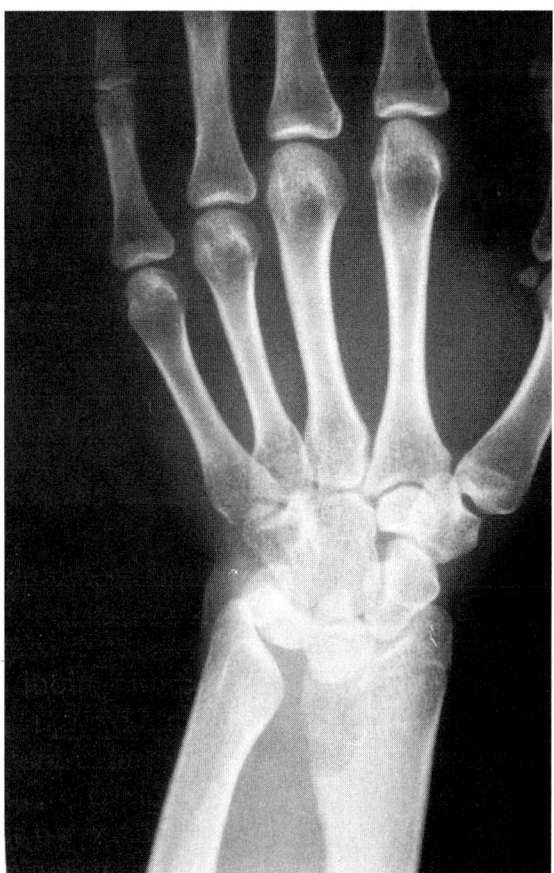

QUESTION

127 The radiographic films shown (*Figures 4-40A and 4-40B*) were taken to evaluate a 45-year-old man who fell after an altercation with one of the disturbed patients at the health care facility where he worked. What is the nature of this problem, and could this be related to his fall 2 weeks ago?

Fig 4-40 **A**

Fig 4-40 **B**

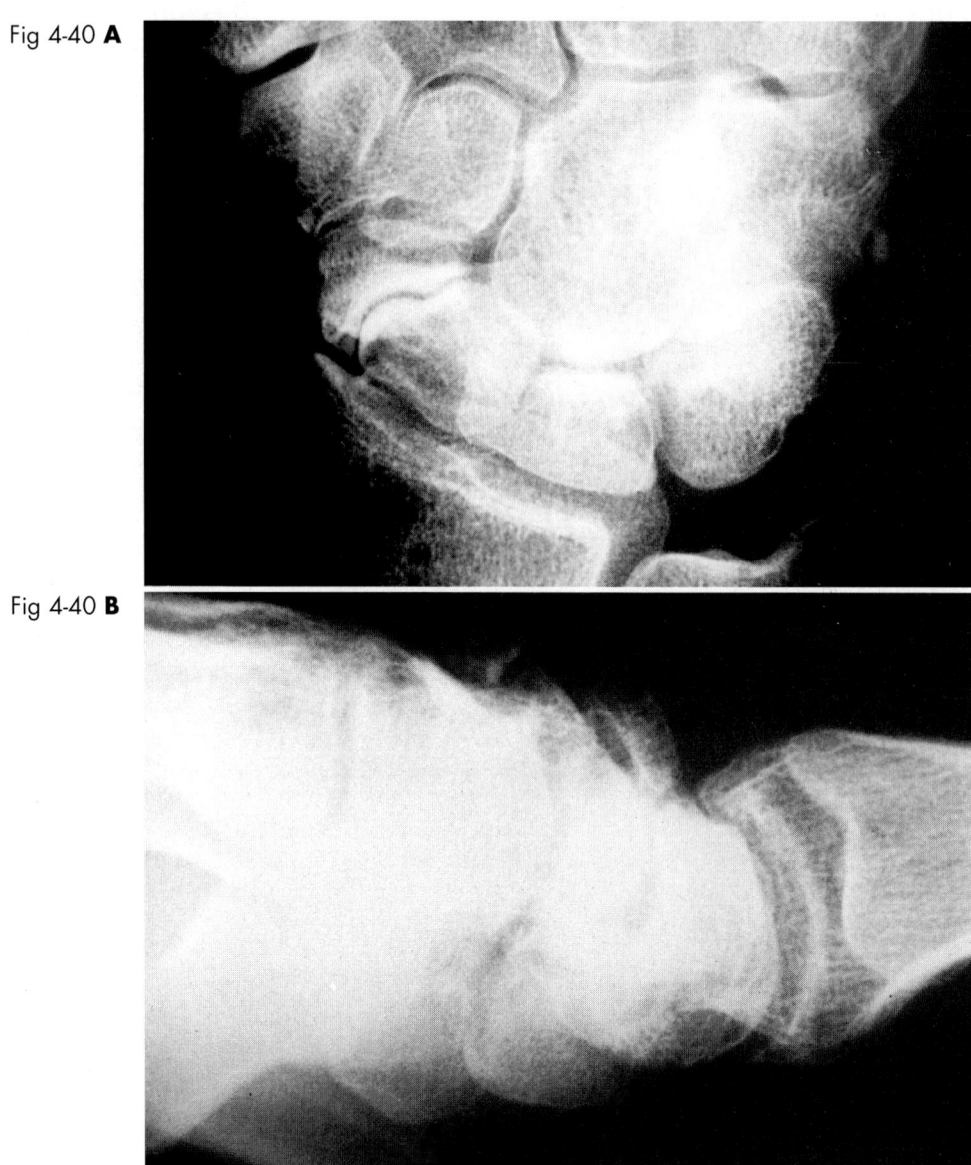

ANSWER

127 This patient has longstanding scaphoid nonunion and has characteristic sclerosis at the nonunion site with other changes that demonstrate this problem to be longstanding. The lateral view demonstrates large osteophytic spurs and a loose body just distal to the lunate, which demonstrate that this condition is not an acute process. The fall 2 weeks ago did not produce these radiographic changes, but arguably it may have exacerbated what was a relatively asymptomatic scaphoid nonunion.

QUESTION

128 Despite the uncertain etiology in this patient's case, the nonunion of the scaphoid was treated with open reduction and internal fixation bone grafting, a radial styloidectomy, and débridement of osteophytes and loose bodies from the dorsal wrist. His scaphoid united well and subsequently he moved to another part of the country. He complained of continued wrist pain, and his new treating orthopedic surgeon elected to perform a wrist fusion. The attempted wrist fusion with hardware failed; the plate was removed by the treating surgeon, and a cast was applied for 3 months. The patient returned to your care, and on physical examination, he has severely painful, limited wrist motion. A radiographic film is shown (*Figure 4-41*). What is the source of his pain, and how should it be addressed?

Fig 4-41

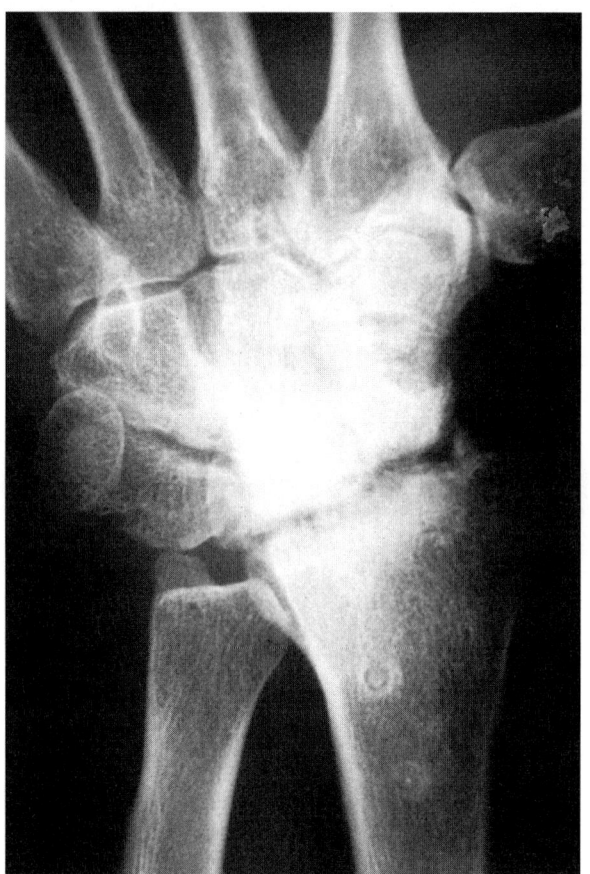

ANSWERS

129 The radiographic film demonstrates scapholunate advanced collapse pattern of arthritis of the wrist. In addition to the scaphoid nonunion, one sees an ossicle distal to the radial styloid with a large cyst in the body of the capitate with erosion of the capitate-scaphoid joint. Because of the involvement of the capitate and arthritic change at the radioscaphoid interface, simply addressing the scaphoid nonunion is insufficient to help this patient. Options for treatment should include scaphoid excision with a capito-lunate-triquetrum-hamate arthrodesis, complete wrist arthrodesis, scapho-capitate-lunate arthrodesis with radial styloidectomy, or a prosthetic or tendinous scaphoid replacement.

130 This is advanced trapeziometacarpal arthrosis.

131 Despite severe radiographic appearance, many of these patients can be managed with a program of nonsteroidal antiinflammatory medication and intermittent splint usage. Occasionally, intraarticular steroid injection can reduce acute inflammation and alleviate severe symptoms. Surgical options include trapezial-metacarpal arthrodesis or one of the many trapezial-metacarpal arthroplasties, using tendon suspension and prosthetic replacement.

QUESTION

132   A 23-year-old college soccer player injured his wrist last season and has had the diagnosis of scaphoid fracture made. He played the majority of the season in an athletic splint so that he could continue to participate; he spent the rest of the offseason in a cast. He returned home for summer vacation and came to your office for follow-up care. He has been in a short-arm, thumb spica cast with an electrical stimulator applied for the past 3 months. He wants to be ready to play the coming season in September. A radiographic film taken in your office is shown (*Figure 4-44*). These radiographic films show no change from those taken 3, 6, and 9 months earlier. What is your recommendation for further treatment?

Fig 4-44

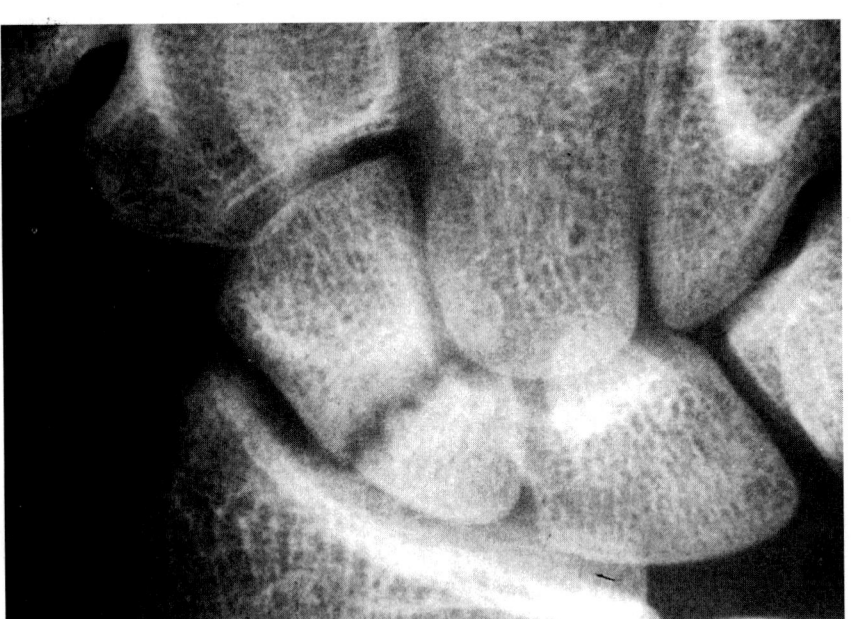

ANSWER

132 To have this patient ready for the next season with no change in the radiographic appearance of his fracture over a 9-month period, one would plan either a closed pinning of the fracture or open reduction with internal fixation and bone grafting.

QUESTION

133 This 53-year-old woman is referred to you because of deformity and ulnar wrist pain. She was managed by her hometown physician for a fractured radius in a cast for 6 weeks and is referred because of continued problems. Radiographic films are shown (*Figures 4-45A and 4-45B*). What is your treatment recommendation?

Fig 4-45 **A**

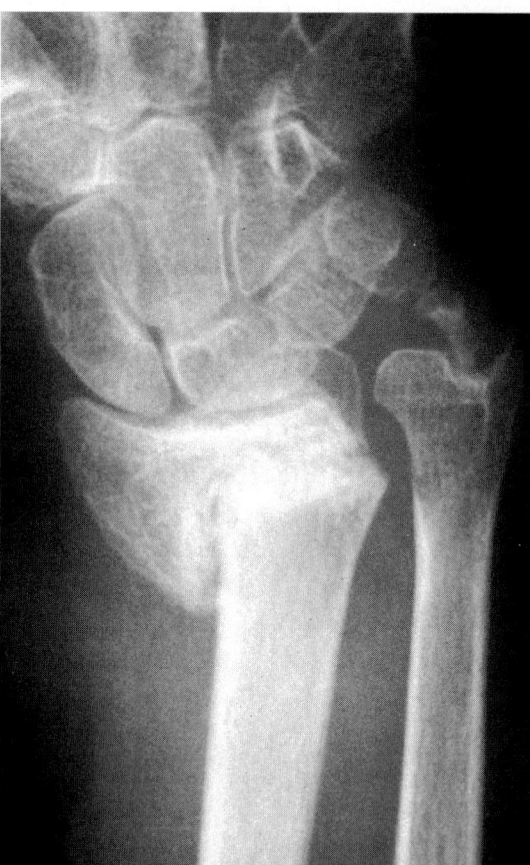

Fig 4-45 **B**

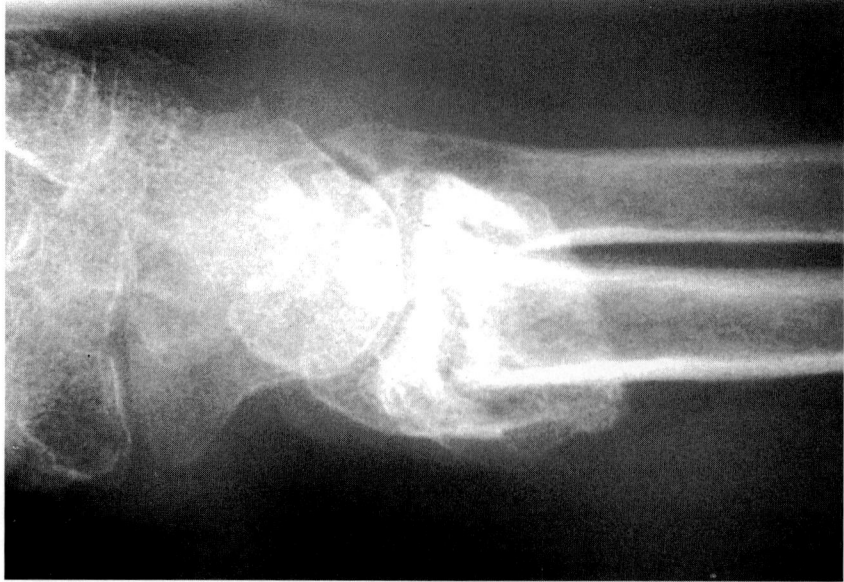

ANSWER

133 This patient has a significant malunion of the distal radius with severe shortening and dorsal angulation. Recommended treatment for a patient of this age is a corrective osteotomy with iliac crest bone graft.

QUESTIONS

134 A 28-year-old factory worker is sent to your office by his company because of bilateral hand complaints. He states that during the course of his shift, his hands become clumsy and weak, and he has difficulty with dropping objects. He has noted problems with holding the newspaper and driving the car and, when he goes to bed at night, he is intermittently awakened by his hands falling asleep. He has to shake his hands to obtain relief. What is his differential diagnosis, and what is the most likely diagnosis?

135 Assuming this is carpal tunnel syndrome, what clinical tests should you perform to confirm the diagnosis?

136 Assuming the patient has clinical evidence of carpal tunnel syndrome but has no interest in surgical intervention, what conservative measures would you suggest that might help decrease his symptoms?

ANSWERS

134   The most likely diagnosis is carpal tunnel syndrome. The differential diagnosis for this patient includes compressive neuropathies including cervical radiculopathy, thoracic outlet syndrome, pronator syndrome, cubital tunnel syndrome, radial tunnel syndrome, and, most frequently, ulnar tunnel and carpal tunnel syndrome. One would also have to consider the possibility of nerve trauma as seen with hypothenar hammer syndrome and vascular disorders such as Raynaud's phenomena.

135   The most frequently used tests to confirm diagnosis of carpal tunnel syndrome include Phalen's test, reversed Phalen's test, median nerve compression test, Tinel's sign over the median nerve at the level of the wrist, as well as motor testing of the abductor pollicis brevis (APB), inspection for atrophy of the APB, and abnormalities in two-point discrimination in the distribution of the median nerve.

136   The use of wrist splints, carpal tunnel injection with corticosteroid, modification of work activities, vitamin B6 therapy, and nonsteroidal antiinflammatory medication have all been employed with varying degrees of success.

Upper Extremity

LTC D.E. Casey Jones

QUESTION

1   Figures 5-1 and 5-2 show the shoulder radiographic films of an 81-year-old woman who has chronic, unremitting shoulder pain, but is otherwise in good health. Her condition has not responded to a course of nonsteroidal antiinflammatory drugs (NSAIDs), or intraarticular corticosteroid injection, and it interferes with both function and sleep. Examination reveals abduction to 100°, flexion to 100°, internal rotation of 45°, external rotation of 30°, and extension of 15°. There are no clinical signs of subacromial impingement nor clinically significant pathology at the acromioclavicular joint. Crepitation is felt with any glenohumeral motion. What are the appropriate age parameters for consideration for shoulder implant arthroplasty? In this case, should consideration be given to other lesser procedures such as a joint débridement or resection arthroplasty?

Fig 5-1

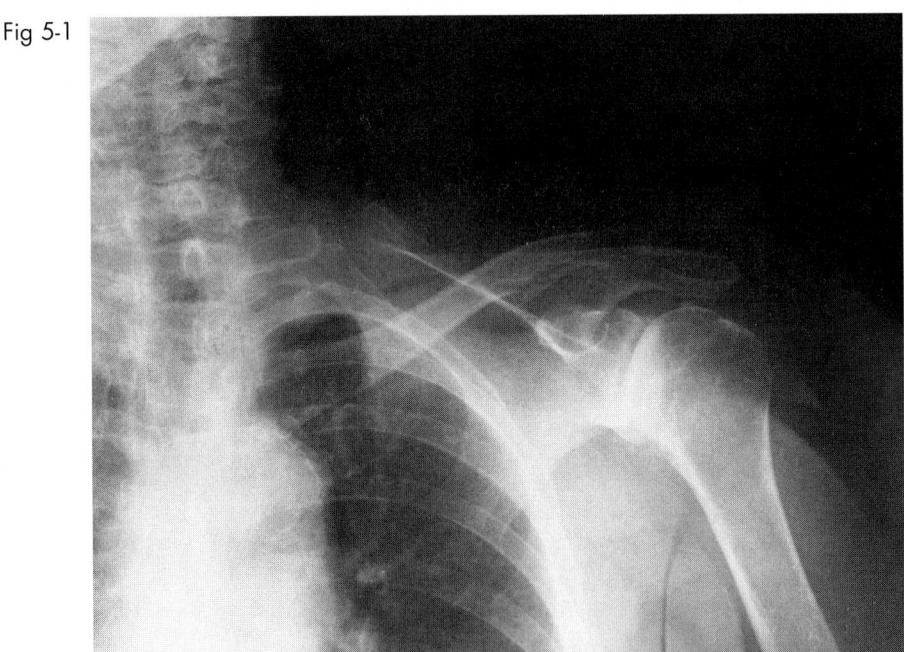

Fig 5-2

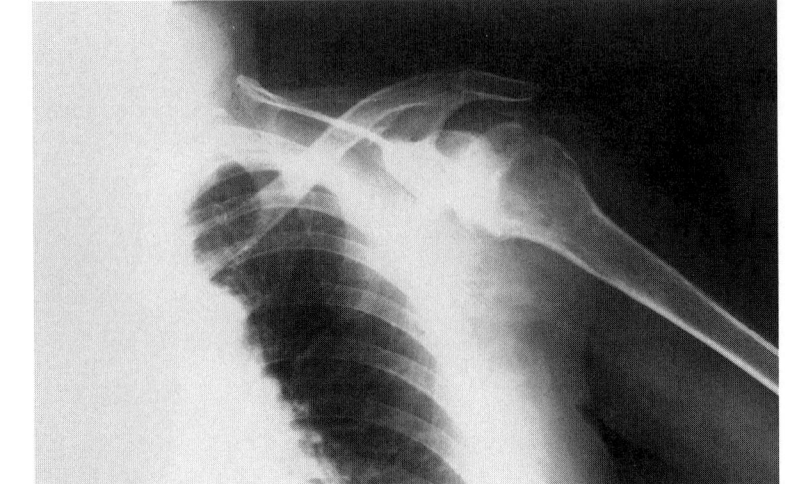

ANSWER

1   There is no upper age limit when considering shoulder implant arthroplasty. The limiting parameter is the general health of the patient and his or her ability to tolerate the surgery. Joint debridement is sometimes indicated in young patients with osteophytes or loose bodies or in some patients with rheumatoid shoulders, but joint debridement is a temporizing measure and is seldom definitive. Resection arthroplasty, a treatment for severe shoulder arthropathy in the preprosthetic era, is now generally reserved for septic or otherwise failed implant arthroplasties. The lower age limit for shoulder implant arthroplasty is not clearly defined. However, in this non–weight-bearing joint, implant arthroplasty at a younger age is generally considered to be a more viable alternative than it would be for a weight-bearing joint, if other reasonable options are not available.

QUESTIONS

2 Is shoulder implant arthroplasty indicated primarily for loss of motion, for relief of pain, or for improvement in strength and function?

3 In considering shoulder implant arthroplasty, of what importance is the status of the rotator cuff—its presence, its clinical function, and its repairability if torn?

4 If it is decided to perform an implant arthroplasty, should it include both the humeral and glenoid sides or the humeral side only? What factors need be considered in such a decision?

5 If you decide to do a TSA, what factors determine whether you will cement the glenoid component or the humeral component?

6 What long-term results can you tell your patient he or she may expect? How do these results compare with the results of total joint arthroplasty (TJA) in weight-bearing joints such as the hip and knee?

7 If you perform a TSA, should you plan to use a constrained prosthesis, a semiconstrained prosthesis, or a nonconstrained prosthesis?

ANSWER

2 The primary indication for shoulder implant arthroplasty is pain relief. Motion improvement is unreliable and is dependent on multiple factors that include the condition of the rotator cuff, the condition prompting the surgery, the general condition of the patient, and the surgical technique and postoperative rehabilitation. Improvement in motion can generally be expected; however, this improvement is secondary to pain relief and osteophyte removal. Improvement in postoperative strength is similarly dependent on multiple factors and is, as a result, unreliable. However, the subjective patient assessment of strength may increase if pain relief is good.

ANSWERS

3   The condition of the rotator cuff may be the *single* greatest determinant of postoperative motion, stability, and strength. An intact rotator cuff is ideal, a repairable rotator cuff is desirable, and an unrepairable rotator cuff is a relative contraindication to shoulder implant arthroplasty. In the face of a marginally repairable or unrepairable rotator cuff, the patient must be counseled regarding the more limited expectations of surgery.

4   There are strong advocates of replacing only the humeral side of the arthritic glenohumeral joint. Failure by loosening virtually always occurs by a failure of the glenoid side, and lucent lines around the bone-cement interface at reasonable follow-up (5 years) probably exceed 50%. However, radiographic lucency does not necessarily correlate with clinical symptoms or failure. Pain relief may be slightly better with total shoulder arthroplasty (TSA) rather than with shoulder hemiarthroplasty, but long-term success of TSA probably requires more optimal conditions of shoulder balance than hemiarthroplasty to prevent nonconcentric loading and other glenoid stresses. In this case, with little apparent glenoid deformity and a clinically intact rotator cuff, either choice is reasonable.

5   Noncemented glenoid components are rarely considered. In rare cases of unusually young patients with excellent bone, a noncemented glenoid component may be an option. On the other hand, humeral components can most often be press fit. Cement on the humeral side is usually reserved for those cases where bone quality is poor and where press fitting will not result in a stable prosthesis.

6   Significant pain relief after shoulder implant arthroplasty reaches 90%. Long-term results compare favorably with lower extremity TJA revision rates. At 10 years old, shoulder arthroplasty revision rates are reported in various studies as being between 10% and 25%. Motion and strength results are less predictable. Motion and strength are dependent on multiple factors as noted, but these results can be excellent. The best *general* predictor of postoperative strength and motion is preoperative strength and motion.

7   Constrained prostheses, which figured prominently in the early history of TSA, have a high failure rate and are now used only on a limited basis for salvage. Semiconstrained prostheses are available, especially for use with massive, unrepairable rotator cuff lesions. The standard prostheses used today in shoulder implant arthroplasty are nonconstrained.

QUESTIONS

8 The postoperative radiographic films (*Figure 5-3*) shows the result of the surgery performed for the patient described in Q1. As previously mentioned this 81-year-old woman is healthy, apart from her osteoarthritis. Although physiologically younger than her chronological age, she is still a low demand patient. Her bone quality at surgery was such that the humeral prosthesis required cement fixation. Intraoperative radiographic films were not taken. Is the abnormality seen on the radiographic film a projection artifact?

Fig 5-3

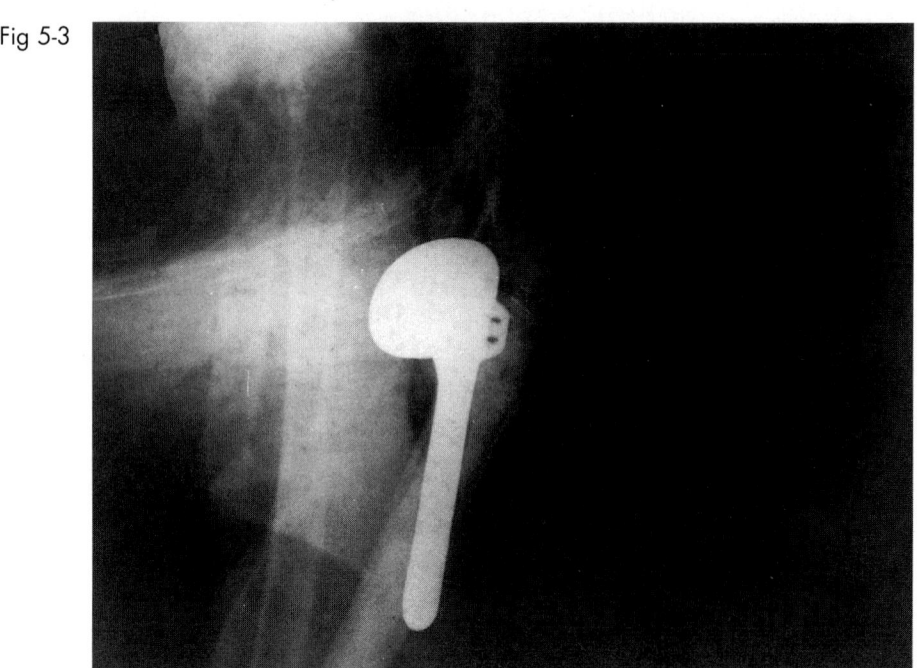

9 Did this problem occur intraoperatively, somewhere between the operating table and the recovery room, or as a result of a postoperative fracture?

10 At this point, is your best option to revise the current prosthesis to a long-stem, cemented prosthesis, remove the current prosthesis and leave a resection arthroplasty, or follow and treat only if clinical problems arise?

ANSWERS

8 The stem of the prosthesis is *clearly* penetrating the humeral cortex.

9 There is no doubt that this complication occurred intraoperatively. Intraoperative, periprosthetic fractures may occur as a result of less than ideal exposure, a poorly planned initial humeral cut, and poor quality bone. In difficult cases one is advised to obtain intraoperative radiographic films before taking steps that commit to a specific course.

10 In the present case, additional and immediate surgery is as likely to compromise the result as it is to improve it. The cortical penetration by the stem of the prosthesis is certainly a stress riser and, as such, increases the likelihood of fracture. An attempt to revise the prosthesis to one with a longer stem would present a risk of fracture of an obviously fragile humerus, the same complication you are operating to prevent. Resection arthroplasties are generally unsatisfactory and would pose the risk of fracture of the humerus, further compromising the situation.

It is imperative to be honest with the patient in such a case and involve them in further planning. However, given a low demand, elderly patient, it may be more advisable to follow and treat expectantly.

QUESTION

11   A 68-year-old man is referred for loss of motion and chronic pain in his right shoulder. He is a retired truck driver who remains active with low demand hobbies. His referring physician has had him on NSAIDs for several years, but his pain and motion loss have progressed despite the medication. He is now unable to engage in his avocations and awakens several times each night as a result of shoulder pain. His examination demonstrates active abduction to only 40°, active flexion to 65°, weak and deficient active internal and external rotation, and pain on virtually all motion. His initial radiographic films are shown (*Figures 5-4 and 5-5*). There are several contraindications and relative contraindications to TSA. Are any of these evidenced by the radiographic films seen in Figures 5-4 and 5-5? Would shoulder fusion be a more reasonable alternative for function and pain relief?

Fig 5-4

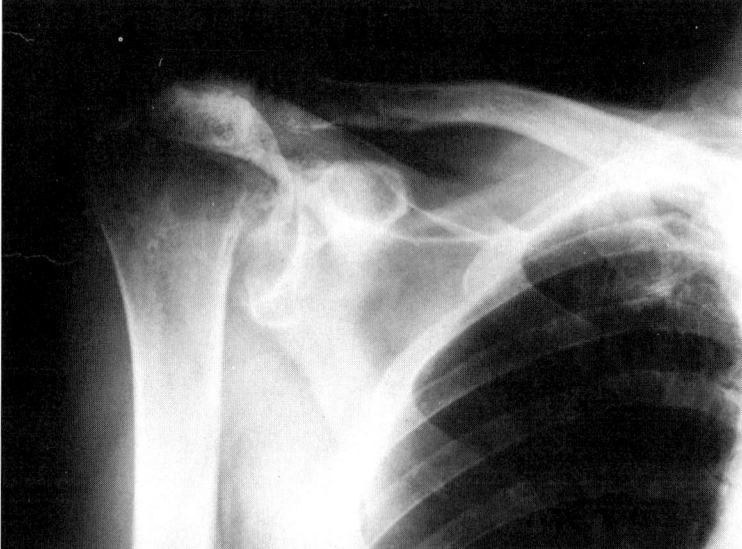

Fig 5-5

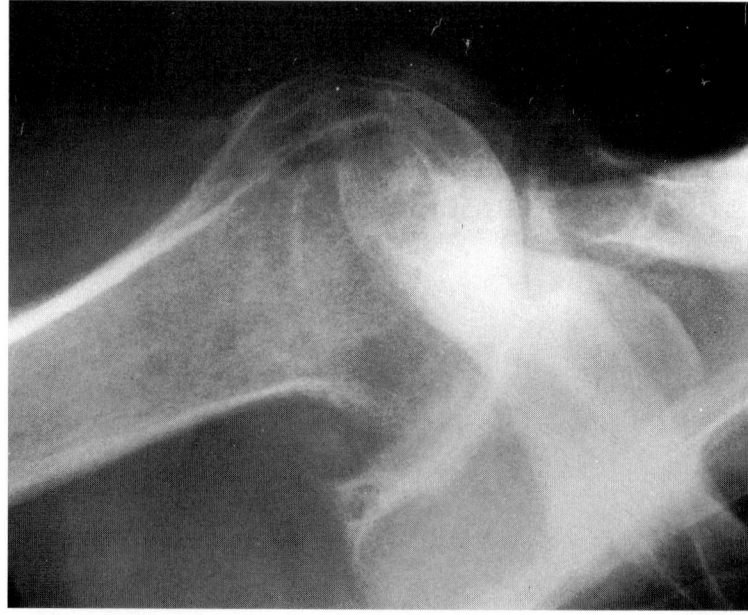

ANSWER

11   Contraindications or relative contraindications to TSA include a history of sepsis, a neuropathic joint, and paralysis or loss of effective deltoid and rotator cuff function. Because these radiographic films give evidence of rotator cuff pathology, a fusion would be a reasonable consideration. Another option might be TSA or tendon transfer to close the cuff defect and then treat with "limited goals" rehabilitation.

QUESTION

12   What is the likely condition of the rotator cuff? Is it repairable?
Would this shoulder require a constrained prosthesis?

ANSWER

12   Because the humeral head is articulating with the acromion, there is
obviously a massive rotator cuff defect that may not be amenable to
repair or effective reconstruction. This patient might be best served
by glenohumeral arthrodesis. More marginal considerations include
shoulder implant arthroplasty with a superiorly constrained glenoid
prosthesis or humeral replacement with an oversized or bipolar prosthesis. As indicated earlier, constrained prostheses have limited indications, and are usually for salvage revision.

ANSWER

After detailed discussion with the patient, the shoulder shown in Figures 5-4 and 5-5 was treated by shoulder implant arthroplasty using an oversized humeral head and no glenoid component. The rotator cuff was judged to be unrepairable at surgery; the patient has some, though not complete, relief of pain. He is now able to perform most desired activities and is not awakened by shoulder pain. He requires only occasional, nonnarcotic pain medication for discomfort caused by heavy use of his arm. His only complaint is an inability to fully abduct actively, though he can hold his arm in an overhead position once it has been assisted to this position by the other arm. Other active motion is nearly equal to the contralateral unaffected shoulder. His current radiographic films are shown (*Figures 5-6 and 5-7*).

Fig 5-6

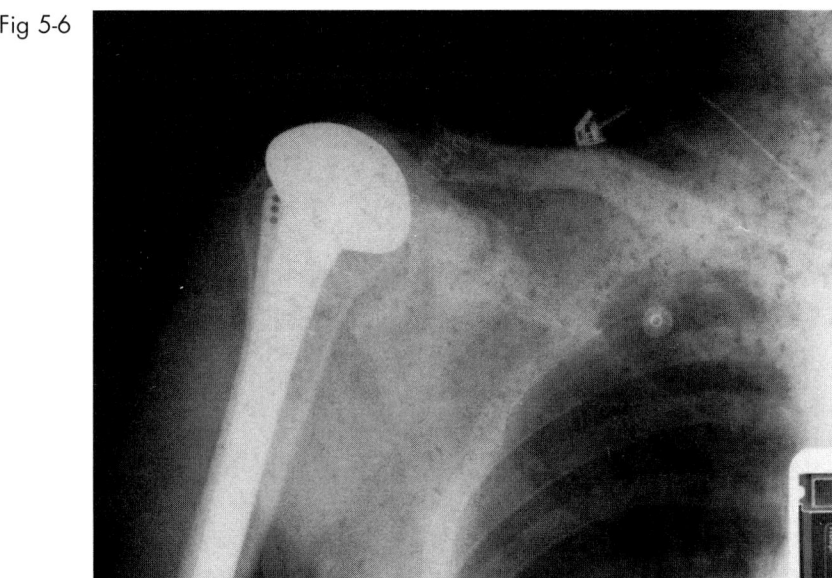

Fig 5-7

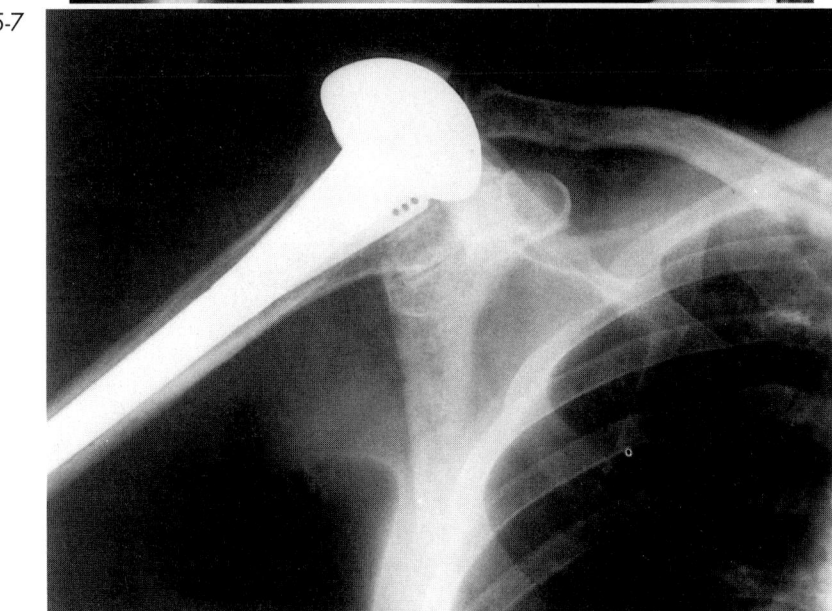

QUESTIONS

13 Is the cephalad migration of the humeral head that is seen in the radiographic films unusual? Does it require treatment? Is it the cause of the deficit in active abduction?

14 Should this shoulder now be fused or should it be revised to a superiorly constrained prosthesis?

15 Should an attempt be made to reconstruct the rotator cuff?

16 You are consulted by a medical oncologist regarding a patient with a 17-year history of renal cell carcinoma and who has, of late, experienced steadily increasing bone pain. A bone scan has demonstrated multiple areas of increased uptake. A plain-film survey of these areas reveals the radiographic lesion shown (*Figures 5-8 and 5-9*). The oncologist informs you that the patient's current life expectancy is 6 to 12 months. Your examination reveals a frail but still ambulatory patient who is living at home with his wife and remains capable of managing his own activities of daily living. His shoulder and elbow motion are full, but motion causes pain in the midbrachium area. This is a pure lytic lesion radiographically. Is the risk for this type of lesion different than for other types?

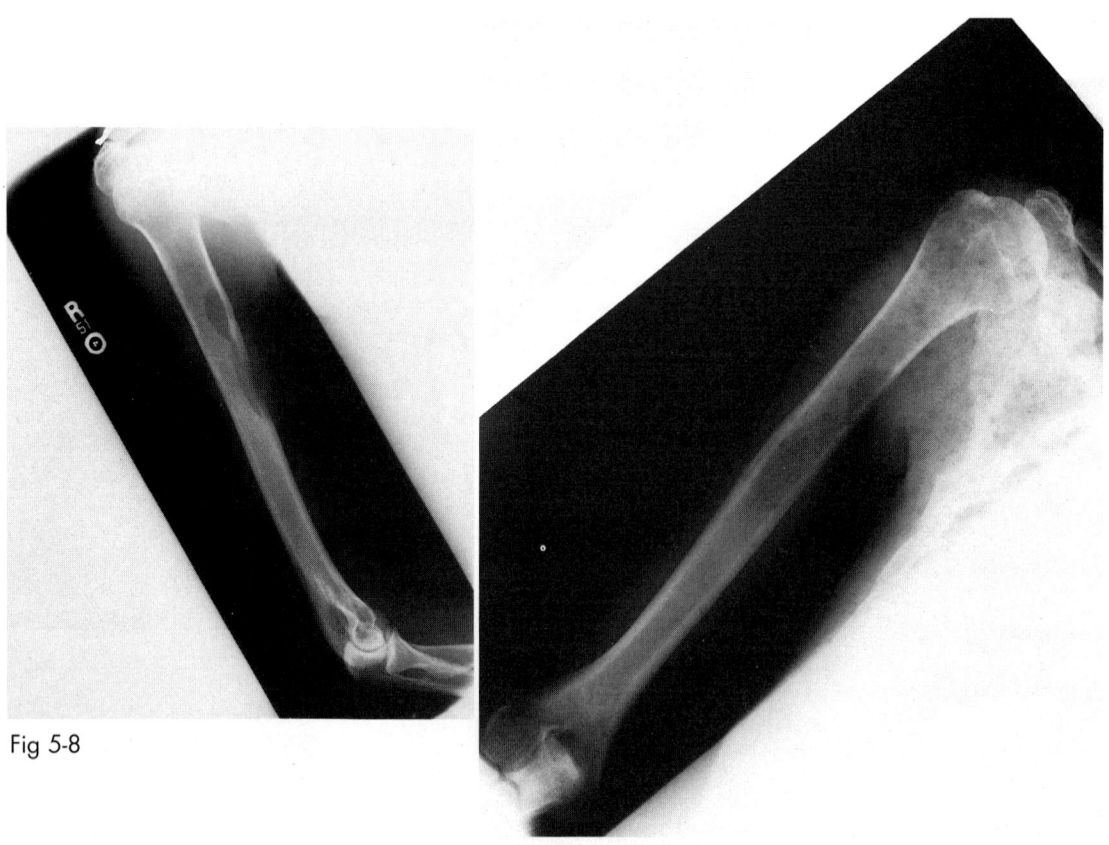

Fig 5-8

Fig 5-9

ANSWERS

13 Cephalad migration of shoulder implant arthroplasty occurs in approximately one fifth of cases and does not necessarily preclude an acceptable clinical result. In this case the humeral head was articulating with the acromion preoperatively. This actually represents less a case of superior migration than it does an expected result, given the preoperative situation and inability to repair the rotator cuff. An oversized humeral head was used in an attempt to achieve an acceptable clinical result. A semiconstrained prosthesis *might* have prevented cephalad migration. The lack of full active abduction is presumably a result of the massive rotator cuff deficiency, although there may be some additional subacromial impingement and thus some limitation of abduction with the use of the oversized humeral head.

14 Despite the radiographic appearance, the surgery has largely accomplished the goal of pain relief. Motion is actually good. Results cannot be measured solely in radiographic terms. There is no *clinical* indication for further surgery at this point. Fusion is unlikely to produce significant benefit if pain relief is already good. It would be more appropriate to consider using a semiconstrained prosthesis at or before the time of surgery rather than postoperatively.

15 If the determination at the time of surgery was not to use a glenoid component, and if cuff repair or reconstruction was not feasible, making a postoperative decision to the contrary carries with it a potential for hazard. Because the patient is largely satisfied with the result and is doing reasonably well clinically, the prudent course is probably good follow-up and expectant treatment.

16 It is traditionally believed that pure lytic lesions pose a greater threat for pathologic fracture than mixed or blastic lesions, although some authors have found no difference in fracture rate by lesion type. K.D. Harrington has pointed out that blastic lesions are not made up of structurally normal bone and that pathologic fractures readily occur through blastic lesions.

QUESTIONS

17   Are size of lesion and risk of fracture associated?

18   Because this is a non–weight-bearing bone, is there risk of fracture?

19   How does the quality of pain (minimal, rest pain, or functional pain) relate to the probability of fracture?

20   Does your advice to the consulting physician include longevity and social situation considerations?

21   What role should radiation therapy play in the treatment of metastatic bone lesions?

22   If this lesion is surgically treated, what factors would you consider in choosing a specific surgical option?

ANSWERS

17   Lesion size is relevant because the greater the size of the lesion, the greater the likelihood that it has compromised the structural integrity of the cortex. In Harrington's system for assessing the risk of pathologic fracture, a lesion greater than 2.5 cm in diameter is believed to cause an increased risk, but the actual determinant is the percent of loss of cortical bone. Harrington uses 50% as the critical value for circumferential cortical loss. Whereas Harrington's system is widely known and used, the author believes that Mirels' scoring system for impending pathologic fracture, using several parameters to reach a score (including location, quality of pain, proportion of cortical destruction, and type of lesion), has a sounder basis.

18   Non–weight-bearing bones are at less risk for developing pathologic fracture than weight-bearing bones. However, because torque is often the mechanism of failure through pathologic lesions, upper extremity bones are certainly at risk and merit careful assessment. In patients requiring the use of ambulatory assistive devices, the upper extremities become weight bearing, which puts them at greater risk of fracture.

ANSWERS

19 The quality of pain is addressed in both Harrington's and in Mirels' systems for assessing the risk of pathologic fracture. Pain on stress (i.e., functional pain or, in the case of a lower extremity, pain while weight bearing) is the most ominous and is felt to represent likely microfractures, implying imminent pathologic fracture.

20 Determinations of longevity are necessarily imprecise. In the case of the patient terminally residing in a care facility, enough should be done to minimize suffering, facilitate nursing care, and minimize the likelihood of potentially greater intervention later. The costs and risks of prophylactic treatment are usually less in appropriately selected patients than the costs and risks of treating a pathologic fracture. Most patients prefer to remain as functional and independent as possible for as long as possible. Intervention must be tailored on a case-by-case basis.

21 Radiation therapy can be used before or after prophylactic surgical stabilization in lesions likely to respond. For smaller lesions with a low likelihood of fracture, radiation therapy may prevent further cortical destruction, relieve pain, and avoid the necessity for future surgery. Lesions with a high likelihood of pathologic fracture should be stabilized. The choice of preoperative versus postoperative irradiation should be made in conjunction with the patient's oncologist, bearing in mind that radiation therapy initially weakens the bone and may increase the probability of fracture. Consideration should also be given to the fact that irradiation can compromise options for surgery or impair wound healing. It is therefore desirable, when possible, to plan incision sites away from the sites of irradiation. Whereas irradiation might be of some benefit, renal cell carcinoma, as in this case, is typically not highly sensitive to radiation therapy.

22 The first surgical consideration is stabilization. Tumor type, the desirability of surgical debulking, and planning surgery compatible with radiation therapy (if it will be used pre or postoperatively) are other important considerations. For some lesions it is desirable to debulk the tumor and then add to the bony stability with the use of methyl methacrylate in conjunction with metal implants. Intramedullary stabilization may allow surgical access using incisions remote from the lesion, enhancing radiation therapy options and potentially decreasing the likelihood of wound problems. Remote access may also avoid hard to control bleeding in the case of highly vascular tumors.
In this case, as the tumor is relatively radioresistant, the following treatment should be recommended:
(1) Tumor debulking for pain relief
(2) Intramedullary (IM) rodding plus methyl methacrylate for bone stabilization

QUESTIONS

23 A 57-year-old school teacher fell from a chair while changing a ceiling light and injured her arm. You are called to the emergency room to evaluate and treat this patient after the radiographic films ordered by the emergency room physician reveal the fracture shown (*Figures 5-10 and 5-11*). Your examination reveals no obvious deficits of either sensory or motor function in the median, ulnar, or radial nerve distributions. The biceps, triceps, and deltoid fire, but the patient resists moving the shoulder or elbow because of pain. Distal pulses are strong, and capillary refill is less than 3 seconds. There is crepitation and pain on movement around the shoulder, and you note a prominent indented area anterolaterally, proximal to the insertion of the anterior deltoid. You assess that the distal fracture spike has impaled the overlying soft tissue. Measurement of the radiographic films show the apical anterior angulation to be 47°. Using Neer's classification, what type of fracture is this?

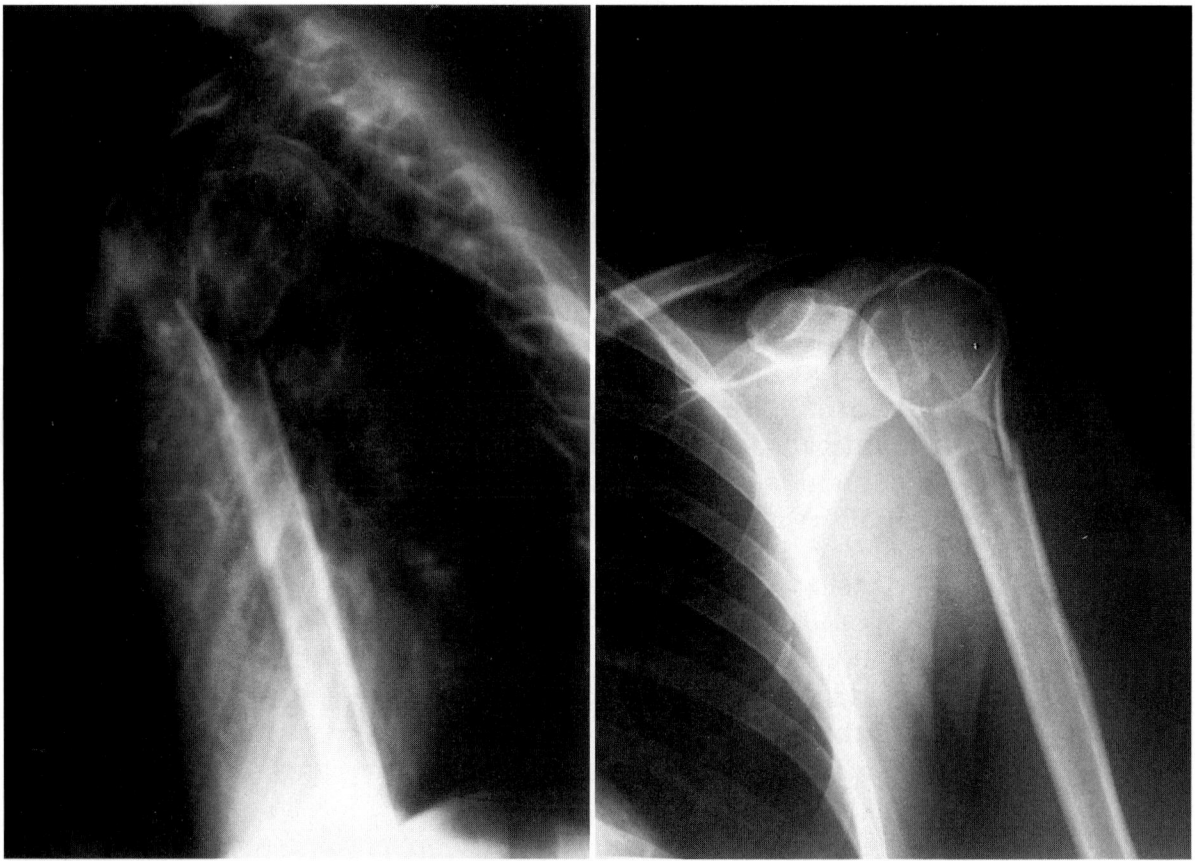

Fig 5-10   Fig 5-11

24 Does this fracture pose a great risk of avascular necrosis of the humeral head?

25 Is the degree of angulation of this fracture acceptable? Would healing in this position result in significant motion deficits or in cosmetic deformity?

ANSWERS

23   This is a two-part surgical neck fracture. Neer's system is the most commonly used classification system for proximal humeral fractures and has demonstrated clinical relevancy over time. To be considered a significant fracture line in the Neer classification, parts must be displaced by a centimeter or more or angulated not less than 45°. The four major fracture fragments in Neer's classification are based on earlier work by Ernest Amory Codman. They are the humeral head (articular portion), the greater and lesser tuberosity fragments, and the humeral shaft. The importance of the system, other than being a fairly comprehensive classification, is in its focus on the blood supply of the head fragment. There are other classification systems for fractures of the proximal humerus that are worthy of note, although less commonly used. The AO classification is more detailed and therefore more cumbersome. It has not become widely used, and its greatest value may be as a research tool.

24   A not uncommon and potentially devastating complication of proximal humeral fractures is avascular necrosis of the head. Disruption of the blood supply to the head (articular portion) is more often associated with three-part fractures and is most often associated with four-part fractures. These fractures have a greater risk of disrupting the arcuate artery, which is the major blood supply to the head and which arises from the ascending portion of the anterior humeral circumflex artery. It typically enters the bone in the intertubercular area. The risk of avascular necrosis in *this* fracture is low.

25   Because of the generous soft tissue coverage of the humerus, even this degree of angulation would likely be cosmetically unnoticeable. The tremendous range of motion of the glenohumeral joint coupled with the contributions of the scapulothoracic joint is also rather forgiving of residual angulatory deformity. The generally accepted parameter for residual angulation is 45° or less. Healing in this degree of apical anterior angulation is not likely to result in significant flexion deficit or impingement.

QUESTIONS

26 Does the obvious soft tissue interposition in this fracture require an open surgical procedure?

27 What muscle forces are acting on this fracture to cause displacement and angulation? Will surgical stabilization be necessary to overcome the deforming forces?

28 Failing to relieve the soft tissue interposition and reduce the angulation, would you advise surgical treatment? If so, what surgery?

ANSWERS

26 Soft tissue interposition may impede fracture reduction and can be the cause of nonunion. Interposed soft tissue, frequently consisting of the biceps tendon, is not uncommon in two part surgical neck fractures. Closed reduction can be successful in dislodging soft tissue from the fracture site and bringing the fracture fragments into contact. In this case the distal spike is likely impaling the deltoid, and acute spasm of the muscle may be pulling the distal fragment proximally, causing continued impalement. Manual or mechanical traction in the well-sedated and relaxed patient may overcome the spasm and allow the deltoid to be disimpaled.

27 Because the tuberosities are not fractured, subscapularis and the balance of the rotator cuff muscles remain attached and are above the fracture site. The proximal part should remain neutral. The major deforming forces are pectoralis major, which inserts distal to the fracture and pulls the distal fragment medially, and deltoid, which causes a proximal and lateral force on the proximal fragment. Skeletal traction is a consideration, but is somewhat impractical considering the other available forms of treatment. A reduction maneuver with sedation or anesthesia could disimpale the deltoid and reduce the fracture. Another option would be to achieve traction with a hanging arm cast. This is a well-accepted and proven method, perhaps more commonly used in humeral shaft fractures, which necessitates careful monitoring to avoid the well-known complications that can attend the use of a hanging arm cast. Once acceptable reduction is achieved, two-part surgical neck fractures can most frequently be successfully managed closed.
This fracture was initially treated in a hanging arm cast, which disimpaled the deltoid and reduced the angulation to acceptable limits. After 5 days the cast was removed and a coaptation splint and sling and swath were applied. The fracture healed uneventfully.

28 Soft tissue interposition that blocks reduction or failure to achieve or maintain acceptable angulation by closed means are indications for surgical intervention. If, after removing the interposed soft tissue and reducing the fracture, internal stabilization is advisable, a number of accepted options exist. There are several intramedullary devices available, and those that interlock have the advantage of affording rotational stability. One may use tension band wiring or a combination of an intramedullary device with a tension band wire. There are plates designed for use in proximal humeral fractures, but these require considerable soft tissue stripping and may increase the possibility of vascular injury to the head. When considering a method for internal fixation, it must be remembered that the incidence of this fracture is much greater in individuals with osteoporosis; therefore, in any surgical treatment of this fracture there is a fair probability that you will be dealing with poor quality bone.

QUESTIONS

29 An active, healthy, 67-year-old man sustains the fracture shown (*Figures 5-12 and 5-13*) in a low-speed motor vehicle accident. He has no injuries other than this closed fracture. He is vascularly intact but has a complete motor and sensory radial nerve palsy. Does the nerve injury necessitate exploration or rigid stabilization of the fracture?

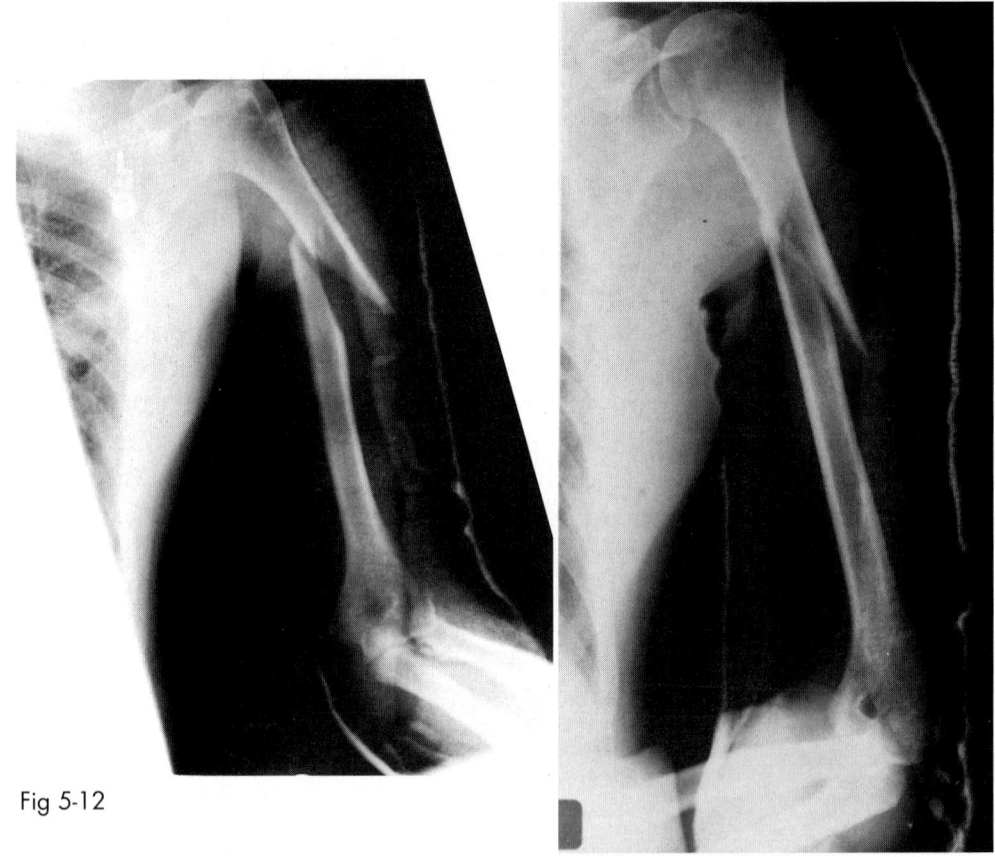

Fig 5-12

Fig 5-13

30 If this were a type II open fracture, being debrided in the operating room, should the radial nerve be explored as part of the surgery?

31 At 4 months from the time of injury, the patient has painless, gross motion at the fracture site, and no significant callus formation is seen on radiographic films. The patient has been treated in a well-fitting fracture brace. His radial nerve palsy has resolved completely. At what point in treatment can this be classified as a nonunion?

32 At this point would you advise the patient to undergo internal fixation, internal fixation with grafting, or continued nonsurgical treatment?

ANSWERS

29 Various sources report that from 5% to 18% of patients with humeral shaft fractures have some radial nerve injury. Traditionally, some types of humeral fractures (Holstein), when associated with complete radial nerve palsy, were believed to require exploration. Secondary radial nerve palsies were also believed to be an indication for immediate exploration. More recent study has shown that the vast majority of radial nerve injuries associated with humeral fractures are injuries in continuity and will resolve without exploration. Those injuries that do not, will, in most cases, do as well with late nerve repair as with immediate nerve repair. There are some data that indicate that some nerve injuries in continuity actually yield worse long-term clinical results if immediately explored. Injuries in continuity do not require rigid fracture stabilization to resolve.

30 Exploring the radial nerve for palsy, when done in conjunction with humeral fracture surgery performed for other reasons, is the one instance in which there is general agreement that such exploration is indicated.

31 Four months is usually the least amount of time required to establish a diagnosis of humeral nonunion.

32 At least two series have reported fracture bracing for humeral shaft fractures to yield a high rate of union. Average time to union for closed fractures treated in a fracture brace is less than 12 weeks. Assuming good compliance and no treatment difficulties and given the findings noted, this case could be classified as a nonunion. Some authors recommend continued nonsurgical treatment; however, it is reasonable at this point to discuss with the patient options for treatment of nonunion. Electrical stimulation has not enjoyed great success or popularity in the treatment of humeral nonunion. Reamed and unreamed, locking and nonlocking intramedullary devices have been used in the treatment of this problem. The best and most consistent results to date have been obtained using meticulous AO/ Association for the Study of Internal Fixation (ASIF) technique for compression plating with concurrent, *cancellous* bone grafting. Locking intramedullary devices have been reported to yield good results, but experience with these devices is less extensive than with compression plating and cancellous grafting.

QUESTIONS

33 While standing next to a lift stanchion, a 28-year-old skier was run into by an out-of-control snow boarder. He was struck from the side and pinned between the stanchion and the snow boarder, compressing his shoulders transversely. In the emergency room he is complaining of pain at the base of his neck anteriorly and difficulty swallowing. A chest radiographic film shows no pneumothorax. Your examination reveals asymmetry of the medial ends of the clavicles and marked tenderness at the left sternoclavicular joint. There seems to be less fullness at the left sternoclavicular joint, and you believe you can palpate the superomedial corner of the manubrium on the left. His anteroposterior radiographic film is shown (*Figure 5-14*). Do you have sufficient information to make a diagnosis and to initiate treatment? What is the diagnosis?

Fig 5-14

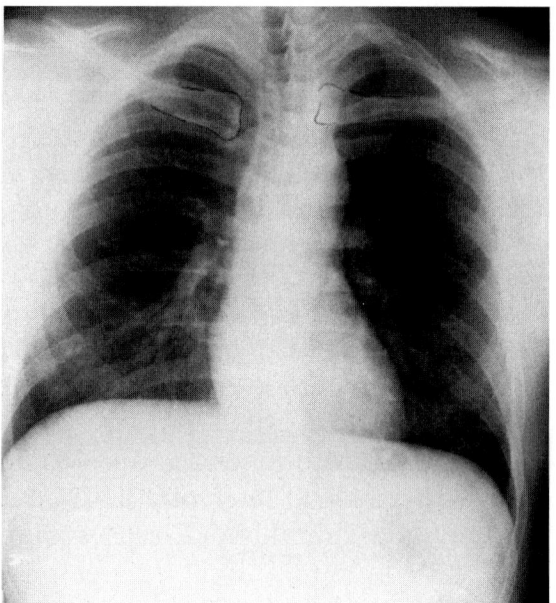

34 Should the diagnosis be made with special plain radiographic films, tomograms, computerized axial tomography (CT), or magnetic resonance imaging (MRI)?

ANSWER

35 The correct diagnosis is posterior sternoclavicular dislocation. Though the ratio of posterior to anterior dislocations of the sternoclavicular joint has not been clarified, posterior dislocations are far less common than anterior dislocations.

Fig 5-17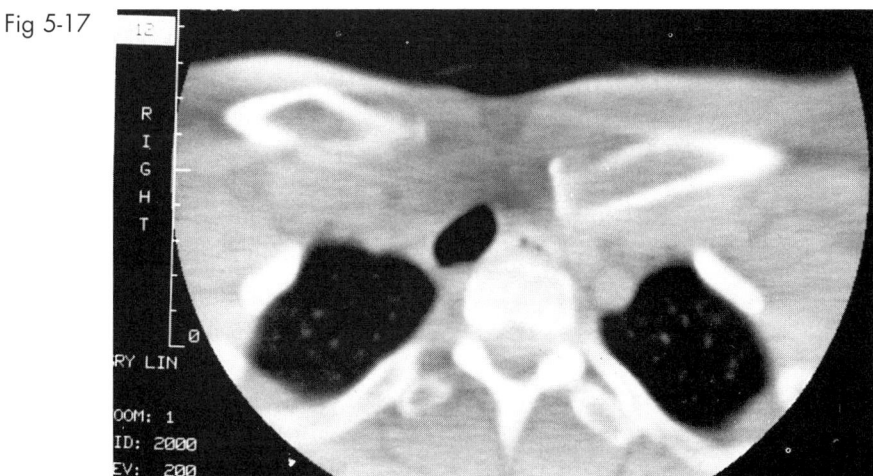

QUESTIONS

36 Does this require treatment? Will this patient's dysphagia resolve spontaneously? Do any consequences attend a chronically unreduced posterior sternoclavicular dislocation?

37 Should this dislocation be reduced closed? Should the procedure be performed in the emergency room or clinic or in the operating room?

38 What treatment would you recommend for an unstable sternoclavicular dislocation?

39 A 37-year-old police officer injured his right shoulder when he fell off a rope slide during training. He landed with his proximal anterior brachium impacting against the corner of a low brick wall. A shoulder trauma series that is ordered when he is seen in the emergency room does not show any fracture or dislocation; however, examination reveals that he is unable to abduct the shoulder more than minimally, and external rotation is markedly weak. You can detect no muscle tone in any part of the deltoid on attempted abduction, but supraspinatus fires. What is your clinical diagnosis?

40 At this point should you explore the axillary nerve, consider tendon transfers for the deltoid paralysis, order electrodiagnostic tests, or treat expectantly?

41 At 1 month you obtain electrodiagnostic tests, which show fibrillation potentials in teres minor and all three parts of the deltoid. What implication does this have?

42 Although you continue physical therapy, 3 months later the patient is still unable to abduct more than minimally, and external rotation remains weak and questionably functional. Flexion is present actively, but beyond 60° the patient has difficulty preventing the brachium from going into internal rotation. Electrodiagnostic testing continues to show fibrillation potentials. Can return of active abduction ever be expected if the deltoid remains paralyzed?

43 Should the shoulder now be fused or the axillary nerve explored?

ANSWERS

36 Unreduced, posterior dislocations of the sternoclavicular joint can compress vessels to the head or to the ipsilateral arm causing vascular compromise. They can also cause dysphagia and breathing problems or can compress the thoracic outlet. Posterior sternoclavicular dislocations should be reduced.

ANSWERS

37 Although some authors advocate reduction maneuvers in a clinic or emergency room, most recommend closed reduction under general anesthesia. Before reduction, a careful assessment should be carried out to determine the status of major vessels and pulmonary structures. It is probably wise to have a surgeon available who can deal with injury to these structures should any become apparent during closed or open reduction.

38 *Anterior dislocations* of the sternoclavicular joint are often unstable and difficult to hold using a figure-of-eight sling or a shoulder harness. They often do not cause clinical symptoms if left unreduced. Given the potential complications of stabilization procedures, anterior dislocations should probably be allowed to heal in the unreduced position if they cannot be held using closed means. Anterior dislocations can be treated late if they cause unacceptable, chronic symptoms. *Posterior dislocations* are usually stable following reduction. If surgical stabilization is desirable for an anterior or posterior sternoclavicular dislocation, either biological or synthetic materials can be used to stabilize the joint. The use of metal implants at the sternoclavicular joint has resulted in horrendous complications including death and is to be condemned.

39 Traumatic axillary nerve palsy.

40 The injury to the axillary nerve may be any magnitude, from a traction neurapraxia to an avulsion of the nerve from the muscle. *Immediate* exploration is difficult to justify. Tendon transfer for a deltoid palsy is a legitimate treatment for this condition, but not before the nature or the permanency of the injury is determined. Electrodiagnostic tests are unlikely to yield useful information until 3 to 4 weeks following injury. Support or immobilization for comfort followed by physical therapy are probably the best early treatment.

41 Fibrillation potentials are indicative of denervation. The posterior branch of the axillary nerve supplies teres minor and the posterior portion of deltoid. The anterior branch supplies the middle and anterior portions of deltoid.

42 In some cases, intact rotator cuff muscles will abduct the glenohumeral joint. Failure to achieve active abduction after 4 months of physical therapy makes it unlikely that this patient will achieve active abduction without deltoid recovery.

43 It is desirable to maintain mobility of the glenohumeral joint if possible. Fusion for a paralytically unstable shoulder is an option, but an attempt to return motion by repairing or reconstructing the nerve or by tendon transfers is probably a better consideration at this point.

QUESTIONS

44 If on exploration the nerve is found to be divided in midsubstance, what options are available for surgical treatment of the nerve?

45 Upon exploration of the axillary nerve you find that it has been avulsed from teres minor and deltoid. What are your options for restoring function and stability to the shoulder?

46 After considering all options, the patient elected to undergo a glenohumeral fusion. What is the optimal position for shoulder arthrodesis?

47 Of these position parameters (abduction, flexion, internal rotation), which is the most critical?

48 What are the minimal scapular motors required to achieve a clinically successful glenohumeral arthrodesis?

49 What is the preferred technique for shoulder arthrodesis?

50 A 55-year-old man, who was unaware that the suitcase he was removing from a high shelf was full, sustained a sudden pronounced load on his flexed, abducted shoulder. He had immediate shoulder pain that has not resolved in the intervening month. He complains of an inability to elevate his arm and persistent pain that disturbs his sleep. On examination he has a positive impingement sign and a positive drop arm test. Which of the two shoulder outlet views shown (*Figures 5-18 and 5-19*) are more likely to be associated with the problem you suspect?

Fig 5-18

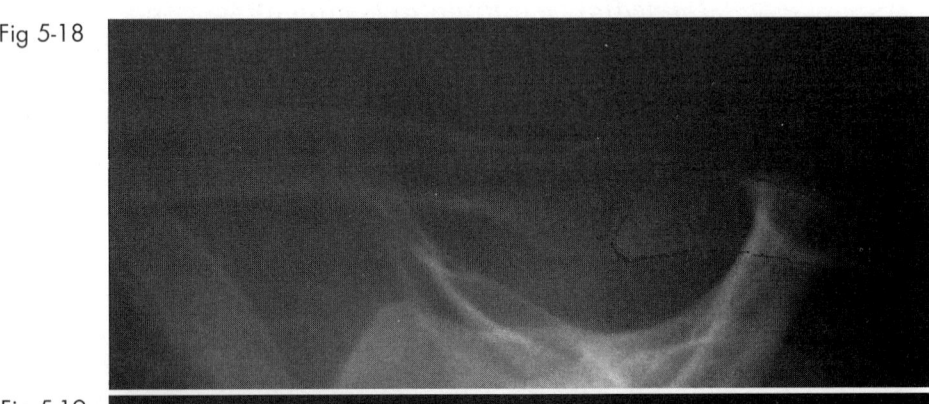

Fig 5-19

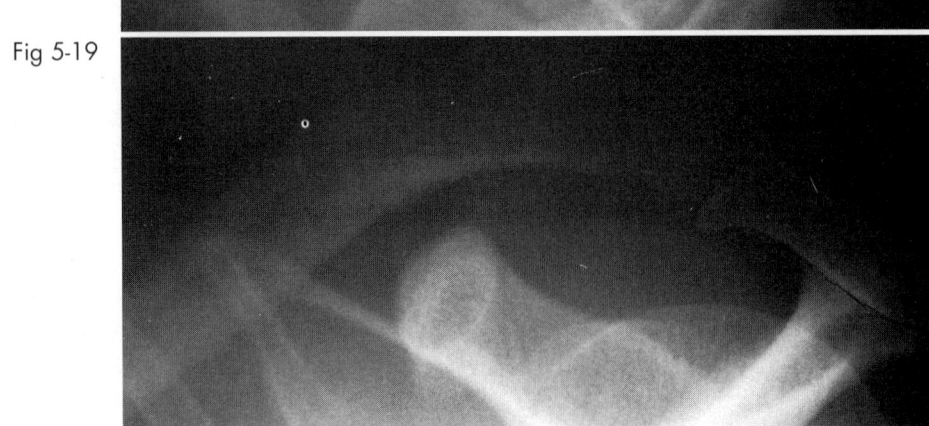

ANSWERS

44   Direct nerve repair is preferred if it can be done without undue tension. If there is a gap that cannot be closed by local mobilization or without undue tension, the use of nerve graft is indicated. Neurotization could be used if the proximal part of the nerve were avulsed from the posterior cord in a way that made repair technically difficult; however, such a case would be rare, and function of the muscle innervated by the donor nerve would have to be sacrificed making this an unattractive option.

45   The option of first choice is to restore motion by tendon transfer. The most common transfer for restoration of deltoid function is transfer of the trapezius to the proximal humerus. Because this patient also has clinical problems with active external rotation, a L'Episcopo procedure, or some variant, would likely be required. Unfortunately, should the transfers fail to provide acceptable motion and stability, the use of trapezius as a transfer precludes salvage by glenohumeral fusion. Overall, using tendon transfer to treat axillary nerve palsy has been disappointing because of poor results. Shoulder fusion would obviously provide stability, but motion would be limited to that afforded by the scapulothoracic joint and, in this patient with relatively functional rotator cuff, he may be best served by an unfused shoulder, retaining some rotation of the humerus and accepting the loss of elevation.

46   There continues to be some debate regarding the best position for shoulder fusion. Most texts recommend 20° to 30° of abduction, 20° to 30° of flexion, and 25° to 40° of internal rotation. An easy-to-remember rule of thumb is 30-30-30.

47   In a review of patients with fused shoulders at the Mayo Clinic, R.H. Cofield and B.T. Briggs found the amount of internal rotation to be the most critical determinant of functional success.

48   Trapezius and serratus anterior.

49   There are numerous techniques for shoulder fusion. Many of these techniques were developed during the era of tuberculous shoulder infections and before the era of sophisticated internal fixation devices. Because of the lack of need for remaining extraarticular in most present day shoulder fusions, and because of the availability of a variety of reliable implants, some variant of a compression arthrodesis with plating is probably the method of choice.

50   The outlet view (*Figure 5-19*) shows a type III hooked acromion. The radiographic film shown (*Figure 5-18*) shows a type II curved acromion. Although rotator cuff tears may occur with any acromial pattern, they are more commonly associated with type II acromions than with type I acromions, and they are most commonly associated with type III acromions.

QUESTIONS

51 You have diagnosed a rotator cuff tear in a patient whose symptoms have not improved over a period of 1 month. What should you advise—surgery, pharmacological treatment, or physical therapy?

52 After a 3-month trial of nonsurgical treatment, your patient is still unacceptably symptomatic. Should you recommend an acromioplasty, a rotator cuff repair, or both?

53 In counseling your patient regarding rotator cuff surgery, what likely outcomes can you predict regarding pain relief and strength and motion?

54 Following repair, what is the likelihood of a recurrent defect in the rotator cuff?

55 Does failure of a rotator cuff repair generally cause a recurrence of pain symptoms?

ANSWERS

51 A.F. DePalma found that approximately 90% of patients diagnosed as having a rotator cuff tear will have adequate resolution of their symptoms without surgery. NSAIDs can benefit as can subacromial steroid injections using local anesthetics or steroids. Physical therapy and activity limitation, or a combination of these, will often resolve symptoms and deserve a trial before considering surgery.

52 With a type III acromion, most authorities would recommend an acromioplasty for this patient, whether or not a rotator cuff repair is performed. Controversy exists regarding the necessity of rotator cuff repair. Some prominent shoulder surgeons believe that the pain associated with cuff tear responds well to acromioplasty alone and that cuff repair adds little to the result. Neer has described "cuff arthropathy," which may lead to destruction of the glenohumeral joint and is an argument in favor of rotator cuff repair.

53 Acceptable levels of pain relief (greater than 50%) are reported to be achieved up to 95% of the time. Various authors have indicated strength recovery of 75% to 90% after rotator cuff repair. Some have related success to the length of time between injury and surgery, indicating that a delay in repair compromises the results. Other authors find no such correlation. Several authors have related success regarding motion and strength to the size of the rotator cuff lesion. Motion is generally less in virtually all planes than in a normal shoulder. Recovery of motion and strength is significantly dependent on both patient motivation and postoperative rehabilitation program and may require as long as 6 to 12 months for maximal improvement.

54 Harryman, et al. found that 65% of 105 rotator cuff repairs remained intact at an average 5-year follow-up. The probability of remaining intact was inversely proportional to both age of the patient and size of the tear.

55 If there has been sufficient subacromial decompression, most patients continue to have satisfactory pain relief despite recurrence of a cuff defect. Some have used this as an argument in favor of decompression without repair. Function, however, seems to be better with an intact cuff repair.

QUESTION

56 A 20-year-old college student fell while snow boarding and landed on her right elbow suffering immediate pain. She was radiographically examined in a clinic near the ski resort. Her radiographic films are shown (*Figures 5-20 and 5-21*). Her examination reveals a swollen and ecchymotic elbow with no skin breaks. Any motion at the elbow is painful and not tolerated. Wrist and digital motion seem unimpaired and nonpainful. There are no apparent vascular or neurologic deficits. She is otherwise healthy. Describe and classify this fracture.

Fig 5-20

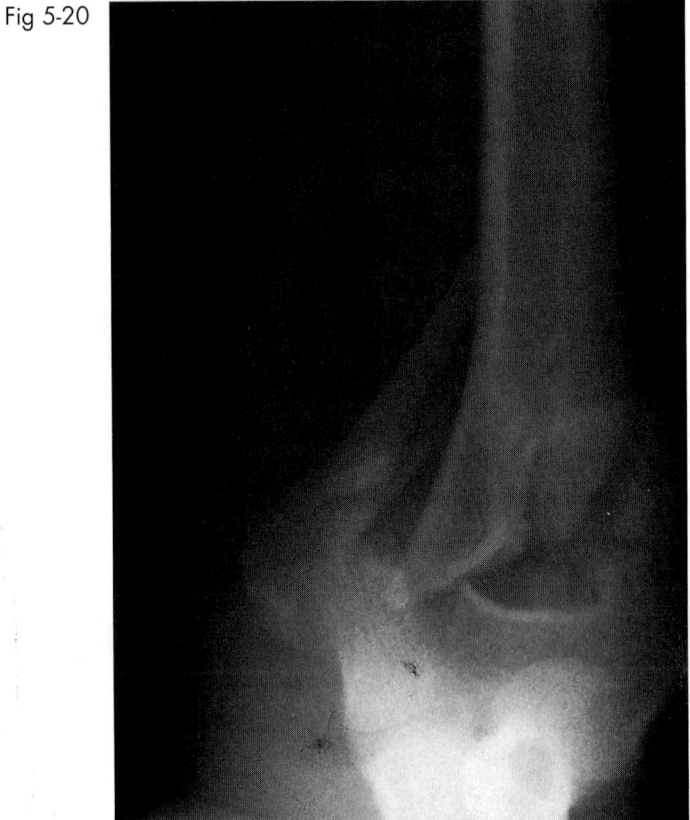

Fig 5-21

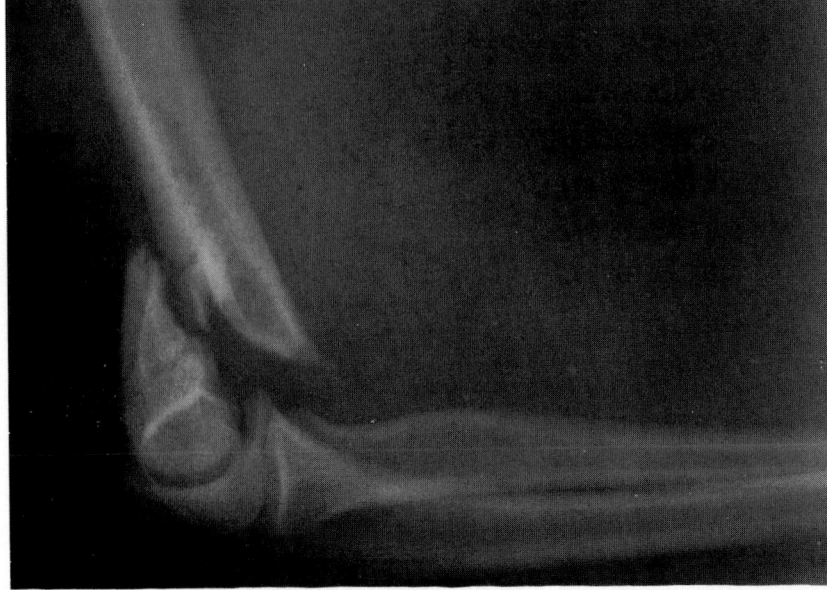

ANSWER

56   This fracture is a displaced and comminuted intercondylar fracture of the distal humerus in a skeletally mature individual. There are several accepted systems by which this fracture could be classified. Müller's system for classification of distal humeral fractures is reasonably comprehensive and would label this a C3 distal humerus fracture (bicondylar, comminuted); however, the more accepted system for classification of humeral intercondylar fractures is that proposed by E.J. Riseborough and Radin. In their system this would be a type III fracture (T-intercondylar with displacement and rotation).

QUESTIONS

57 Would you advise closed treatment, the "Bag of Bones Technique" of Eastwood, or traction?

58 Should internal fixation of this fracture be accomplished by percutaneous pinning, by open pinning, or by open anatomic reduction and rigid fixation?

59 What approaches are reasonable for exposure of this fracture?

60 What nerves are at risk in the surgical treatment of this fracture?

ANSWERS

57 Before the advent of modern implants and surgical techniques, fractures such as this did poorly with open treatment; consequently, many authors recommended closed management for all distal humeral fractures. However, at this point the principal of early motion in the treatment of elbow fractures is widely espoused and should be the primary goal in the management of elbow fractures. Most closed means of treating this fracture would require an unacceptable length of immobilization. An exception to this would be the "Bag of Bones Technique" of Eastwood. This technique involves a collar and cuff (initially keeping the elbow in marked flexion) and a rapidly advanced program of elbow motion. This method is generally recommended for elderly patients with type III and IV fractures, a group in whom the results of open treatment have been less than satisfying; it is also recommended for patients in whom, for other reasons, surgery is not an option. Traction is an acceptable alternative, allowing initiation of early motion and reportedly yielding reasonable results, requiring prolonged hospitalization and bedrest. Results are probably inferior to optimal internal fixation and early motion, although no comparative studies have been done.

58 Again the key principal in treating elbow fractures is early motion, which is best accomplished by rigid internal fixation. This involves restoring the articular surface and the continuity of the medial and lateral columns. Smooth or threaded pins will not generally provide sufficient stability or strength to allow early motion in adult intercondylar fractures. Although pins are used to provide temporary fixation during open reduction, the intercondylar portion of the fracture is probably best held with cannulated or solid screws and the medial and lateral columns with plates as shown (*Figures 5-22 and 5-23*).

ANSWERS

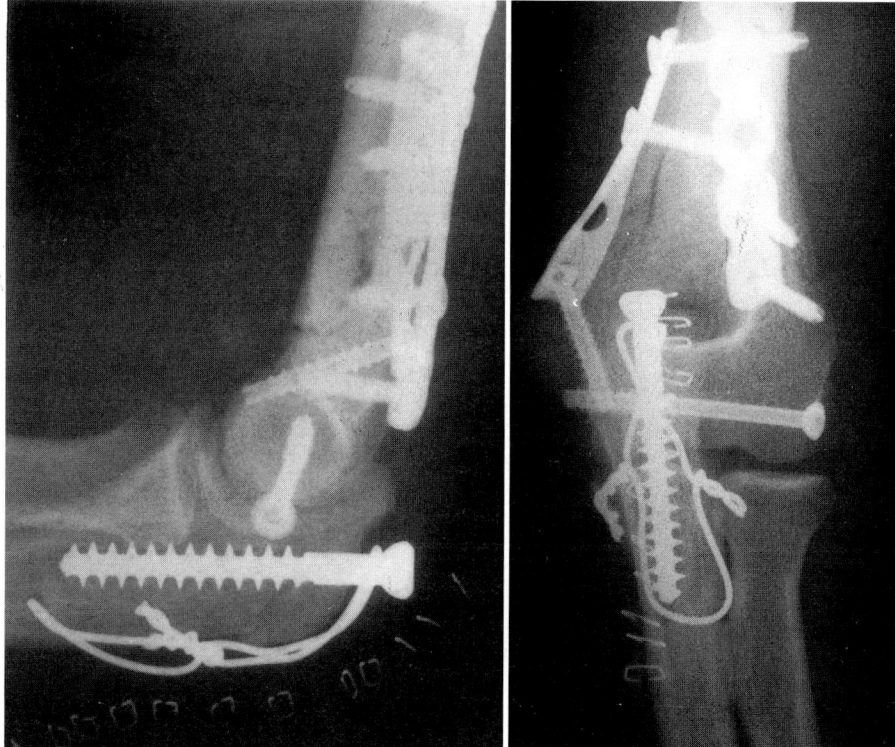

Fig 5-22   Fig 5-23

59   An anterior approach has been described but has never enjoyed wide advocacy. Several posterior approaches exist and have their proponents. Campbell's approach, as described by Van Gorder, involves dividing the triceps tendon as a distally based tongue. This approach has the disadvantage of requiring protection while the soft tissue repair heals. A popular alternative is the triceps sparing approach. This involves an incision along the medial border of the triceps extending distal into the posterior forearm fascia and subperiosteally dissecting this flap away from the bone in continuity as described by Bryan and Morrey. The advantage of this approach is nondisruption of the triceps mechanism. It may require resection of the tip of the olecranon. The recommendation of the AO group is an olecranon osteotomy. Several variations of this procedure exist. All allow predrilling of the olecranon for later fixation. The advantage to this approach is broad exposure and no necessity for tendon-to-tendon healing. The disadvantage of this approach is the creation of another "fracture."

60   The obvious nerve at risk is the ulnar nerve. To allow its protection, it should be visualized in the dissection, and it may need to be transposed anteriorly. The radial nerve is at risk if the fracture or the dissection extend proximally.

QUESTIONS

61 A 36-year-old athletic woman complains of elbow "dislocation" every time she fully extends her elbow. This condition was the result of an injury sustained 4 years earlier while she was engaged in a karate practice session. During this session there was a collision of the ulnar border of her forearm with her opponent's foot, causing a severe valgus stress at her elbow. At the time she was not noted to have a fracture or dislocation and was treated in a sling for comfort. Recovery took several weeks. Since that injury, she has had a feeling of elbow instability, which has prevented vigorous activity involving the affected arm. Your examination does not demonstrate dislocation on extension but does show gross valgus instability. Radiographic films are remarkable for an old radial head injury that healed with mild deformity. Of the structures shown in Figure 5-24, which is the primary valgus stabilizer of the elbow?

Fig 5-24

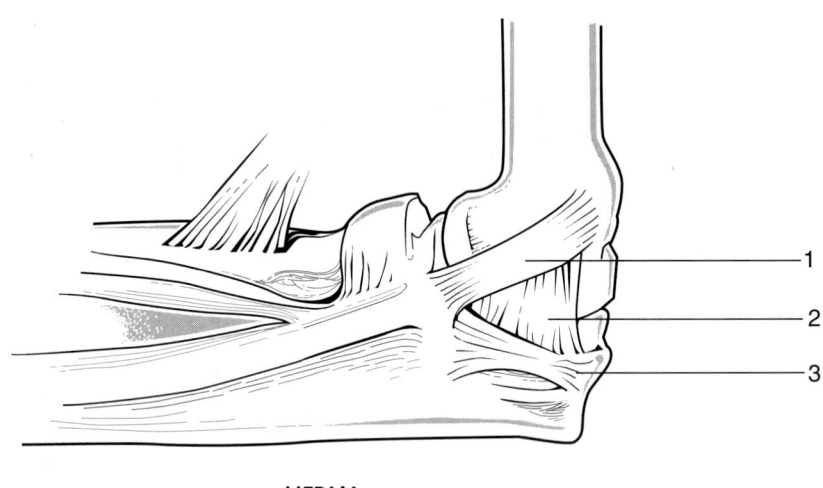

MEDIAL

62 What is the most important secondary valgus stabilizer of the elbow?

63 What are the relative contributions of soft tissue and bony valgus stabilizers at this joint?

64 What long-term problem may result from valgus instability of the elbow?

65 Would radial head replacement afford relief from this patient's valgus instability?

61 Structures 1, 2, and 3 constitute the medial collateral ligament of the

ANSWERS

61   Structures 1, 2, and 3 constitute the medial collateral ligament of the elbow. Of these, the transverse portion (3) contributes little stability. The anterior oblique bundle (1) is the most active in the functional range of motion at this joint and is considered to be the primary valgus stabilizer of the elbow.

62   The radial head is the predominant secondary valgus stabilizer of the elbow.

63   According to Morrey et. al., the medial collateral ligament (MCL) complex accounts for 54% of stability against an applied valgus stress in flexion. The osseous articulation, predominantly the radial head, accounts for 33%. The majority of the balance of stability is from the joint capsule.

64   The most notable long-term sequela from chronic valgus instability at the elbow is ulnar neuropathy.

65   Although there is a clear relationship between MCL and radial head injury in creating valgus instability at the elbow, radial head replacement has been used for valgus stabilization only of acute elbow trauma and is now recommended only when no other options are available. Jobe has described both MCL repair and reconstruction as yielding good results in chronic valgus instability at the elbow.

QUESTIONS

66 A 38-year-old man complains of numbness and weakness in his right hand. He does not relate the problem to a traumatic event and notes its onset to have been gradual over a period of several months. He notes his symptoms are more pronounced when his elbow is flexed, such as when he is holding a newspaper. He is sometimes awakened at night with marked numbness in his little finger. On questioning, he indicates that during childhood, he had a fracture around the right elbow that was "set" and then treated in a cast. On examination, you find that he has full and symmetrical flexion and extension of the elbow and wrist. There is a mild but definite increase in cubitus valgus at the right elbow. Distally, there is 6 mm static two-point discrimination (2PDS) in the ulnar one and a half digits of the right hand compared with 4 mm 2PDS in the remainder of the right hand and all of the left. There seems to be some weakness of abduction and adduction in the right hand compared with the left hand. There is some decrease of first dorsal interosseous mass on the right despite it being the dominant hand. There is a positive Tinel's sign just posterior to the medial epicondyle and also just distal and radial to the pisiform, though this is much less prominent. You diagnose an ulnar neuropathy. At what level is ulnar nerve compression most likely?

67 With your clinical diagnosis and examination findings, should you proceed with further diagnostic testing or treat the patient on the basis of your current evaluation?

68 What diagnostic test(s) will most likely confirm your diagnosis?

69 If you choose to treat this problem nonsurgically for a time, what treatment would you recommend?

70 What is the recommended surgical treatment for cubital tunnel syndrome?

71 What theoretical advantages do decompression and epicondylectomy have over transposition of the ulnar nerve?

72 What are the disadvantages of decompression and epicondylectomy when compared with anterior transposition?

ANSWERS

66   The most common site of compression of the ulnar nerve is the cubital tunnel. This patient's history of childhood elbow fracture with a presumably resultant cubitus valgus also suggest the elbow is the likely site of compression, because chronic cubitus valgus has been associated with an increased likelihood of tardy ulnar nerve palsy.

67   Although the history and examination strongly suggest a cubital tunnel syndrome, Guyon's canal is another potential area of compression. Other unusual causes of peripheral nerve compression (tumor, vascular anomaly) can exist virtually anywhere along the course of the nerve. Because of the existence of atrophy, expectant treatment is not prudent, and further diagnostic evaluation is indicated.

68   The accepted method to confirm a compressive ulnar neuropathy at the elbow is electrodiagnostic testing. Eversmann has stated that slowing nerve conduction velocity greater than 33% across the elbow is always significant. Electromyographic testing of ulnar enervated muscles helps to confirm the diagnosis. In cases where a mass is suspected of causing compression, CT or MRI may be helpful. X-ray film of the right elbow permits objectively measuring cubitus valgus and looking for bony elements impinging at the cubital tunnel.

69   Specific options for the nonsurgical treatment of cubital tunnel syndrome include elbow pads, avoidance of prolonged elbow flexion, and elbow extension night splints. The rationale for these treatments is the relative superficial course of the ulnar nerve as it courses behind the medial epicondyle and the decrease in the cross sectional area of the cubital tunnel as the elbow flexes. Considering the presence of intrinsic atrophy in this case, prolonged nonoperative treatment is probably not indicated, and surgery is the treatment most likely to either halt or reverse the clinical deficits.

70   Several surgical options have been described for the treatment of this problem. Although different authors advocate different operative procedures, simple decompression, medial epicondylectomy, and anterior transposition (subcutaneous, submuscular, or partially submuscular) are all accepted treatments.

71   In both decompression and epicondylectomy, the ulnar nerve is not disturbed from its bed and, therefore, is not put at vascular risk by partial skeletonization. Additionally, anterior transposition risks kinking the nerve.

72   Simple decompression can fail to expose or treat the site of actual compression of the ulnar nerve. In addition, the nerve continues to course behind the medial epicondyle and is stretched when the elbow flexes. Epicondylectomy has been criticized for removing the osseous protection of the ulnar nerve afforded by the medial epicondyle.

QUESTIONS

73 What preoperative findings are of predictive value in determining the likelihood of a poor operative outcome?

74 An early middle-aged grocery store checker complains of elbow pain. The onset of the pain was gradual and seems to be related to work. There is no numbness, but the patient does complain of weakness, perhaps related to pain. Your examination discloses no obvious distal neurovascular abnormalities. There is marked tenderness just distal and anterior to the lateral epicondyle, and there is an exacerbation of pain when wrist extension is blocked with the elbow in extension. The tendinous origin of which muscle (*Figure 5-25*) is the most common site of pathology in the condition suggested by the history and examination?

Fig 5-25

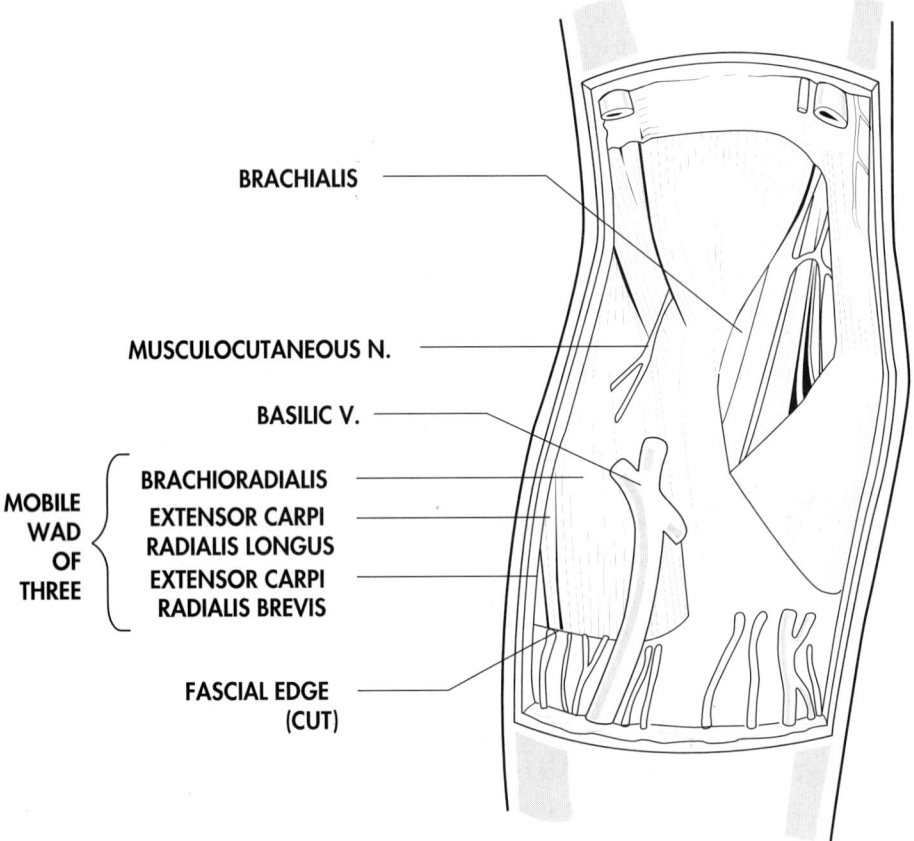

BRACHIALIS

MUSCULOCUTANEOUS N.

BASILIC V.

MOBILE WAD OF THREE

BRACHIORADIALIS

EXTENSOR CARPI RADIALIS LONGUS

EXTENSOR CARPI RADIALIS BREVIS

FASCIAL EDGE (CUT)

75 Would the presence of calcification in the extensor origin seen on a radiographic film impact your recommended treatment?

76 What condition is reported to be the most common coexistent or alternate diagnosis associated with the clinical symptom complex typical of "tennis elbow" syndrome, and what condition is suggested as the diagnosis in cases of "tennis elbow" that are resistant to treatment?

77 What initial, nonsurgical treatment would you recommend for this patient?

ANSWERS

73 R.S. Adelaar, et al. showed a statistically significant correlation between preoperative muscle atrophy and poor outcome and a correlation between the presence of preoperative and postoperative fibrillation potentials and a poor surgical outcome.

74 Microtears or macrotears in the tendinous origin of the extensor carpi radialis brevis are currently the most accepted cause of lateral epicondylitis, or "tennis elbow."

75 Such calcifications are seen in approximately 25% of cases of lateral epicondylitis. They have no prognostic significance and should not alter your planned treatment.

76 Radial tunnel syndrome, or posterior interosseous nerve compressive neuropathy, although less frequent than "tennis elbow" syndrome, has been associated with it in multiple reports. Radial tunnel syndrome may exist in up to 5% of cases diagnosed as "tennis elbow."

77 "Tennis elbow," or lateral epicondylitis, is most often sports or occupationally related. The primary treatment is to remove or modify the activity that is inciting the symptoms. Other treatments may include NSAIDs, physical therapy (heat, ice, ultrasound, and diathermy have all been suggested, as well as cautious stretching and strengthening exercises), manipulation, and "tennis elbow" straps.

QUESTIONS

78 Should steroid injections be considered as an initial treatment for this condition?

79 What percent of patients will require operative intervention for "tennis elbow" symptoms? Should surgical treatment ever be considered primarily?

80 What are the indications for surgery to alleviate "tennis elbow" symptoms?

81 Is surgery for "tennis elbow" extraarticular or intraarticular?

ANSWERS

78   Several studies have indicated success in relieving "tennis elbow" pain by the use of steroid injections, but recurrence of symptoms is approximately 20% to 50%. The use of injected steroids is probably not curative and should be coupled with additional rehabilitation. Although steroid injection is an accepted treatment for this condition, most current authors consider it a second echelon treatment rather than a first.

79   The majority of patients will respond to nonsurgical treatment for "tennis elbow." Probably less than 5% and no more than 10% will require surgery. Virtually all authors who write about this condition agree that a prolonged course of nonsurgical management is indicated in all cases before consideration for surgery.

80   Refractory cases that persist beyond 6 to 12 months despite proper nonoperative treatment may be candidates for surgery. As discussed earlier, other conditions may be the cause of symptoms that persist in the face of appropriate nonoperative treatment for "tennis elbow." These conditions must be ruled out before surgery.

81   Some controversy exists regarding the operative management of "tennis elbow," and some current texts still recommend intraarticular procedures. Most leading authors agree that unless specific intraarticular pathology can be demonstrated preoperatively, extraarticular procedures, especially those focused on the tendinous origin of extensor carpi radialis brevis, are the procedures of choice.

QUESTION

a history of elbow fracture when the boy was 9 years old, which required manipulation and casting in an operating room. The injury was then treated in a cast for several weeks after which her son began range-of-motion exercises. He did not regain full motion for a number of months. When he did, he was noted to have an elbow deformity. The parents were told by the treating physician that the deformity would correct with time, but after 3 years, they can detect no improvement. Clinically, he appears as shown (*Figures 5-26 and 5-27*). His current radiographic films are seen in Figures 5-28 and 5-29. How likely is it that this 12-year-old boy with open physes will yet remodel his distal humerus and correct his deformity?

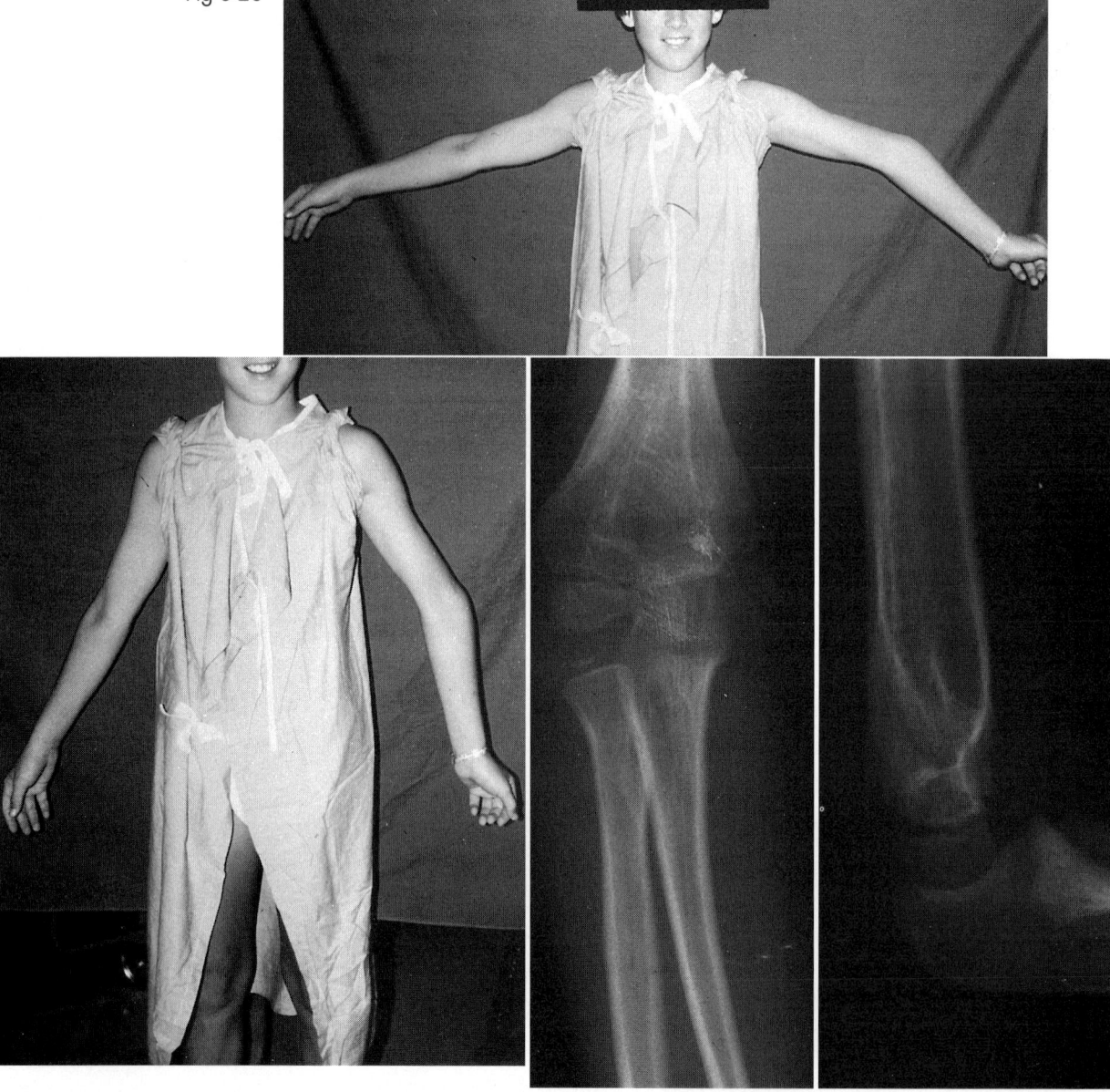

Fig 5-26

Fig 5-27

Fig 5-28

Fig 5-29

ANSWER

82   Several studies have confirmed that after supracondylar humeral fracture, even in skeletally immature patients, the varus-valgus configuration of the elbow does not change or remodel.

QUESTIONS

83 The elbow fracture is likely what specific type of fracture?

84 In children, what other fractures of the distal humerus, if any, can produce cubitus varus?

85 Is the likely cause of the deformity in this case a vascular injury to the physis causing premature closure, vascular stimulation of a portion of the physis causing lateral overgrowth, or postreduction collapse of the medial cortex?

86 Can cubitus varus be avoided by reduction under anesthesia with intraoperative pinning?

87 How are childhood supracondylar fractures classified?

88 What is the incidence of vascular complications in this fracture?

89 What nerve injuries have been reported in association with childhood supracondylar fractures?

90 What nerve is most commonly injured with childhood humeral supracondylar fracture?

91 A number of pin configurations have been advocated for stabilization of type III fractures. Has any of these been shown to be superior to the rest?

ANSWERS

83 The most common type of fracture around the elbow in skeletally immature individuals is the supracondylar fracture. A well-recognized complication of this fracture is cubitus varus (gunstock deformity). Men and boys predominate in this type of fracture. The ratio of male to female is 2 to 1. The fracture occurs most frequently in children in the 3- to 10-year-old age group. The highest probability is that the injury was a supracondylar fracture.

84 Cubitus varus is the most common osseous deformity produced by both medial and lateral humeral condylar fractures in children. Although both medial and lateral condylar fractures can produce valgus, both more commonly result in varus. In medial and lateral condylar fractures of the immature distal humerus, the varus that may be produced is usually mild and rarely requires treatment.

ANSWERS

85   All of the above explanations of cubitus varus resulting after supracondylar humeral fractures in children have been proposed. However, the weight of current evidence and opinion is that this deformity is the result of inadequate reduction.

86   The incidence of varus deformity after childhood supracondylar fracture of the humerus is less, but not zero, in series that employ pinning for type III fractures than in those relying exclusively on cast immobilization. Reports ranging from less than 10% to more than 50% incidence of cubitus varus, using cast immobilization alone, have been presented. The incidence of this deformity in series of cases stabilized with pins is generally less than 5%. Failure to avoid this complication in cases treated with pin stabilization is due to pinning in an inadequately reduced position.

87   A number of classifications have been proposed, but the most commonly used classification separates these fractures into flexion type (5% of supracondylar fractures) and extension type (95% of supracondylar fractures). These fractures are further classified as type I, nondisplaced; type II, angulated but with an intact cortical hinge; and type III, completely displaced. Type III extension fractures are then usually subclassified as posteromedial or posterolateral. Of these, posteromedially displaced fractures account for 75% of cases.

88   Although the incidence of Volkmann's ischemia is much lower, the overall incidence of vascular compromise in humeral supracondylar fracture is approximately 5%. Posterolateral type III extension injuries are particularly prone to put the brachial artery at risk.

89   All the major nerves traversing the elbow have been reported to be injured in association with this fracture. Spinner has also documented several instances in which the anterior interosseous nerve was injured in conjunction with supracondylar fracture.

90   The radial nerve is injured with the greatest frequency. This is reasonable when one considers that posteromedial, type III extension injuries are the most common type III injuries and are the type to most likely put the radial nerve at risk.

91   Herzenberg et al. has shown the medial and lateral crossed pin technique to be the most stable configuration biomechanically. However, the critical element for success remains the adequacy of reduction before pinning.

QUESTIONS

92 Have either closed reduction and percutaneous pinning or open reduction and pinning demonstrated benefits over the other technique?

93 For the patient described in Q92, what exercises or braces are likely to be of benefit to correct the deformity?

94 What long-term sequelae or functional deficits are likely to result should this deformity be left untreated?

ANSWERS

92   Full open reduction and pinning more often result in permanent loss of motion or myositis ossificans or growth disturbance than closed reduction and percutaneous pinning. Indications for full open reduction are open fractures, fractures that are irreducible or inadequately reducible by closed means, and fractures associated with vascular injury.

93   Nonsurgical treatment is ineffective in treating posttraumatic cubitus varus. Osteotomy, using some variation of a lateral closing wedge, or a dome osteotomy are the standard surgical approaches to this problem.

94   Whereas long-term cubitus valgus deformities have been associated with tardy ulnar nerve palsy, the functional deficits associated with cubitus varus are minimal and are limited to highly specific activities. Although some authors have suggested a loss of strength with cubitus varus, it is generally conceded to be a purely cosmetic deformity. Surgical correction is done for cosmesis alone.

QUESTION

95 A 28-year-old man is a passenger in the front seat of a vehicle that is involved in a head-on collision. Although restrained, he describes putting his hands out to the dashboard to brace himself just before impact. His only major complaint in the emergency room is pain in his left elbow. The elbow is swollen, and motion is severely limited by pain. You obtain the radiographic films shown (*Figures 5-30 and 5-31*). With the obvious radial head injury, what ipsilateral injuries must concern you in deciding on the most appropriate management of this radial head fracture?

Fig 5-30

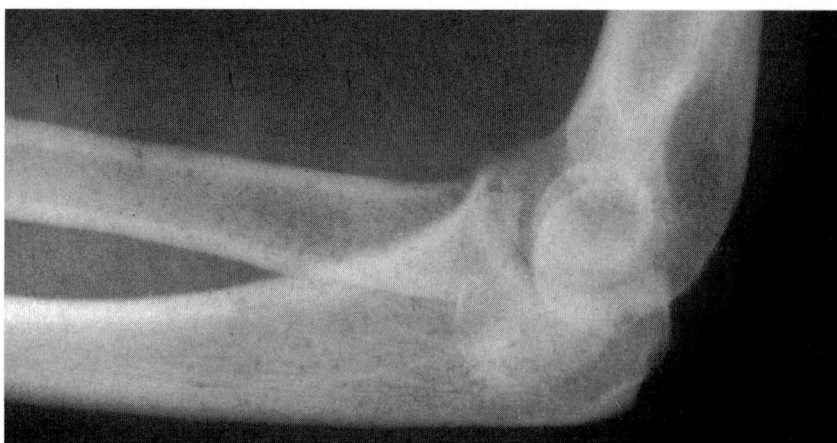

Fig 5-31

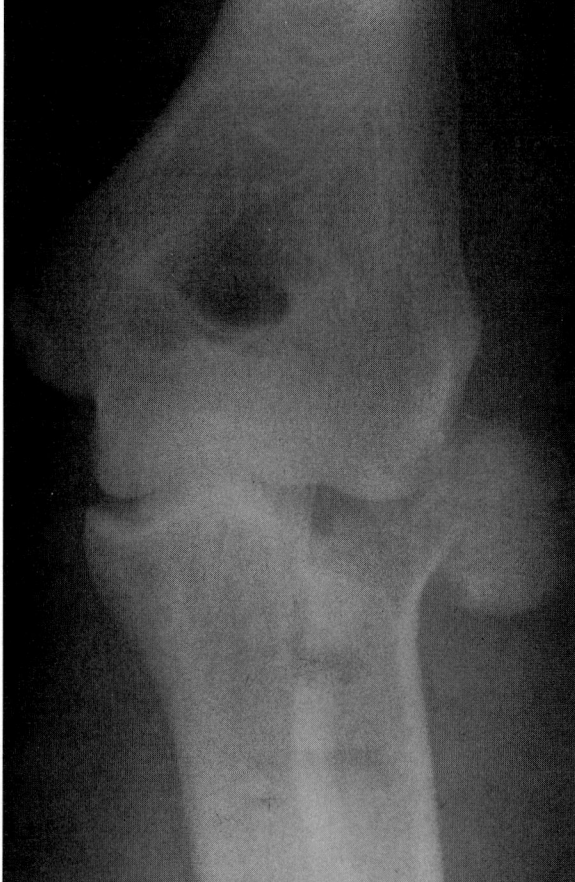

ANSWER

95 Because the radiocapitellar joint is a secondary valgus stabilizer of the elbow, the primary valgus stabilizer (the MCL complex) must be carefully assessed. Because of both the mechanism and the nature of the injury, the patient's wrist and forearm should also be evaluated for signs of an Essex-Lopresti injury (acute longitudinal radioulnar dissociation [ALRUD]). Both of these injuries may significantly influence your management of this condition.

QUESTIONS

96 What system is most commonly used to classify radial head fractures?

97 In the fracture previously shown (*Figures 5-30 and 5-31*), you suspect some degree of ALRUD. Is the most appropriate treatment for this fracture closed reduction, excision, open reduction, open reduction with internal fixation, or silastic radial head replacement?

ANSWERS

96   The system that Mason proposed in 1954 is currently the most widely used. It uses an anatomic classification of three types of radial head fracture to which a fourth type was added in 1962 by Johnston.

97   There is an increasing appreciation of the desirability of maintaining the radial head whenever possible. Your best hope is open or closed reduction with or without internal fixation, as required. Even if the radial head can be maintained, thought should be given to pinning the distal radioulnar joint with the forearm in supination. (*Figures 5-32 and 5-33*). Excision in the face of ALRUD leads to disaster, which is difficult to overcome. The efficacy of silastic radial head replacement as both a valgus and as a longitudinal stabilizer has been seriously challenged and should be considered only where no other treatment is appropriate.

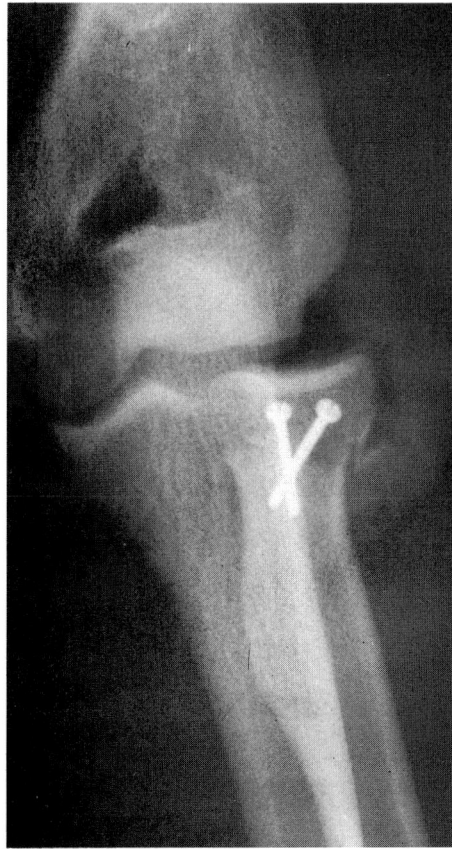

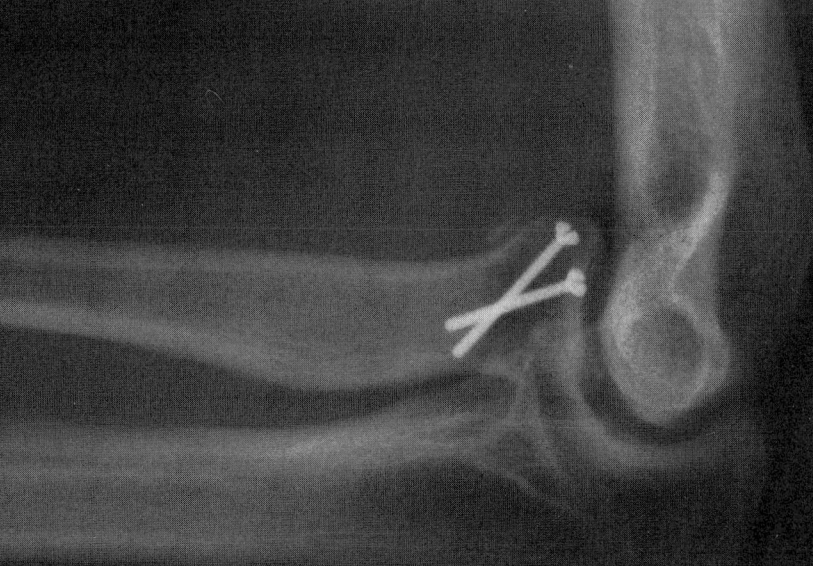

Fig 5-32   Fig 5-33

QUESTION

98   Is the best means of internal fixation for this fracture pins, screws, or a small, low-profile plate?

ANSWER

98 Pins provide tenuous fixation and are prone to backing out. A plate, no matter how low its profile, would almost certainly impinge at the proximal radioulnar joint. Screws are the optimal means of internal fixation, if internal fixation is found to be necessary. Standard small screws, such as shown (*Figures 5-32 and 5-33*) are acceptable as long as they do not impinge on the proximal radioulnar joint. The use of self-compressing, completely intraosseous screws of several varieties (*Figure 5-34*) for the internal fixation of radial head fractures has obvious advantages and continues to gain popularity.

Fig 5-34

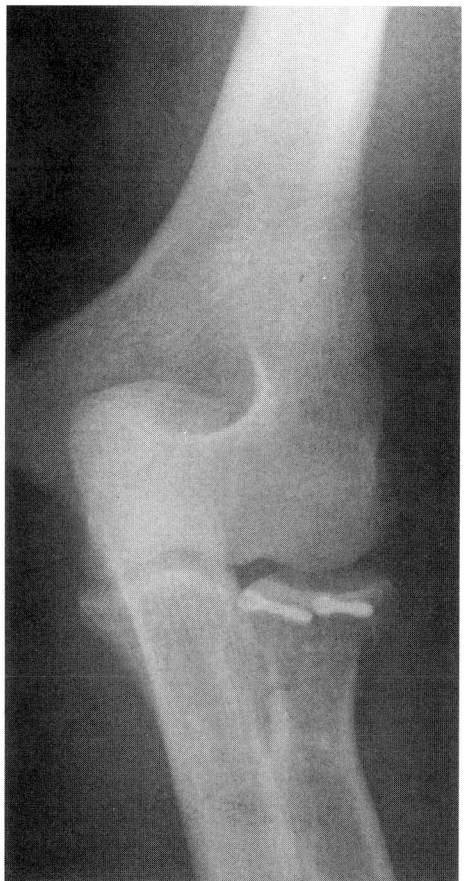

QUESTIONS

99 A pediatrician colleague refers a patient for treatment of a fracture of the right forearm. The child has an obvious congenital abnormality as well. Radiographic films of both forearms are shown (*Figures 5-35 and 5-36*). Is this type of deficiency hereditary or teratogenic?

Fig 5-35

Fig 5-36

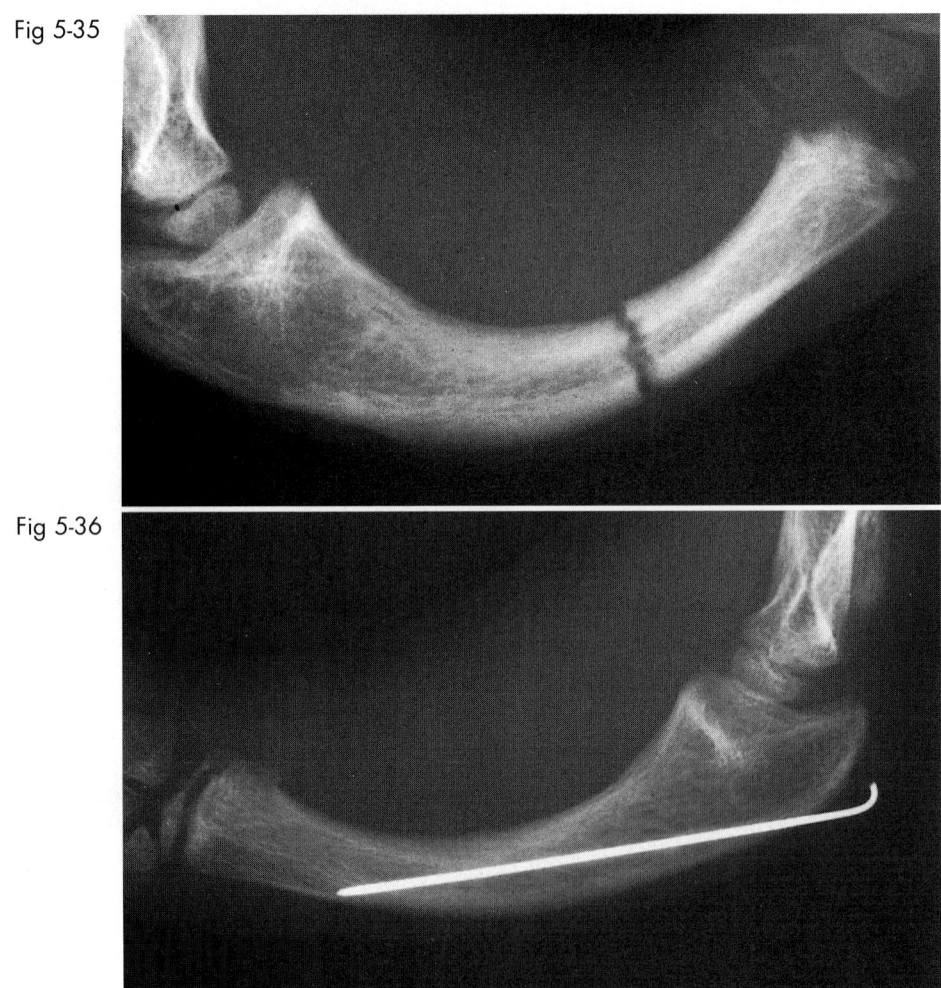

100 At what period during embryogenesis would an insult have to occur to produce this deformity?

101 What are the major classes of upper extremity congenital abnormality? Into which category would this abnormality fall?

102 Which is the most common of the four types of radial deficiency?

103 Are radial deficiencies always bilateral and symmetric as in this case?

ANSWERS

99 Although there are recognized genetic causes of malformations, most radial deficiencies are considered to be sporadic, and the etiology is not clear. The experience with thalidomide in the late 1950s and early 1960s suggests environmental factors may be causative. Current thinking tends to implicate such things as infections, ionizing radiation, or chemicals (drugs).

100 The limb bud appears at about the fourth week following fertilization, and the hand outline is complete by the seventh week. Whereas some types of transverse deficiency may be a result of later intrauterine insult, longitudinal deficiencies would have to occur during the fourth to seventh week after fertilization.

101 The current, accepted system for classifying upper extremity congenital abnormalities is a modification of that proposed by Swanson. It is endorsed by the American Society for Surgery of the Hand and the International Federation of Societies for Surgery of the Hand. The major classifications are:
  I. Failure of formation of parts
  II. Failure of differentiation of parts
  III. Duplication
  IV. Overgrowth
  V. Undergrowth
  VI. Congenital constriction band syndrome
  VII. Generalized skeletal abnormalities

This deficiency would be classified as category I—failure of formation of parts, longitudinal deficiency.

102 Bayne divides radial deficiencies into four categories:
  I. Short distal radius
  II. Hypoplastic radius
  III. Partially absent radius
  IV. Totally absent radius

Type IV, the totally absent radius, is the most common.

103 Radial deficiencies are reported to be bilateral in 50% of cases, but some authors observe that in unilateral cases there is a high incidence of contralateral thumb abnormalities. This implies a higher incidence of *asymmetric* radial deficiency than may have been previously appreciated.

QUESTIONS

104 With what associated congenital abnormalities do you need to be concerned with when evaluating a neonate with a radial deficiency?

105 What surgery is most often recommended in total radial deficiencies with marked radial deviation and radial bowing of the ulna?

106 A 12-year-old patient had bilateral centralization and ulnar straightening within her first year of life. On the right side the centralization has partially failed, and the radial bow of the ulna has recurred bilaterally. Ignoring her fracture for the moment, should she be advised to consider further surgery to straighten the ulnar bowing and to recentralize the right hand?

107 A 20-year-old roofer receives a direct blow to his forearm from a load of materials on the end of a hoist. He is unable to work and comes to your office. His examination reveals no breaks in the skin or any tenderness along the radius. There is moderate swelling, tenderness, and ecchymosis around the middle and distal thirds junction of the ulna. There is pain on attempted pronation and supination. Radiographic films are shown (*Figures 5-37 and 5-38*). What is the usual mechanism for this injury?

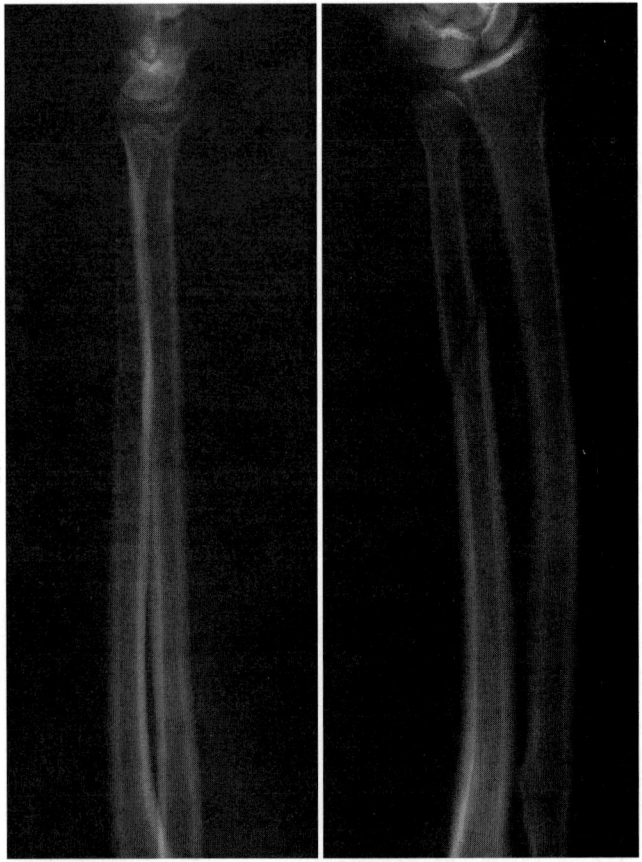

Fig 5-37   Fig 5-38

ANSWERS

104 Cardiac abnormalities are not uncommon in radial deficiency, and VATER-associated abnormalities have also been reported. The awareness of hematologic abnormalities that may be associated with radial deficiencies is critical, to include thrombocytopenia-absent radii (TAR) syndrome and Fanconi's anemia (FA). The latter has especially severe implications and is often not diagnosed in a timely manner. Fifty percent of patients with FA will evidence some degree of upper extremity preaxial dysplasia.

105 The current recommendation of most authors for this problem would be centralization of the hand over the end of the ulna, combined with a procedure to straighten the ulna and a pollicization.

106 Most adolescent and adult patients with radial deficiencies have adapted to their impairment and are not greatly benefited by additional surgery. Unless there is some **clear** benefit to be achieved, most older patients should not be considered for additional corrective surgery.

107 Isolated fractures of the ulna are usually the result of a direct blow. They are also known as "nightstick" fractures.

QUESTIONS

108 Assuming radiographic films of the elbow to be negative, should this fracture be treated closed or with internal fixation?

109 Should external immobilization for a single bone forearm fracture extend above the elbow?

110 Are there any single-bone ulna fractures that are not suitable for closed treatment?

111 Would the fracture shown in Figures 5-37 and 5-38 be considered to be displaced?

ANSWERS

108 For relatively stable, isolated fractures of the ulna, the bulk of current evidence indicates that closed treatment results in healing in a high proportion of fractures. Various authors have advocated cast or fracture brace treatment of these injuries or no immobilization at all, although the latter is not widely practiced.

109 As implied in A108, there is controversy regarding the vigor of immobilization necessary for these fractures. A reasonable general rule would be to use a long arm device (cast, cast brace) for a fracture of the proximal half of the ulna, whereas a fracture of the distal half might be expected to do well in a short arm device. As forearm rotation is motion of the *radius* around the ulna, consideration for a long arm device for initial immobilization should be given to practically all single bone radius fractures, regardless of location.

110 Fractures with significant displacement (defined as greater than 10° angulation in any plane or displaced greater than 50% of the diameter of the ulna) should not be treated closed, and several authors have pointed out that a Monteggia's fracture cannot be treated using external immobilization.

111 Displacement in isolated ulnar fractures may be defined as angulation greater than 10° or displacement of greater than 50% of the diameter of the bone.

QUESTIONS

112 A general surgery colleague consults you regarding a multiple trauma victim, asking for evaluation of an injury of the patient's forearm. The patient will require surgery for other injuries including head and chest trauma. After a thorough musculoskeletal evaluation, you determine that the only orthopedic injury is the one displayed radiographically (*Figures 5-39 and 5-40*). You have determined that the patient has no nerve or compromising vessel injury. There is a 1 cm laceration over the ulnar fracture site. It appears to be a type I, open injury. Would you recommend débridement and casting, intramedullary fixation, or plate fixation?

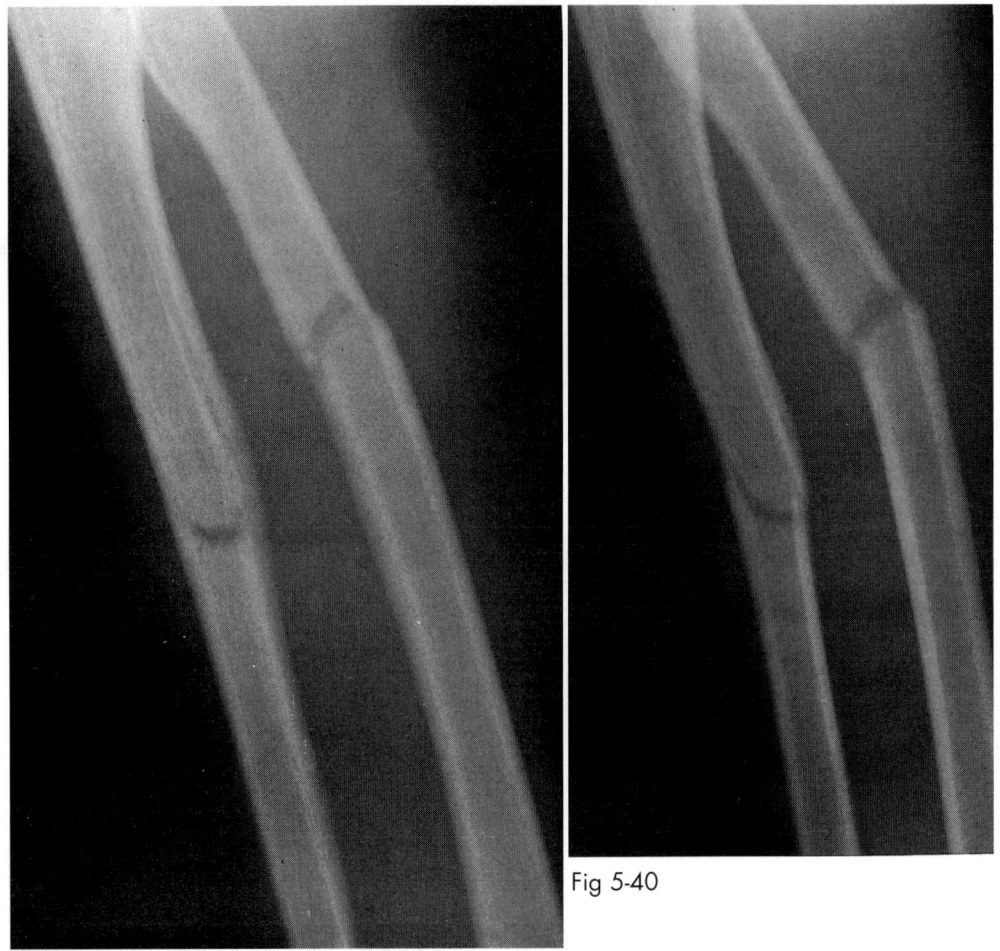

Fig 5-40

Fig 5-39

113 What difficulties might you expect to attend the use of intramedullary fixation?

114 What degree of rotation or angulation is acceptable in the treatment of radius and ulna diaphyseal fractures in adults?

115 Would it be advisable to débride and wash out the laceration over the ulnar fracture and then approach both fractures through a single incision away from the laceration site?

ANSWERS

112 Although there are advocates of cast or fracture brace treatment of adult forearm fractures of both bones, the accepted treatment currently is internal fixation. This procedure is especially true in multiple-traumatized patients. Many current authors recommend immediate fixation in type I and type II open fractures following appropriate debridement. Intramedullary fixation of radius and ulna fractures is acceptable for selected diaphyseal fractures. Devices with a triangle, box, or diamond cross section are preferred. Plate fixation, using a 3.5-mm compression plate is the gold standard.

113 Intramedullary devices for radius and ulna fractures are occasionally difficult to place. Proximally in the ulna and distally in the radius, intramedullary fixation is not stable. In cases where the isthmus is narrow, intramedullary fixation risks fracturing or comminuting the bone. It is necessary to maintain the bow of the radius and to assure rotational reduction in treating both bone forearm fractures. This is at times difficult when using intramedullary fixation.

114 Both clinical and laboratory data show that up to 10° in any plane (including rotation) will result in only minimal loss of pronation and supination.

115 With meticulous care of the wound, the probability of infection is acceptably low; therefore, the ulnar laceration need not be avoided in the approach to the ulna. Open reduction and internal fixation of both bone forearm fractures through a single incision has been associated with an increased incidence of cross union and is not recommended.

QUESTIONS

116 What factors are felt to affect the incidence of cross union in both bone forearm fractures?

117 If a cross union occurs, should it be treated by excision, excision and interposition of silastic, osteotomy for positioning the hand, or not treated?

118 What are the indications for removal of upper extremity hardware?

119 If it is believed desirable, at what point after fracture should upper extremity hardware be removed?

120 Should the forearm be casted following plate removal?

ANSWERS

116 According to Vince and Miller, factors that may affect the incidence of cross union include the following:

(1) Fractures at the same level
(2) Severe local trauma and comminution
(3) Multiple trauma and head injury
(4) Plating both bones through a single incision
(5) Repeated closed reductions
(6) Primary onlay bone grafting
(7) Non-anatomic reduction
(8) Narrowing of the interosseous space
(9) Delayed surgical fixation
(10) Bone fragments in the interosseous space
(11) Overpenetration of screws when using plates

117 Although some authors have reported success in treating cross union surgically, the general experience has not been favorable. Vince and Miller suggest aggressive resection of type II cross unions after the callus demonstrates quiescence, usually between the first and second year after fracture.

118 The general recommendation regarding upper extremity hardware is that it should be left in place unless it is prominent and causing irritation or in cases in which the patient is at risk for further trauma to the area.

119 Refracture after plate removal has been reported in multiple studies. The most recent edition of *Internal Fixation of Small Fractures* suggests that the average interval between fracture and plate removal for forearm shaft fractures should be 24 to 28 months. Rossen et. al. found that bone does not return to prefracture density until 21 months following fracture. Current sources generally recommend not removing forearm plates before 24 months.

120 Protection for a period of 6 weeks following plate removal is recommended.

CHAPTER 6

Lower Extremity

Stanley H. Dysart
Kenneth J. Koval

QUESTIONS

1 A 62-year-old overweight individual complains of right groin pain with ambulation. Radiographic films demonstrate degenerative arthritis of the hip. What nonoperative measures might be considered before performing a total joint replacement?

2 A 75-year-old man has been referred for a hip replacement because of complaints of groin pain when ambulating and because of radiographic films that demonstrate degenerative arthritis. Additional history reveals that he has bilateral thigh and calf pain when walking distances greater than one block and that discomfort is relieved by sitting. What additional evaluation should be considered before performing a total joint replacement?

3 A 26-year-old heavy laborer has extensive post-traumatic hip arthritis and concentric joint space loss. He has failed nonoperative therapy and would like to proceed with operative therapy. He would like to continue in his current occupation after the procedure. What surgical option is best?

4 What clinical factors are considered important when considering a femoral osteotomy for a patient with localized arthrosis?

5 A 35-year-old office manager has been diagnosed with traumatic hip arthritis and has progression of pain and limitation of activities of daily living despite adequate nonoperative management. Radiographic films show extensive involvement of the joint. The patient has a history of low back pain that is chronic and has required one previous hospital admission. What is the best surgical option for this young patient?

6 What alterations in cement technique have resulted in lower femoral loosening rates?

ANSWERS

1 Activity modification, use of nonsteroidal antiinflammatory drugs (NSAIDs), weight reduction, and use of a cane in the left (opposite) hand when ambulating. Use of a cane in the contralateral hand reduces hip contact force. Hip replacement is reserved for failure of nonoperative therapy.

ANSWERS

2 The patient's symptoms are compatible with spinal stenosis; therefore, an evaluation of the lumbar spine with radiographic films and a computerized tomographic (CT) or magnetic resonance imaging (MRI) scan should be considered. A careful physical examination is necessary to evaluate vascular compromise because symptoms of leg pain with ambulation may be caused by vascular claudication.

3 Hip arthrodesis is the option most likely to produce pain-free function of long duration. Although hip replacement is an option for the younger individual with degenerative arthritis, it is not recommended in the individual who is a heavy laborer. A patient engaged in heavy labor or with extensive degenerative changes is a poor candidate for femoral osteotomy. The positioning of the hip is important for maximal postoperative function. Neutral rotation, neutral abduction and adduction, and 30° of hip flexion are considered ideal. Internal rotation and hip abduction are to be avoided. Slight hip adduction (10°) and up to 5° of external rotation are well tolerated.

4 Important factors to consider include the age, weight, and occupation of the patient. The obese patient and the patient in labor-intensive occupations are poor candidates. Leg length discrepancy must be considered because varus osteotomy may shorten the limb 1.5 cm. The status of the ipsilateral knee must be considered because the osteotomy must be performed so that the mechanical axis passes through the center of the knee. An ideal candidate should have a flexion arc of hip motion of at least 80° and at least 15° of abduction and adduction arc. Preoperative radiographic studies should confirm that hip congruency is obtained by varus, valgus, extension, or flexion positioning.

5 A total joint replacement is the best option for this patient. The patient's history of low back pain contraindicates hip arthrodesis. A successful hip arthrodesis exposes the lumbar spine and ipsilateral knee to increased stress. Long-term follow-up of successful hip arthrodesis demonstrates ipsilateral knee and back pain in 60% of patients. A femoral osteotomy would be appropriate in the patient with more localized arthrosis.

6 Pulsatile femoral lavage, plugging of the femoral canal, centrifugation or vacuum mixing of cement, retrograde injection of cement with a cement gun, and pressurization have resulted in a lower rate of loosening. These techniques result in more even cement distribution in the femoral canal and deeper cement intrusion into bone, yielding a stronger cement bone interface. The strength of the cement bone interface correlates with the depth of cement penetration; 4 mm of penetration is desirable. Centrifugation or vacuum mixing of cement reduces the porosity and increases the fatigue resistance of cement.

QUESTIONS

7 What factors are associated with an increased rate of loosening of the femoral component?

8 What factors are associated with increased rates of dislocation after hip replacement surgery?

9 What is the primary indication for conversion of hip arthrodesis to total hip replacement? What are the expected clinical results after this procedure?

10 In the patient with advanced osteonecrosis of the hip, pain is most reliably relieved by what surgical procedure?

11 What is the effect of hip arthrodesis on oxygen consumption and gait efficiency when compared with the normal hip? Is energy consumption greater when compared with a total hip replacement?

12 What is the most frequent long-term complication of cemented total hip arthroplasty?

ANSWERS

7   Factors associated with loosening of the femoral component include young age, heavy weight, male gender, increased level of activity, stems placed in varus, curved stems with a narrow medial edge, suboptimal cement technique, and poor bone stock.

8   Factors associated with increased rates of dislocation include use of the posterior approach and revision hip surgery. Avulsion of the greater trochanter in the patient undergoing a lateral transtrochanteric approach has an increased rate of dislocation. Malposition of components, neuromuscular disease, or shortening of the limb also result in higher rates of hip dislocation.

9   Ipsilateral knee pain and disabling back pain are the primary indications for conversion. The expected clinical results are less back and knee pain, improved ability to sit, and improvement in leg length discrepancy. Limp, secondary to weakness of the hip abductors, may be present, and some patients require the use of a cane or other walking aid. The patient in whom the hip biomechanics are more completely restored has less residual limp and is more likely to have stronger abductors.

10   Total hip arthroplasty most reliably relieves pain and improves function. Resurfacing arthroplasty has not been reliable in the treatment of osteonecrosis. Bipolar hemiarthroplasty is more reliable, but results have not been as reliable as with total hip arthroplasty. A recent evaluation of bipolar arthroplasty in the patient with aseptic necrosis demonstrated only 48% satisfactory results 4 years after the procedure. Femoral osteotomy may be indicated in less advanced disease where joint space congruency and unloading of an osteonecrotic segment can be obtained. Core decompression has not been reliable in the patient with advanced disease.

11   In a study of energy expenditure after hip arthrodesis, mean oxygen consumption was 32% more than normal, gait efficiency was 53% of normal, and energy consumption was greater than that reported after total hip arthroplasty.

12   Aseptic loosening represents the most frequent long-term complication of total hip arthroplasty. In a recent review of cemented total hip arthroplasty using first generation cementing techniques, the probability of loosening of the femoral or acetabular component increased from 13% at 5 years to 32% at 15 years. Second generation techniques for cemented femoral and acetabular components show a definite improvement in femoral loosening rates but no improvement in acetabular fixation. In a recent review of a series of 100 hip arthroplasty procedures performed with second generation cementing techniques, only one stem was definitely loose at 10 years; however, 24.5% of acetabular components were loose by radiographic criteria.

QUESTIONS

13 What size of femoral head is associated with increased acetabular revision rates for total hip arthroplasty?

14 When considering cemented total hip arthroplasty, what is the importance of porosity reduction in cement, and how is porosity reduction best achieved?

15 A 55-year-old asymptomatic man comes for routine follow-up 5 years after uncemented total hip arthroplasty. Radiographic films reveal a large area of osteolysis adjacent to zones two and three of the acetabular component. Laboratory evaluation is normal, and the patient does not have an elevated erythrocyte sedimentation rate (ESR). What is the likely etiology of this problem, and what will histologic examination of the area most likely reveal? (*Figure 6-1*)

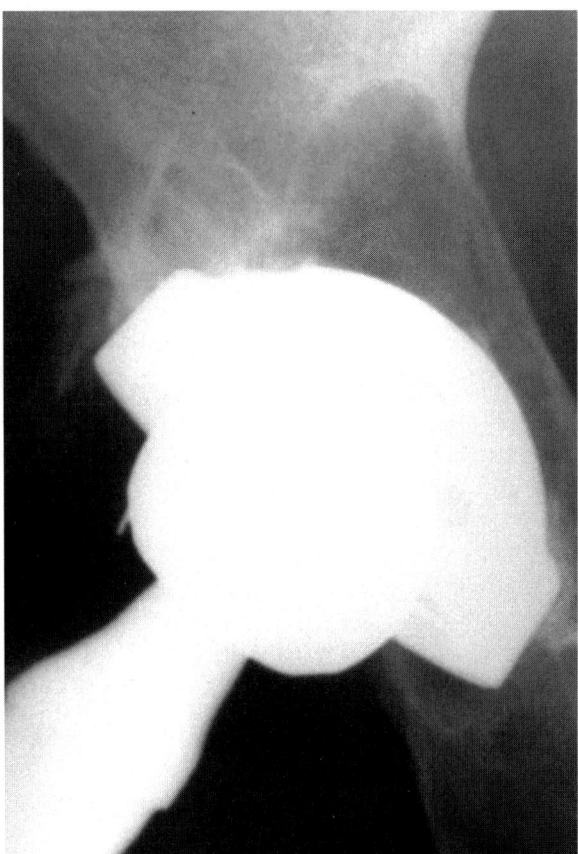

Fig 6-1

ANSWERS

13   Acetabular revisions are more frequent with 32-mm acetabular heads. Charnley's first principle was to achieve low friction arthroplasty. The 32-mm head reduces the rate of hip dislocation, but increased friction forces result in increased volumetric polyethylene wear, increased polyethylene mean wear rates, and increased acetabular revision rates.

14   The presence of cavitation voids, air entrapment during the mixing of cement, and void generation caused by evaporation and boiling of the monomer contribute to the porosity of cement. Entrapment of air during the mixing process is the most common contributor to porosity, and methods devised to reduce this source of porosity include mixing in a partial vacuum and centrifugation after mixing. Porosity reduction is greatest with mechanical mixing in a vacuum. Porosity reduction improves the tensile and fatigue strength of the cement and is an important adjunct to second and third generation cementing techniques.

15   The patient has osteolysis secondary to polyethylene wear debris. Histologic examination is likely to reveal a foreign body inflammatory response, and diffuse infiltration of foamy macrophages, histiocytes, and multinucleated foreign body giant cells. Birefringent particles can be identified under polarized light.

QUESTIONS

16 The greatest volumetric wear and the greatest mean volumetric wear of polyethylene are seen with what size femoral head?

17 When compared with a femoral stem with a low modulus of elasticity, how will a stem with higher modulus affect stress in the stem and in the cement?

18 A 75-year-old otherwise healthy man with osteoarthritis of the hip requires total hip arthroplasty. What is the preferred technique for component fixation?

19 What are considered increased risk categories for heterotopic ossification after total hip replacement? What is the most effective postoperative adjuvant method recommended to decrease the risk of heterotopic bone in high risk patient undergoing total hip arthroplasty?

20 A 65-year-old otherwise healthy man complains of pain 5 years after successful hybrid (uncemented acetabulum and cemented femur) total hip arthroplasty. Radiographic films demonstrate circumferential lucency around the femoral component, and hip aspirate yields methicillin-sensitive staph aureus. What method of management is preferred?

21 What factors are associated with sciatic nerve palsy after total hip arthroplasty?

ANSWERS

16 The 32-mm head is associated with the greatest volumetric wear and mean volumetric wear. The 28-mm head is associated with the least rate of linear wear, whereas the 22-mm head is associated with the greatest mean rate of linear wear.

17 A femoral component of higher modulus of elasticity will increase stresses in the stem and decrease stresses in the cement.

18 A cemented femoral component is considered most appropriate in this age group. A noncemented metal-backed acetabular component is preferred over a cemented metal-backed acetabulum. A cemented all-poly acetabulum is appropriate for the less active older patient.

ANSWERS

19 The increased risk categories for development of postoperative heterotopic ossification include ankylosing spondylitis, diffuse idiopathic skeletal hyperostosis (DISH syndrome), the patient undergoing revision surgery, the patient with ectopic bone formation on the contralateral hip and male osteoarthritics with extensive osteophyte formation. Postoperative adjuvant methods advocated to reduce the risk of ectopic bone in the high risk patient are low-dose radiation, diphophonates, and NSAIDs. The most effective form of treatment is low-dose radiation administered within a few days of the arthroplasty procedure. If uncemented arthroplasty has been used, the areas of potential bone ingrowth should be shielded. The major disadvantage of this technique is the concern over using ionizing radiation in a patient without a malignancy. Reports on the use of diphosphonates have been mixed regarding efficacy. Although diphosphonates inhibit mineralization, there is no evidence that diphosphonates inhibit the formation of osteoid matrix. Mineralization of the matrix occurs when the diphosphonate is discontinued. NSAIDs have been found to be effective; however, disadvantages include patient compliance and the potential adverse pharmacologic effect on the bone prosthesis interface in uncemented bone ingrowth arthroplasty.

20 The lowest rates of recurrence are achieved with removal of the prosthesis and all cement, débridement of devitalized tissue, and treatment with 6 weeks of antibiotics achieving a minimum postpeak serum bacteriocidal level of 1:8 against the infecting organism. If bone stock and soft tissues are adequate and if the patient is appropriate for rehabilitation, a reimplantation is recommended. The use of antibiotic cement during reimplantation should be considered. The rate of recurrence of infection after one-stage reimplantation is higher than that of two-stage reimplantation and is not generally recommended in this clinical setting. Candidates for a one-stage procedure are those in whom the infection is early, the infecting organism is sensitive to intravenous antibiotics, and the treating antibiotic is one that can be added to the cement without loss of efficacy. Antibiotic suppression is generally reserved for the debilitated and severely medically compromised patient; girdlestone arthroplasty without reimplantation is reserved for failures of therapy, for the person with inadequate bone stock, or for the debilitated individual who is not a candidate for rehabilitation.

21 Factors found to increase the risk of sciatic nerve palsy include revision hip surgery, total hip replacement for congenital dislocation of the hip, lengthening of the femur greater than two centimeters in the patient with long-standing shortening, postoperative hematoma, and postoperative hip dislocation.

QUESTIONS

22   Acetabular revision in a patient with adequate bone stock is usually best accomplished by what technique?

23   What is the most important surgical factor associated with recurrent sepsis after removal of a hip prosthesis because of infection?

ANSWERS

22 An uncemented acetabular component is usually the most effective technique. Peripherally threaded acetabular cups have been found to have a high rate of loosening and migration, and a bipolar prosthesis has not been effective in follow-up evaluations. Metal-backed cemented acetabular components have been associated with a high rate of loosening. Cemented polyethylene acetabular components have been associated with increased rates of loosening.

23 Retained cement at the time of initial débridement is the most important surgical factor.

QUESTION

24 An uncemented hip arthroplasty was performed, and minutes after placement of the acetabular component with anterior superior screws the patient became profoundly hypotensive. What is the most likely etiology of hypotension?

ANSWER

24 Injury to iliac vessels from screw penetration is a concern when hypotension accompanies screw placement in the anterosuperior region of the acetabulum. The external iliac vein is in close proximity to the anterior cortex of the acetabulum at the level of the acetabular dome. The external iliac artery is anterior and lateral to the vein at this level and may be found within 1.5 cm of the anterior acetabular wall. Injury to the obturator vessels may occur with screw penetration in the anteroinferior quadrant of the acetabulum. The obturator vein is within 0.3 cm at the level of the inferior quadrilateral surface of the acetabulum. Treatment of hypotension secondary to injury of pelvic vasculature is managed by identification and repair of the lacerated structures. A retroperitoneal approach may be necessary. (*Figures 6-2A, 6-2B, 6-2C, and 6-2D*)

ANSWER

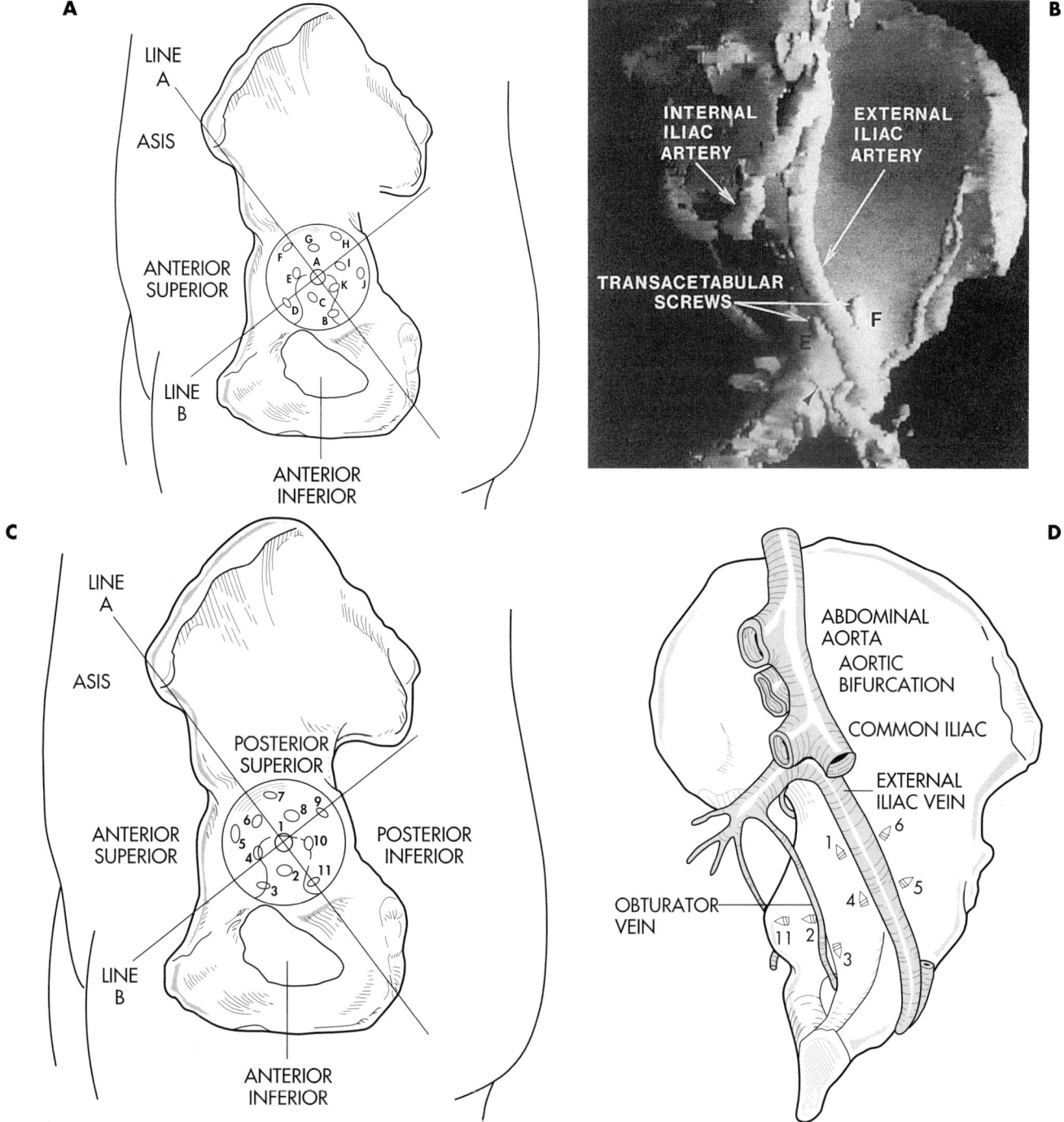

Fig 6-2 Data obtained from the transacetabular placement of screws in a cadaver, with use of arterial opacification: **A**. Schematic drawing showing the acetabular origin of the screws (labeled A through K). ASIS = anterior superior iliac spine. **B**. Three-dimensional reconstruction of a computed tomographic scan showing the location of excessively long screws on the quadrilateral intrapelvic surface relative to the iliac arterial system. Screws E and F are near the external iliac artery; their acetabular origin is the anterior superior quadrant (see A). Data obtained from the transacetabular placement of screws in a cadaver, with use of venous opacification: **C**. Schematic diagram showing the acetabular origin of screws (numbered 1 through 11). ASIS = anterior superior iliac spine. **D**. Schematic diagram showing the location of the screws on the quadrilateral intrapelvic surface relative to the iliac venous system. Screws 1, 4, 5, and 6 are near the external iliac vein; their acetabular origin is the anterior superior quadrant (see C). Screws 2 and 3 are near the obturator vein; their acetabular origin is the anterior inferior quadrant (see C).

QUESTIONS

25 What are the four modes of femoral stem failure? What mode is most often associated with femoral stem fracture? Where, along the stem, is the usual origin of the stem fracture?

26 What is the leading cause of revision in most series of total knee arthroplasty?

27 Five years after total knee arthroplasty a 55-year-old woman complains of pain on ambulation. Radiographic films demonstrate a large cystic area of bone loss in the medial femoral condyle. The patient has no complaints of pain at rest and is not awakened at night with pain. The patient's ESR is 2 mm, her white blood cell (WBC) count is 6.2, and aspiration of the joint reveals no growth on culture, and the fluid is clear. What is the most likely explanation for the radiographic findings? (*Figures 6-4A and 6-4B.*)

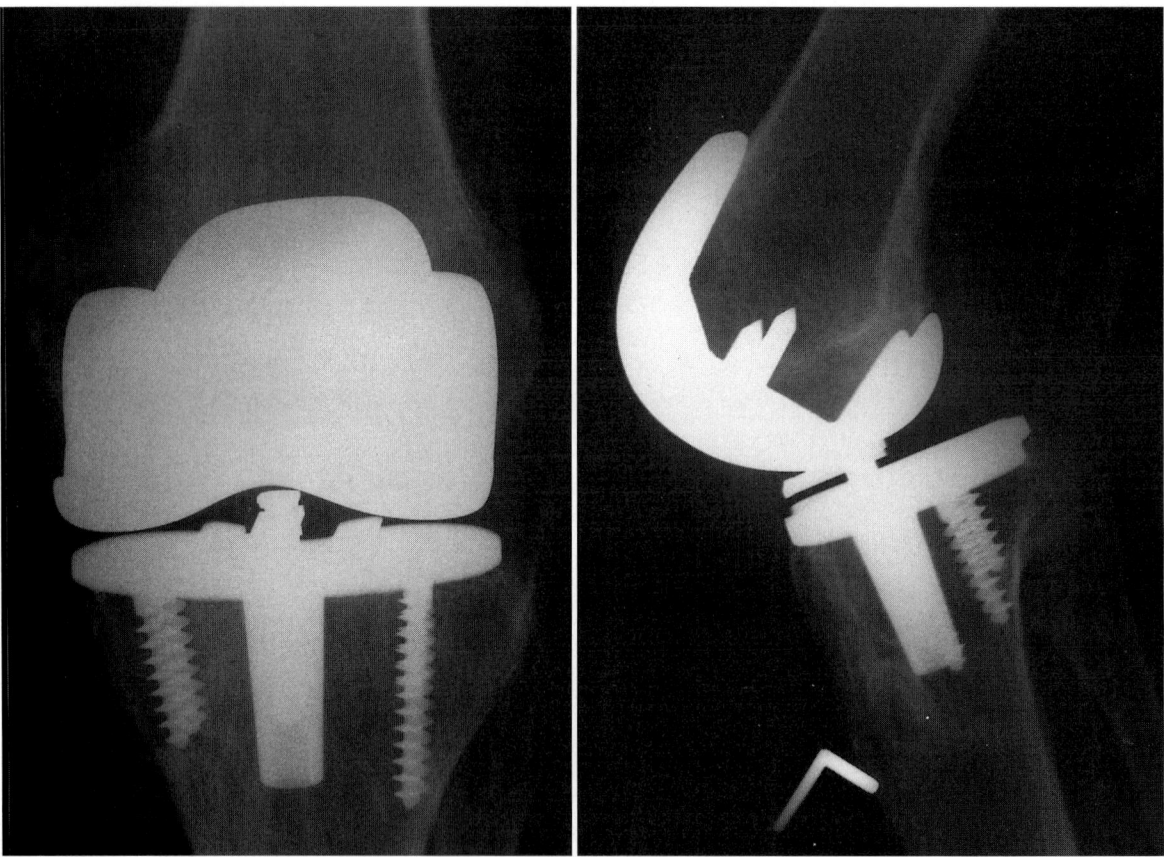

Fig 6-4 **A**   Fig 6-4 **B**

28 A 58-year-old man had an uncemented total knee arthroplasty 4 years ago. He complains of pain with ambulation, and radiographic films demonstrate a 1- to 2-mm lucency beneath the entire baseplate of the tibial component. Laboratory evaluation reveals an ESR of 2 mm, WBC of 6.3, and aspirate reveals no growth, and the fluid is clear. What is the most likely explanation for the findings?

ANSWERS

25 The modes of failure are pistoning of the stem within cement or bone, medial midstem pivot, calcar pivot, and bending cantilever (fatigue). Bending cantilever is most often associated with femoral stem fracture. The anterolateral corner of the stem at its middle third is the usual initial site of stem failure. Femoral stem fracture is more often seen in the heavy, active patient with varus stem positioning without proximal cement or bony support. This complication was seen with stainless steel components and is now only rarely seen with newer alloy femoral components. (*Figure 6-3*)

Fig 6-3

I	**Ia**	PISTONING: STEM WITHIN CEMENT	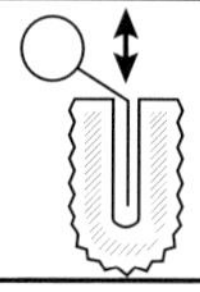
	Ib	PISTONING: STEM WITHIN BONE	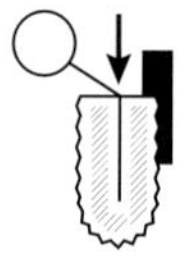
II		MEDIAL MIDSTEM PIVOT	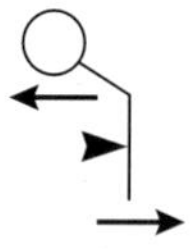
III		CALCAR PIVOT	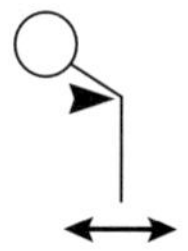
IV		BENDING CANTILEVER (FATIGUE)	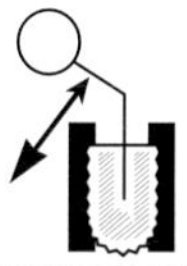

26 Patellar failure is the leading cause of revision.

27 Osteolysis, which has occurred as a response to polyethylene wear debris, is the most likely explanation.

28 Failure of bone ingrowth with micromotion of the tibial component is the most likely explanation.

QUESTIONS

29 What is the benefit of continuous passive motion (CPM) in patients undergoing total knee replacements (TKR)?

30 What is the major determinant of postoperative knee flexion in condylar total knee arthroplasty?

31 What is the major determinant of failure leading to revision after high tibial osteotomy for medial gonarthrosis?

32 What are the risk factors associated with infection after total knee replacement arthroplasty?

33 A 65-year-old otherwise healthy man complains of acute pain 7 years after cemented total knee arthroplasty. Examination of the knee reveals a warm swollen knee that is painful on range of motion. Laboratory evaluation reveals an ESR of 100 mm/hr and a WBC count of 10,000, and a joint culture on aspirate reveals staphylococcus aureus. Radiographic films reveal a lucent line beneath the tibial and femoral components. What is the best management of this problem?

34 What preoperative knee deformity is most commonly associated with postoperative peroneal nerve palsy after total knee arthroplasty?

35 A 66-year-old man complains of pain 2 weeks after cemented total knee arthroplasty. An examination demonstrates a warm swollen knee. Aspirate of the knee reveals a gram-positive organism, and culture shows beta-hemolytic streptococcus. Radiographic films reveal an absence of lucent lines beneath the tibial or femoral components. Describe the management of this problem.

ANSWERS

29 Controlled evaluations have shown that CPM results in a decreased rate of manipulation to achieve motion. There is no evidence that CPM results in increased motion or in increased quadricep strength at long-term follow-up. Hospital stay is also not decreased.

30 Preoperative knee flexion is the major determinant of postoperative knee flexion. This has been found to be more of a determinant than the use of CPM, the use of a cruciate retaining rather than cruciate sacrificing prosthesis, or preoperative or postoperative knee alignment.

ANSWERS

31 Postoperative limb alignment is the major determining factor. The clinical results of high tibial osteotomy for medial gonarthrosis are more dependent on postoperative rather than on preoperative limb alignment. Postoperative limb alignment has been found to correlate more closely with outcome than arthroscopic findings at the time of osteotomy, range of motion of the knee at the time of osteotomy, choice of fixation of the osteotomy, and patient sex or age at the time of osteotomy.

32 In a large series of total knee arthroplasties performed at one institution, the risk of infection was increased significantly in the patient with rheumatoid arthritis, in the patient who had undergone a previous operation of the knee, and in the patient with skin ulcers. A statistically significant correlation was not found with obesity, recurrent urinary tract infection, or use of oral steroids; however, infection occurred more often in association with these conditions. A second series of total knee arthroplasties were evaluated, and the risk of infection in this series was increased with the use of hinged arthroplasty, a diagnosis of rheumatoid arthritis, and a history of previous surgical procedures excluding arthroscopy.

33 Removal of components, 6 weeks of intravenous antibiotics, and delayed reimplantation of the components with antibiotics in the cement is the best management if there is no evidence of continued infection. The time interval to reimplantation is controversial with the most usual recommendations ranging from 3 to 6 weeks. If an organism is unusually resistant to antibiotics, reimplantation is delayed. Débridement with retention of components is best used with infection in the early perioperative period if the components are well fixed and the infecting organism is easily identified and treated.

34 Preoperative valgus and flexion deformities are most associated with postoperative peroneal nerve palsy.

35 Irrigation and débridement of the knee, retention of components, and intravenous antibiotics is the best management option for this scenario. Removal of all components, 6 weeks of antibiotics, and reimplantation at 6 weeks or later is probably not necessary because the infecting organism is very sensitive to antibiotics. There are no lucencies beneath the implant (indicating a stable implant), and the infection is treated soon after implantation.

QUESTIONS

36 How does the mechanical axis of the lower limb differ from the anatomic axis of the lower limb? What is the average angle between the anatomic axis and mechanical axis in men and women?

37 Through what compartment does the majority of the load pass in the normal knee?

38 What are the characteristics of an ideal candidate for a valgus producing high tibial osteotomy?

39 A 55-year-old woman complains of knee pain, and examination demonstrates a genu valgus deformity of 18°. Radiographic films primarily show lateral compartment disease and minimal tibial deformity. If an osteotomy is considered, what is the procedure of choice? Is arthroscopic débridement at the time of osteotomy an effective adjunct to the procedure?

40 A 55-year-old overweight man complains of knee pain with activity; radiographic films demonstrate mild to moderate medial compartment disease. There are no symptoms compatible with a meniscal pathologic condition. What is the most appropriate initial management?

ANSWERS

36 The mechanical axis of the normal limb passes through the center of the femoral head, just medial to the center of the knee and center of the tibial plafond, whereas the anatomic axis passes through the midshaft of the femur and the midshaft of the tibia. The average angle between the anatomic axis and mechanical axis in men is 5° of valgus; in women it is 7° of valgus. (*Figure 6-5*)

ANSWERS

Fig 6-5

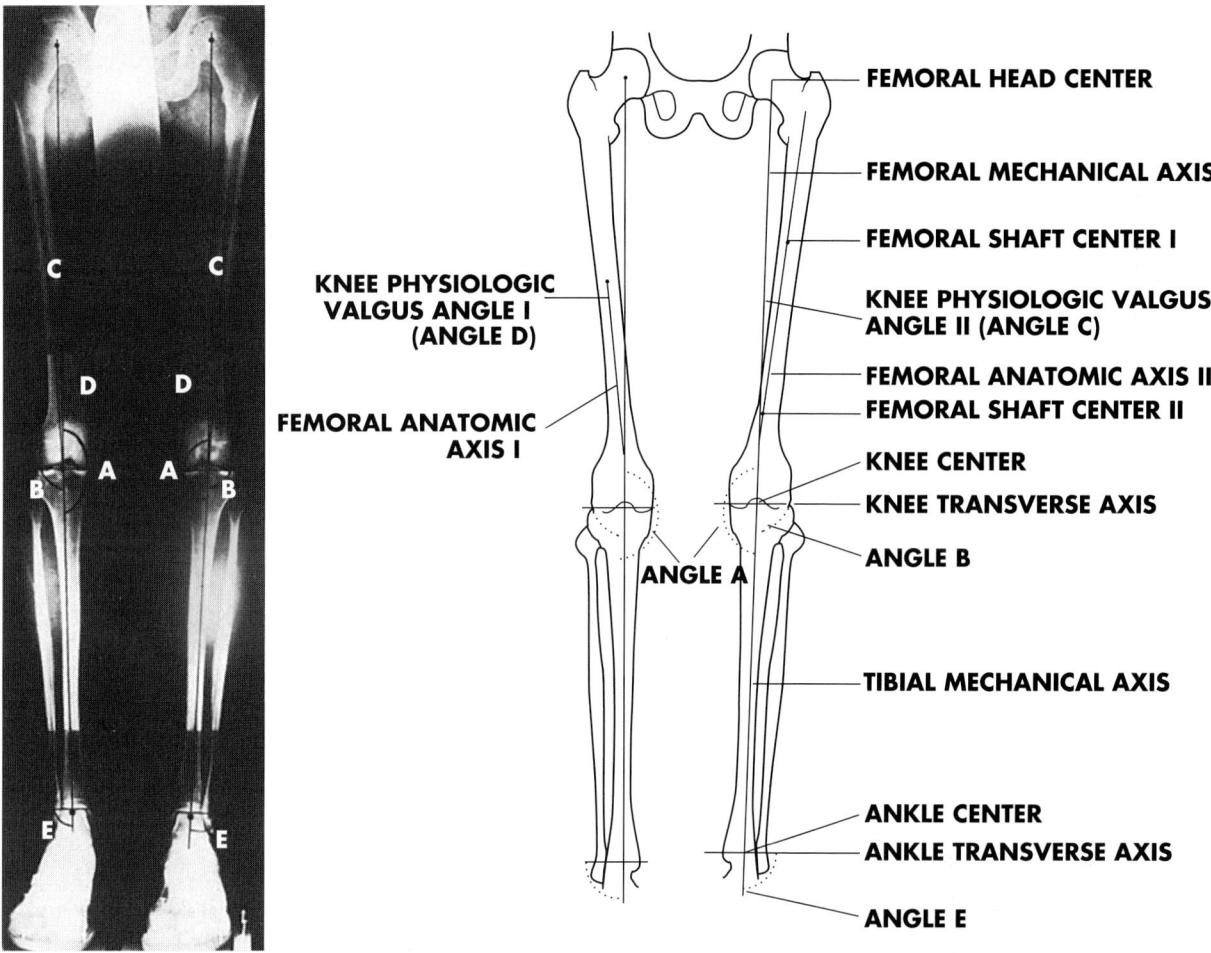

37 Sixty percent of the load passes through the medial compartment.

38 An ideal candidate should be less than 60 years of age, have primarily medial compartment disease, have a flexion arc of at least 90°, and have a flexion contracture of less than 15°. Contraindications include inflammatory arthritis, multicompartmental disease, significant tibial subluxation, and active infection.

39 A varus producing distal femoral osteotomy rather than a high tibial osteotomy is the procedure of choice. If the femorotibial axis is greater than 12 to 15° or if the plane of the joint deviates from the horizontal by more than 10°, a distal femoral osteotomy should be performed rather than a proximal tibial osteotomy. The goal of osteotomy should be a femorotibial angle of 0 to 2° of valgus. Arthroscopic debridement at the time of osteotomy has not been shown to be an effective adjunct.

40 NSAIDs, activity modification, and weight reduction is the most appropriate initial management option.

QUESTIONS

41 A peroneal nerve palsy is noted postoperatively in the recovery room following an uncomplicated total knee arthroplasty. What is the most appropriate initial management?

42 What factors are associated with patellar instability after total knee replacement?

43 An arthrodesis of the knee should be accomplished in what position?

44 What are the differences in infection and loosening rates in constrained knee designs when compared with an unconstrained prosthetic design?

45 Six years after cemented total knee replacement a 65-year-old man complains of anterior knee pain after a fall. Radiographic films demonstrate a patella fracture with 2 mm of displacement and with no obvious loosening of the patellar button. The patient exhibits active knee extension. What is the best initial management of this fracture?

46 A 40-year-old man has failed nonoperative therapy for tricompartmental degenerative arthritis of his knee. He has a history of an inability to actively extend his knee secondary to gross quadriceps weakness; however, he has full passive extension of his knee, and he currently wears a knee brace. He desires operative therapy. What is the best option at this point? Is constrained or unconstrained total knee arthroplasty a useful option?

47 What are the benefits of open synovectomy of the knee in the patient with rheumatoid arthritis?

48 Five years after total knee arthroplasty with a cemented total knee replacement and cemented metal-backed patella, a 65-year-old man complains of pain, swelling, and patellar crepitation on range of motion of his knee. Aspiration of the knee reveals dark debris, and radiographic films reveal patellar tilt. What is the most likely explanation of this patient's problem?

ANSWERS

41 Flexion of the knee and removal of compressive dressings is the most appropriate initial management option. Peroneal nerve palsy is usually associated with correction of the knee with a preoperative flexion and valgus deformity. This complication occurs in less than 3% of cases and has also been associated with external compression, com-

ANSWERS

pression secondary to a hematoma, and intraoperative traction. Initial management should include flexion of the knee and removal of compressive dressings. In one study only 35% of patients with an initial complete palsy recovered completely, whereas 84% of patients with a partial peroneal nerve palsy recovered completely.

42   The factors are excessive internal rotation of the femoral component, excessive internal rotation of the tibial component, and preoperative valgus limb alignment.

43   Position is 10 to 15° of flexion and 5 to 10° of valgus.

44   When compared with unconstrained designs, a constrained knee prosthesis has increased loosening and infection rates.

45   Nonoperative treatment in an extension orthosis for 6 weeks followed by range of motion is the best initial management option. In most clinical situations revision of the patellar component is reserved for failure of nonoperative management, displacement of the patellar component, or loss of extensor mechanism function.

46   Arthrodesis is the best surgical option because of this patient's gross quadriceps weakness. Contraindications to total knee arthroplasty generally include active sepsis, a neuropathic joint, gross quadriceps insufficiency, and a painless, well functioning arthrodesis. A constrained total knee arthroplasty in this clinical setting would not produce a functional knee.

47   The benefits of open synovectomy of the knee in rheumatoid arthritis include diminished pain and swelling and no change or slight decrease in range of motion of the knee. There is usually no increase in range of motion postoperatively, and there is no appreciable prevention of joint deterioration.

48   Failure of the patellar polyethylene with an exposed metal backing is the most likely explanation. Failure of metal-backed patellar components has been reported with multiple patellar designs and is associated with wear of the polyethylene, where it is most thin at the edge of the prosthesis. This failure is followed by fracture and dissociation of the polyethylene with exposure of the metal backing. An exposed metal backing articulating with a metallic femoral prosthesis produces wear debris and a metallic synovitis. In most patients the clinical onset of failure is dramatic with the onset of pain, swelling, and a sensation of grating. Several current designs have attempted to solve this potential problem by implanting the metal backing in patellar bone. Using a cemented all-poly patella avoids this particular complication.

QUESTIONS

49 What is the most appropriate treatment in a patient with failure of a metal-backed patella?

50 What clinical and surgical factors are associated with periprosthetic fractures of the femur after total knee arthroplasty?

51 What is the most important factor influencing the union rate of knee arthrodesis after failed, infected total knee arthroplasty?

52 In terms of morbidity and mortality, what is the difference of bilateral simultaneous total knee arthroplasty when compared with staged bilateral total knee arthroplasty performed during separate hospitalizations?

53 When considering a total knee arthroplasty, how are contact stresses between the femoral component and polyethylene reduced?

54 A 68-year-old active, healthy woman with genu valgum and osteoarthritis underwent total knee replacement. Follow-up standing radiographic films performed 6 months postoperatively demonstrated genu valgum and a widened medial joint space. The patient complains of a feeling of instability with ambulation. Examination demonstrates two to three plus medial laxity and no lateral laxity. The components are in appropriate orientation. What is the best solution for this problem?

55 In performing a total knee arthroplasty, what structures are surgically released to correct for:
A.   Valgus deformity
B.   Varus deformity
C.   Flexion deformity

ANSWERS

49 The most appropriate treatment is revision patellar arthroplasty with removal of the patellar component, placement of a cemented all-polyethylene patellar component, a thorough synovectomy, and a revision of the femoral component if the wear is severe. It is important to correct any patellar malalignment that might have contributed to patellar maltracking. The rotational alignment of the tibial and femoral components should be assessed.

ANSWERS

50 Osteoporosis, notching of the femoral cortex, revision knee arthroplasty, and stress risers from screw holes are factors associated with periprosthetic fractures. One case reports of a supracondylar femur fracture that occurred in an uncemented total knee arthroplasty associated with a large polyethylene wear-induced osteolytic defect in the femur.

51 The extent of bone loss before knee arthrodesis has been found to be the most important factor. The presence of active infection does not preclude union.

52 There is no statistically significant difference in terms of morbidity and mortality. The bilateral simultaneous procedure is more cost effective.

53 Increasing the thickness of the polyethylene and use of a more conforming femorotibial articulation, particularly in the medial-lateral direction, will reduce contact stresses between the femoral component and polyethylene and will reduce stress in the polyethylene. Polyethylene thickness of 6 to 8 mm has been recommended to reduce polyethylene wear. Use of carbon fiber reinforced polyethylene is not effective in reducing stress and wear.

54 Reoperation with lateral release, attainment of equal and symmetric flexion, and extension gaps and revision of components, if necessary, is the best solution. Use of a more constrained prosthesis to correct for ligamentous laxity without addressing alignment and flexion and extension gaps is of limited effectiveness.

55 **A.** For a fixed valgus deformity, the lateral capsule is incised followed by release of the lateral collateral ligament and popliteus tendon from the lateral condyle of the femur. Alignment is reassessed; if this is not sufficient, release of the iliotibial band is performed. Posterior capsule release is performed if additional release is necessary.
B. A varus deformity is addressed by releasing contracted medial structures. Medial osteophytes are removed, and medial soft tissues consisting of capsule, superficial medial collateral ligament, and insertion of pes anserinus are lifted as a flap from the medial surface of the tibia. If additional correction is necessary, the posterior capsule and semimembranosus insertion can be released.
C. A flexion deformity is addressed by excision of an additional few millimeters of distal femur, and if this is inadequate to correct the deformity the cruciates and posterior capsule are released. The posterior capsule is released with a transverse incision in the capsule under direct visualization.

QUESTIONS

56 In performing a total knee arthroplasty on a knee with very limited flexion, what procedures can be performed intraoperatively to enhance flexion, and limit risk of patellar tendon avulsion?

57 After initial bone cuts have been made for a total knee arthroplasty, the flexion gap is larger than the extension gap. How is this corrected?

58 When performing a revision total knee arthroplasty, a 15-mm distal femoral bony defect is encountered. What are the most appropriate management options for this problem?

59 In what hip position do dislocations occur after an anterior approach in total hip arthroplasty? After a posterior approach?

60 In total hip replacement, what acetabular placement results in a reduction of hip joint contact forces? What effect does an increased femoral shaft-neck angle have on peak joint load?

ANSWERS

56 Exposure is enhanced by performing a rectus snip, a quadriceps turndown, or by performing an osteotomy of the tibial tubercle. A rectus snip is performed by making an oblique incision in the quadriceps tendon at the most proximal extent of the usual incision in the quadriceps tendon. This incision from distal-medial to proximal-lateral extends the incision and relaxes the lateral tissues, enhancing knee flexion and exposure. Repair is not necessary if an adequate repair of the remaining quadriceps tendon and medial tissues is performed. The quadriceps turndown is performed by incising the quadriceps tendon obliquely proximal-medial to distal-lateral, in line with the usual lateral retinacular release. Repair of the quadriceps tendon to vastus lateralis is performed along with the repair of medial structures. The lateral retinacular release is often left open. An osteotomy of the tibial tubercle is made by osteotomizing from medial to lateral a 2- to 3-inch by 3/4- to 7/8-inch fragment of bone, which is levered laterally. The lateral soft tissues are not incised to enhance vascularity. Repair is performed by using screws, wires, or staples as necessary.

57 Resection of appropriate additional distal femoral bone would correct this surgical problem. This problem would not be addressed by resection of additional tibial bone since both gaps would be altered. Ligament balancing by further ligament release of medial and lateral soft tissues with the knee extended would result in larger flexion and extension gaps.

58 Appropriate management options include the use of an augmented femoral component to replace the 15 mm of bone loss or the use of a bone graft. Using a cement column to replace the defect is much less common because of the increasing sophistication of current implants. Placement of the femoral component at the level of the femoral defect with resection of less tibia and the use of a thicker polyethylene is not recommended because of the alteration of patellar mechanics and the creation of patella baja.

59 Extension and external rotation put the hip at risk for dislocation in an anterior approach. Flexion and internal rotation put the hip at risk in a posterior approach.

60 The location of the hip center is the most important factor affecting loads on the hip joint. Placement of the center of the acetabulum medially, inferiorly, and anteriorly as possible in the pelvis results in the greatest reduction in hip joint contact force. An increased femoral shaft-neck angle increases peak joint load secondary to loss of abductor muscle moment arm.

QUESTIONS

61   What is the relationship between stem cross-sectional shape and stresses in the cement for cemented total hip arthroplasty?

62   When considering a porous coated implant for total hip arthroplasty, what is the most important factor for maximizing bone ingrowth into porous surfaces?

ANSWERS

61   Stems with a broad medial surface and a broader lateral surface have the most desirable compressive and tensile stress distributions. Stem cross sections with a small anteroposterior dimension result in large cement compressive stresses. Stems with a narrow lateral anteroposterior dimension result in higher cement tensile stresses. (*Figures 6-6A and 6-6B*)

ANSWERS

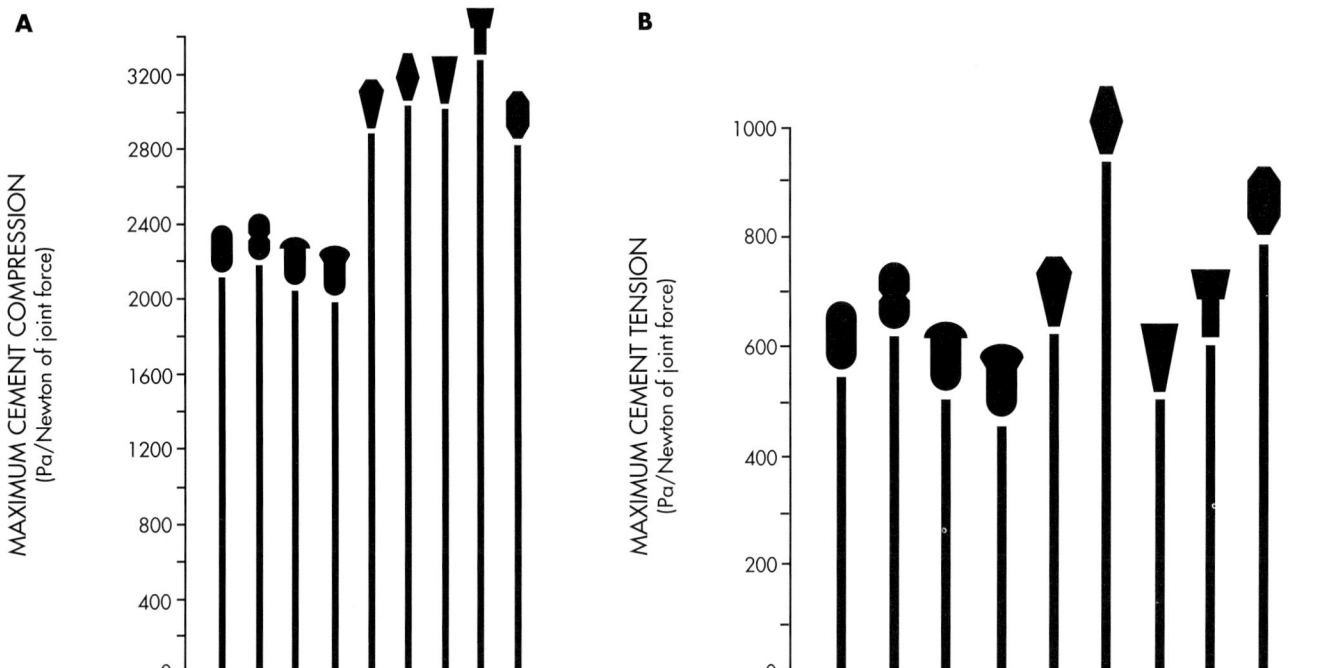

Fig 6-6 **A.** Maximum cement compression (principal stress) resulting from varus stem cross-sectional shapes. Predicted stresses are within the most proximal portion of the structure and result from a one-Newton joint load. **B.** Maximum cement tension (principal stress) resulting from varus stem cross-sectional shapes. Predicted stresses are within the most proximal portion of the structure and result from a one-Newton joint load.

62 The achievement of initial stability between implant and bone is critical and the most important factor for maximizing bone ingrowth. The exact threshold of relative motion for osseous ingrowth has not been determined; however, fibrous fixation has been reported with more than 150 micrometers of motion. The optimal pore size for bone ingrowth into porous surfaces ranges from 100 to 400 micrometers. Short-term enhancement of fixation has been shown to occur with applications of calcium-phosphate to the substrate; however, the appropriate clinical application is still being investigated. The use of autogenous bone graft for routine primary uncemented arthroplasty is not necessary to maximize bone ingrowth.

QUESTIONS

63 When considering total hip arthroplasty for congenital dislocation of the hip, what preoperative prosthetic considerations are important for successful arthroplasty. What complications are increased when compared with routine total hip arthroplasty?

64 An immediate postoperative lucency seen at the cement bone interface in a cemented femoral revision of a previously failed cemented total hip replacement is most likely caused by what?

65 What principles govern the choice of skin incision when revising a multiply operated knee? What attention should be directed to develop skin flaps in this clinical situation?

66 What are the usual pathologic features identified in a symptomatic valgus knee?

67 What are the surgical options for a symptomatic valgus knee with degenerative arthritis?

ANSWERS

63 In the patient with congenital dislocation of the hip, the acetabulum is hypoplastic, the femoral neck is short and anteverted, and a false acetabulum is usually present at the ilium where the femoral head has articulated. Acetabular bone stock may be deficient, particularly along the anterior column. Since bone stock is limited, a small acetabular component should be used, and a 22- or 26-mm head should be chosen to allow for sufficient polyethylene. To permit reduction of the hip after placement of the acetabular component, a femoral osteotomy may be required. An osteotomy performed in the subtrochanteric area will permit correction of excessive femoral anteversion and excessive femoral length. Deformity of the proximal femur may require use of a custom femoral component, and a narrow straight femur may require use of a very narrow femoral implant. Complications of dislocation and sciatic nerve palsy are increased relative to routine total hip replacement.

ANSWERS

64 The lack of cement intrusion into femoral diaphyseal bone is the likely cause. Cemented revision has a higher failure rate when done for a failed cemented total hip replacement because of the lack of intrusion of cement into bone at the time of placement of the component. A lucent line at the cement bone interface is an indication of the lack of microinterlock.

65 Use a preexisting incision whenever possible. The most laterally placed anterior skin incision should be selected when multiple incisions exist in a previously operated knee. Skin necrosis is most likely to occur when a parallel incision is made medial to a previous lateral incision. Usually a well-healed transverse incision can be crossed. A previous direct lateral incision used for collateral ligament repair may be ignored. Where possible, a long anterior incision is generally considered best. Care should be taken to minimize flap dissection and to develop full thickness skin flaps where skin flap dissection is necessary.

66 The usual pathologic findings are contracted lateral structures, which include the lateral and posterolateral capsule, lateral collateral ligament, popliteus, and iliotibial band. The biceps femoris and lateral intermuscular septum may be contracted as well. The medial structures are often attenuated and include the medial capsule and medial collateral ligament. The lateral femoral condyle is often hypoplastic.

67 Arthroscopic débridement is a consideration for minor unicompartmental disease, particularly when mechanical symptoms are present. As expected, the clinical results deteriorate with time, and additional procedures are often required. Osteotomies considered are a varus-producing high tibial osteotomy, a distal femoral varus osteotomy, and a combined distal femoral-proximal tibial osteotomy. The combined osteotomy is appropriate when the projected femoral osteotomy would produce an excessively oblique joint line. Arthroplasty options consist of a unicompartmental arthroplasty or total joint replacement. A hemiarthroplasty is often considered in the patient with unicompartmental degenerative or posttraumatic disease. The patient with inflammatory arthritis or arthritis secondary to hemochromatosis, hemophilia, or chondrocalcinosis is not a candidate. The most suitable candidate for unicompartmental replacement is a thin and relatively sedentary individual that has a knee examination that is without excessive collateral ligament laxity and in whom the valgus can be corrected passively. Total knee arthroplasty is an excellent option in the older, sedentary, symptomatic individual.

QUESTIONS

68   What are the mechanical advantages of ceramic in total hip arthroplasty? What are the disadvantages?

69   What is the treatment of hip dislocation following total hip arthroplasty?

70   What risk factors are associated with thromboembolic disease?

71   What is the most common cause of death in the patient undergoing total hip or knee arthroplasty?

72   What are the current recommendations for prophylaxis of venous thrombosis or thromboembolism in the patient undergoing total hip or knee arthroplasty?

73   What are contraindications to distal femoral osteotomy for the treatment of osteoarthritis and genu valgum deformity?

ANSWERS

68   The advantages are low coefficient of friction and high resistance to wear when ceramic is used as a bearing surface. The low frictional properties reduce volumetric wear in total hip arthroplasty. Ceramic acetabular components have not been uniformly successful. Threaded acetabular designs have largely been a failure. Excessive strain may lead to fracture of the ceramic head.

69   The hip is reduced under general or intravenous sedation. Open reduction is indicated for failure of closed reduction. Placement of the patient in a hip spica or abduction brace for 6 weeks may be indicated. Patient education is an important adjunct to treatment. Recurrent dislocations may be treated by revision arthroplasty, trochanteric advancement, or, in extreme cases, use of a more constrained acetabular component. At the time of revision arthroplasty, component malposition, if present, should be corrected, and soft tissues should be balanced through appropriate neck length and component choice (use of more component offset). The hip should be evaluated for impingement of the prosthetic neck at the range-of-motion extremes. Sepsis must be ruled out in cases of recurrent dislocation. Trochanteric avulsion, if present, should be repaired if possible.

ANSWERS

70 Three general categories of risk factors attributed to Virchow are venous stasis, injury, and hypercoagulability.

Associated with venous stasis are heart failure, immobility, and previous thrombosis. Obesity is considered by some to be a secondary risk factor. Endothelial injury is attendant with many orthopedic procedures and orthopedic trauma. Hypercoagulable states are associated with adenocarcinoma, any congenital or acquired deficiencies of endogenous anticoagulant proteins (including antithrombin 111 and heparin cofactor 11), and congenital abnormalities or deficiencies of plasminogen or fibrinogen.

There is a significant association of venous thromboembolism and the patient undergoing total hip or total knee replacement. If prophylaxis is not used, deep vein thrombosis has been documented to occur in 40% to 60% of patients undergoing total hip or knee arthroplasty. Prolonged venous stasis and endothelial injury are associated with intraoperative limb positioning in total hip arthroplasty. Venous stasis and potential venous endothelial injury are associated with use of the thigh tourniquet and with intraoperative manipulation in the patient undergoing total knee arthroplasty.

71 Pulmonary embolism is the most common cause of death.

72 Low-dose warfarin, adjusted-dose heparin, and low–molecular-weight heparins are considered to be effective prophylaxis for the patient undergoing total hip arthroplasty. Dextran is also effective but is associated with risks of volume overload, bleeding, hypersensitivity reactions, and a relatively higher cost. Aspirin has not been an effective prophylaxis in the setting of total hip arthroplasty.

Effective regimens in the patient undergoing total knee arthroplasty include low-dose warfarin and low–molecular-weight heparin. Pneumatic compression boots are effective in reducing the incidence of proximal venous clots and pulmonary emboli in the setting of total knee arthroplasty. Dextran has not been thoroughly investigated for total knee arthroplasty, and the efficacy of aspirin is questionable.

73 Contraindications to supracondylar femoral osteotomy generally include severe ligamentous instability, a flexion contracture exceeding 30°, significant involvement of the medial compartment, and a flexion arc of less than 80°.

QUESTIONS

74 A 40-year-old active man with posttraumatic ankle arthritis and severe pain with activity has failed nonoperative therapy and desires a total ankle arthroplasty. What considerations are important in determining the treatment of this patient?

75 What are the goals of ankle arthrodesis? In what position should the ankle be fused?

76 What nonoperative options should be considered in a patient with posttraumatic ankle arthritis?

77 Describe the primary vascular supply to the hip.

78 True or false, in adults the artery within the ligamentum teres provides a significant blood supply to the femoral head?

79 Describe the capsular attachments of the hip joint onto the femoral neck.

80 What is the calcar femorale?

ANSWERS

74 This patient is a poor candidate for total ankle arthroplasty because of the high rate of failure for this age group and activity level. Failed previous arthroplasty, avascular necrosis, prior arthrodesis, inadequate peripheral circulation, ankle ligamentous instability, or poor skin coverage are also contraindications for total ankle arthroplasty. The most appropriate candidate for total ankle replacement is the patient with rheumatoid arthritis or the occasional older posttraumatic arthritis patient.

Ankle arthrodesis is the most appropriate definitive procedure for this patient. The majority of patients have relief of pain postoperatively. A satisfactory gait pattern can usually be achieved if the patient has normal subtalar motion and proper alignment of the fused ankle.

75 The fundamental goals of ankle arthrodesis are to achieve painless ankle and a plantigrade foot. The usual position of fusion is neutral flexion, 0 to 5° of valgus and external rotation of the foot equal to the opposite foot (usually 5 to 10°).

76 Alternatives to surgical therapy include use of NSAIDs if there are no contraindications, intraarticular injection with corticosteroids, and modifications of shoe wear. Effective foot wear modifications include use of a rocker bottom sole and a double upright brace.

77 The profunda femoris divides into the medial and lateral femoral circumflex arteries. The ascending branch of the lateral circumflex artery and the medial circumflex artery form an extracapsular ring at the base of the femoral neck. This ring gives rise to ascending cervical arteries that transverse the femoral neck proximally to form a second ring at the base of the femoral head. Branches from this second ring penetrate the femoral head and provide its primary blood supply.

78 False. In adults the artery within the ligamentum teres has only a limited role in providing blood supply to the femoral head.

79 Anteriorly, the capsule attaches to the femoral neck at the intertrochanteric line; posteriorly, the capsule attaches to the midportion of the femoral neck.

80 The calcar femorale is a vertical wall of dense bone that forms an internal strut within the inferior portion of the femoral neck and intertrochanteric region. It is an important conduit for stress transfer in this area.

QUESTIONS

81 What is an acetabular depression fracture?

82 When is the optimum timing for surgical treatment of a hip fracture in the older patient?

ANSWERS

81 An acetabular depression fracture represents a rotated, impacted osteocartilaginous fracture of the posteromedial acetabulum that results from a posterior fracture dislocation of the hip. (*Figure 6-7, arrow*)

Fig 6-7

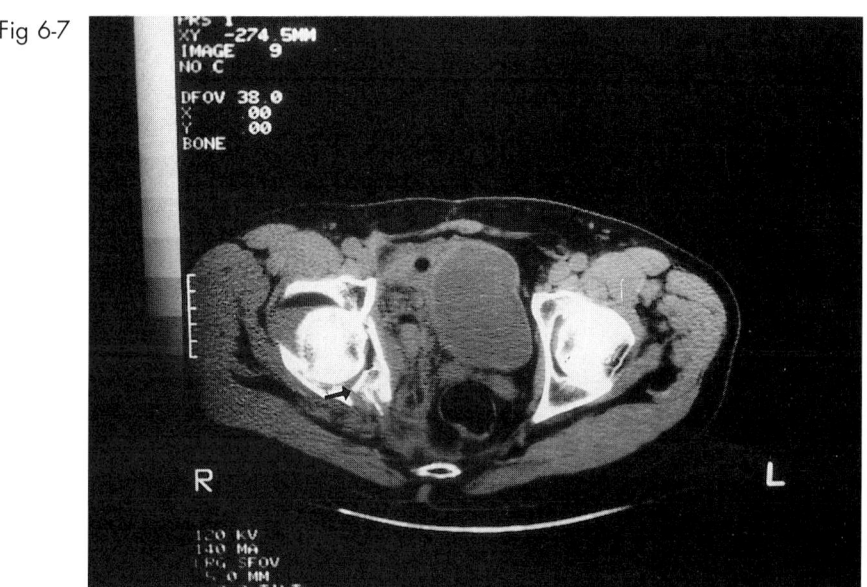

82 After medical stabilization is the optimum time. Surgical treatment of a medically unstable patient significantly increases the mortality risk.

QUESTIONS

83 What is the appropriate work-up of a patient with a suspected hip fracture, not evident of plain radiographic films?

84 How should this fracture be treated? (*Figure 6-9*)

Fig 6-9

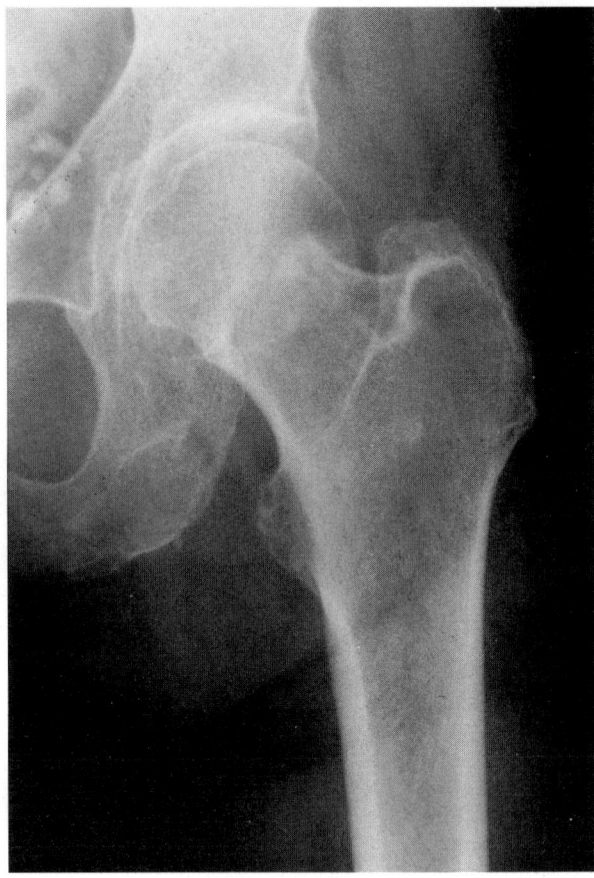

85 What is the risk of fracture displacement with nonoperative treatment?

86 What is the risk of avascular necrosis (AVN) and nonunion with this fracture?

ANSWERS

83   Bone scanning or MRI is the appropriate work-up. In the elderly patient, it may take 2 to 3 days for bone scanning to become positive. MRI has been shown to be sensitive for the detection of occult hip fractures within 24 hours of injury. (*Figure 6-8*—MRI of a left intertrochanteric hip fracture in an 80-year-old woman, taken within 24 hours of injury. The fracture was not apparent on plain radiographic films.)

Fig 6-8

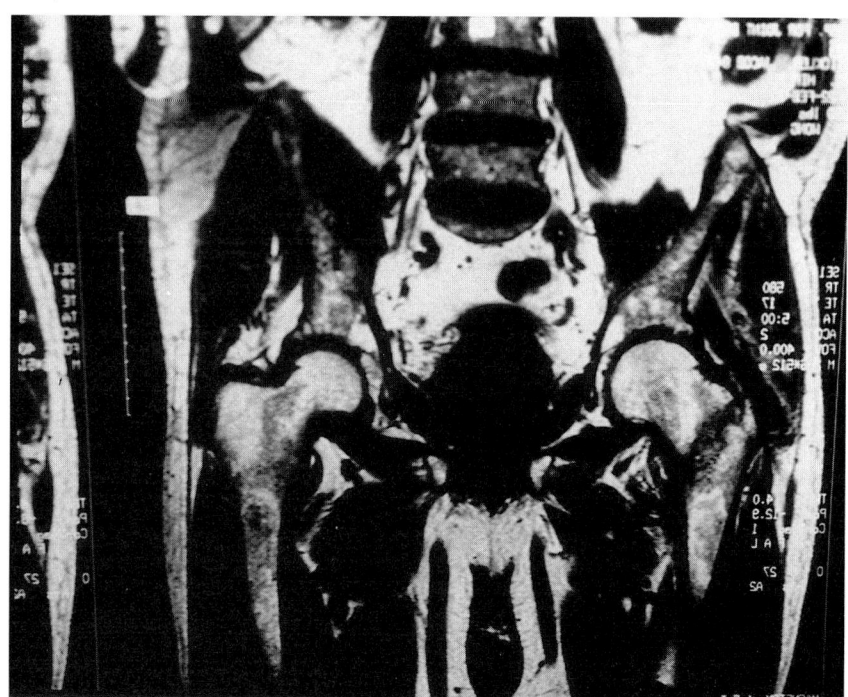

84   Internal fixation with multiple parallel lag screws or pins is the appropriate treatment.

85   Reported rates of disimpaction range between 8% and 15%.

86   With nondisplaced and impacted femoral neck fractures, the rate of AVN is less than 8%, and nonunion is less than 5%.

QUESTIONS

87   What is the most important determinant of healing complications after internal fixation of this fracture? (*Figure 6-10*)

Fig 6-10

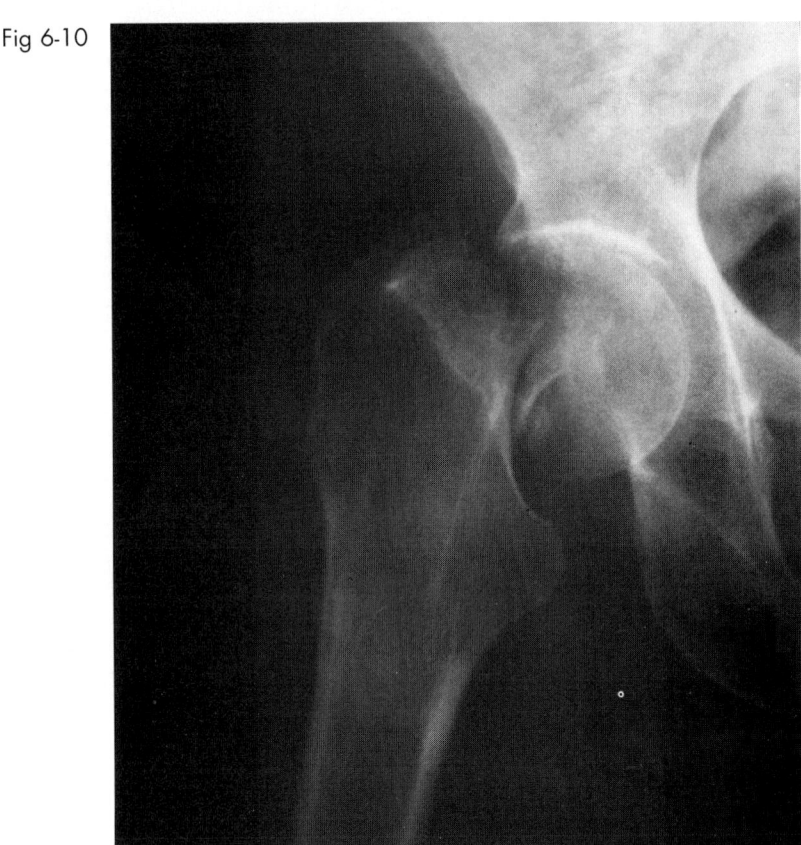

88   What is the theoretical advantage of hip joint aspiration in femoral neck fractures?

89   What are the indications for prosthetic replacement after femoral neck fracture?

90   What are the theoretical advantages of a bipolar prosthesis over a unipolar prosthesis?

91   What determines the stability of an intertrochanteric hip fracture?

92   When used for stabilization of an intertrochanteric hip fracture, what is the advantage of a sliding hip screw over a rigid nail plate?

93   With use of the sliding hip screw, where in the femoral head should the screw be positioned?

ANSWERS

87 The adequacy of reduction is the most important factor. An adequate reduction may have up to 15° of valgus and 10° of anterior or posterior angulation.

88 It is believed that capsular distension and increased intracapsular pressure may decrease femoral head perfusion through the capsular vessels and contribute to the development of AVN.

89 Prosthetic replacement should be considered in the elderly patient with a displaced femoral neck fracture when an adequate reduction cannot be obtained or when severe posterior comminution precludes stable internal fixation.

90 The bipolar prosthesis allows motion between the prosthetic femoral head and polyethylene liner and between the metallic shell and acetabular cartilage. By allowing motion at the inner bearing, this device may cause less acetabular wear.

91 Intertrochanteric fracture stability is determined by the presence or absence of an intact posteromedial cortical buttress.

92 The sliding hip screw allows controlled impaction of the fracture. In addition, the sliding hip screw is load sharing compared with the rigid nail plate, which is load bearing.

93 A central location in the femoral head and neck, within 1 cm of the hip joint is most commonly recommended. If a central position is not possible, the screw should be positioned in the posteroinferior aspect of the head and neck. The anterosuperior aspect of the femoral head should be avoided because the bone is weakest in this area.

QUESTIONS

94   What are the theoretical biomechanical advantages of this device over a sliding hip screw? (*Figure 6-11*)

Fig 6-11

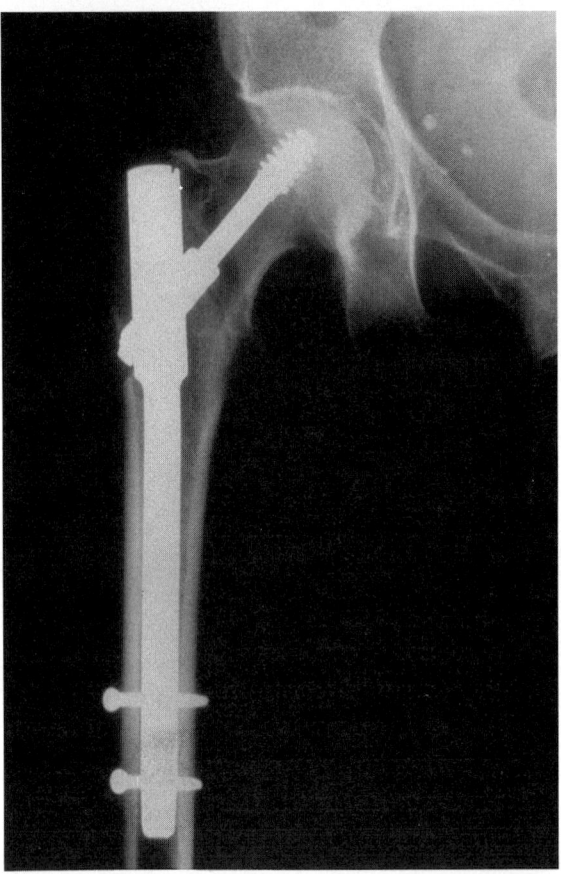

95   In subtrochanteric femur fractures, what is the usual position of the proximal fragment?

96   What is the treatment of choice for femoral shaft fractures?

97   What are the biomechanical advantages of an intramedullary femoral nailing versus a femoral plating?

98   Explain the concept of static and dynamic locking with use of an interlocking nail.

ANSWERS

94 Its intramedullary location results in a shorter lever arm and lower bending moment on the device.

95 Flexion by the iliopsoas, abduction by the gluteus medius, and external rotation by the short external rotators is the usual position.

96 Surgical stabilization with an intramedullary nail is the treatment of choice.

97 Biomechanically, intramedullary femoral nails offer several advantages over plates, screws, and external fixation:
1. The intramedullary canal is closer to the center of motion of the body than the plate position on the lateral surface of the bone; consequently, intramedullary nails are subjected to smaller bending loads than plates and are less likely to result in fatigue failure.
2. Intramedullary nails act as load-sharing devices in fractures that have cortical contact of the major fragments. If the nail is not locked at both proximal and distal ends, it will act as a gliding splint and allow continued compression as the fracture is loaded.
3. Stress shielding with resultant cortical osteopenia, commonly seen with plating, is avoided with intramedullary implants.
4. Refracture after implant removal is rare with the use of intramedullary devices, secondary to the lack of cortical osteopenia and the minimum of stress risers created in the bone.
5. In midshaft femur fractures, large diameter intramedullary devices that fill the medullary canal automatically reestablish the bony alignment.

98 A nail that is statically locked is bolted to both the proximal and distal aspects of the long bone, thereby providing maximal rotational and axial control. A nail that is dynamically locked is bolted to the long bone at either its proximal or distal end or not bolted to the bone at all. Dynamic locking has the potential for fracture shortening and rotation.

QUESTIONS

99 True or false, this fracture can be adequately stabilized with a dynamically locked femoral nail? (*Figure 6-12*)

Fig 6-12

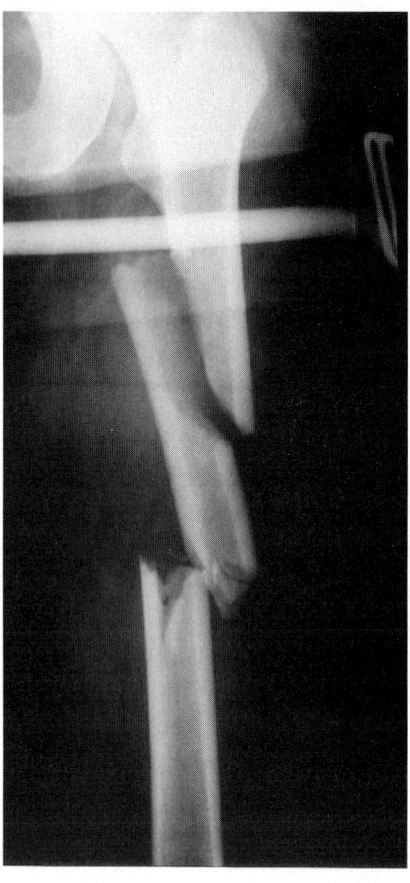

100 In the multiple-injured patient, what is the optimum timing of femoral shaft stabilization?

101 In a supracondylar femur fracture, what is the usual deformity of the distal fragment?

102 What deformity usually occurs after lateral plating of a comminuted distal femur fracture?

ANSWERS

99   False. Comminuted femoral shaft fractures need to be statically locked to prevent fracture shortening and malrotation.

100   Early stabilization of femoral shaft fractures (within the first 24 hr) is desirable in the patient with multiple injuries to decrease the incidence of acute respiratory distress syndrome (ARDS), fat emboli, pneumonia, and pulmonary failure.

101   Flexion, secondary to the pull of the gastrocnemius muscle, is the usual deformity.

102   A varus deformity of the distal femur may occur secondary to loss of the medial femoral buttress. Prevention of this deformity may require use of medial and lateral plates in comminuted distal femur fractures.

QUESTIONS

103 What is the mechanism of injury? (*Figure 6-13*)

Fig 6-13

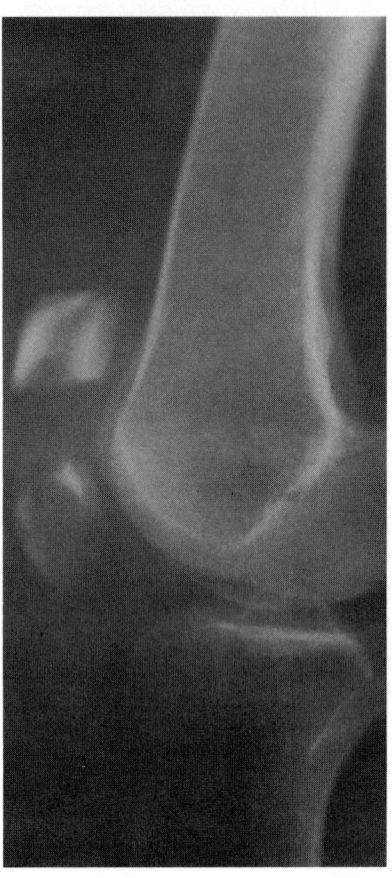

104 What is the treatment of choice?

105 Describe the shapes of the medial and lateral tibial plateaus.

106 Which meniscus is peripherally attached to the knee joint capsule?

107 What is the mechanism of injury for tibial plateau fractures?

108 How are knee dislocations classified?

ANSWERS

103 An eccentric contraction, with active quadriceps shortening while passively being lengthened, is the mechanism of injury.

104 Open reduction and internal fixation using a tension band technique is the treatment of choice.

105 The lateral plateau is convex, and the medial plateau is concave.

106 The medial meniscus. The lateral meniscus is not attached to the capsule at the popliteal hiatus.

107 Tibial plateau fractures result from indirect coronal or direct axial compressive forces, or both. Fracture fragment size, location, and displacement are determined by the magnitude, direction, and location of the generated force, the bone quality, and the degree of knee flexion at the moment of impact. The interplay of varus and compression results in medial plateau fractures, whereas the interaction of valgus and compression produces lateral fracture patterns. The prevalence of lateral plateau fractures is related to the valgus inclination of the anatomic axis and the usual lateral direction of the applied force.

108 Knee dislocations are classified by the relationship of the tibia to the femur. The five major types are anterior, posterior, lateral, medial, and rotatory. Anterior dislocations result from hyperextension of the knee. Posterior dislocations result from a posterior directed force on the anterior aspect of the tibia. Medial and lateral dislocations result from varus and valgus stresses respectively.

QUESTION

109   How should this injury be treated? (*Figure 6-14*)

Fig 6-14

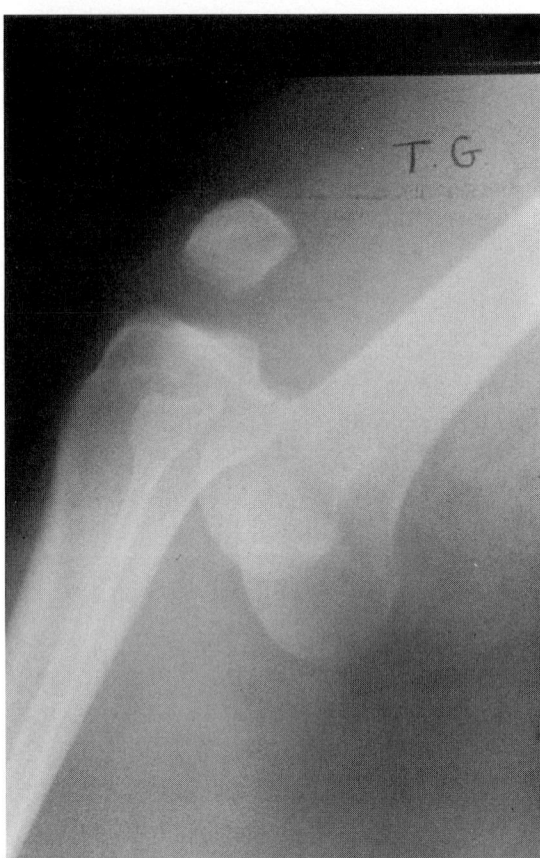

ANSWER

109   Immediate closed reduction and splinting in slight flexion is the treatment of choice. A thorough neurovascular examination is mandatory. Anterior dislocations can cause a traction injury to the popliteal artery, resulting in an acute intimal tear or intraluminal thrombus. Arteriography should be performed in all patients. Ligamentous repair or reconstruction or both is recommended to allow early range-of-knee motion and avoid knee stiffness.

QUESTIONS

110   What is the treatment of choice for this closed isolated tibia fracture? (*Figures 6-15A and 6-15B*)

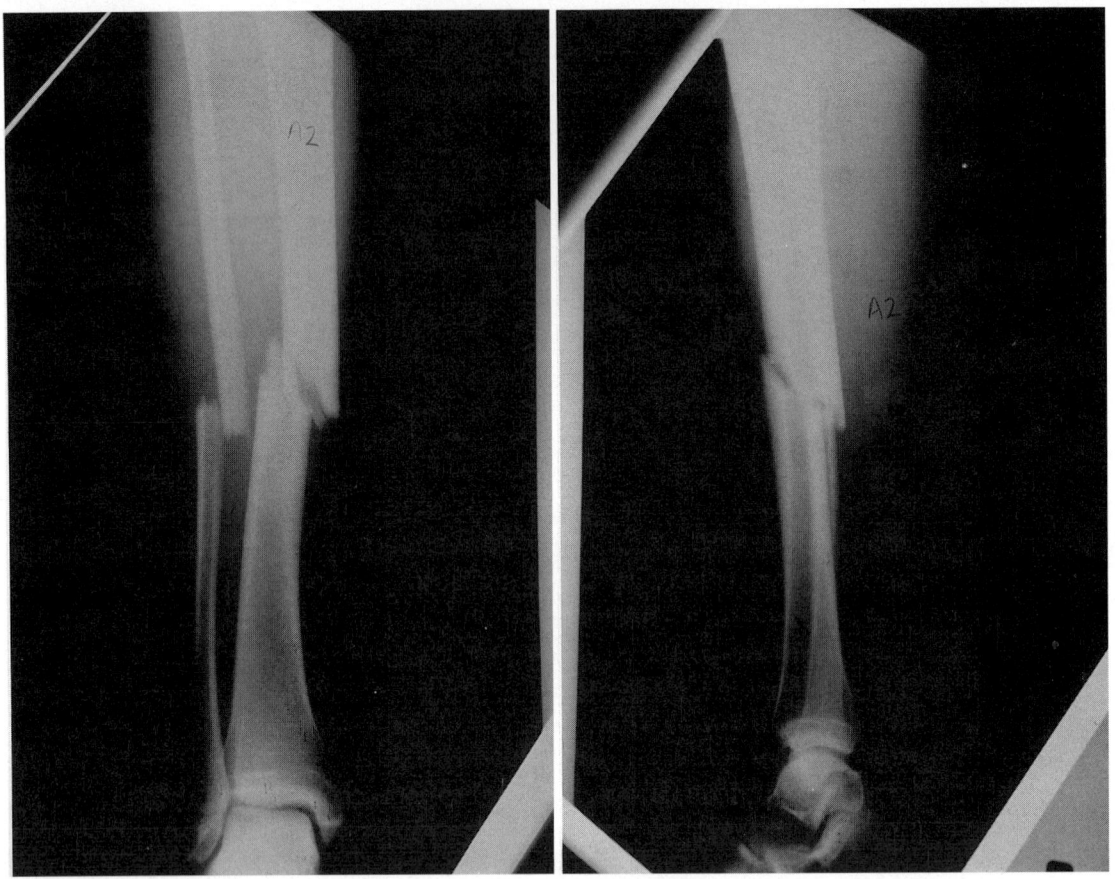

Fig 6-15 **A**   Fig 6-15 **B**

111   With early weight bearing, can this fracture be expected to shorten?

112   In open fractures of the lower extremity, what is the role of débridement in the emergency room?

113   What are the contraindications to pulsed electromagnetic fields in the treatment of a tibial or femoral nonunion?

ANSWERS

110 Closed reduction and application of a long leg cast is the treament of choice.

111 No, tibia shaft fractures do not usually shorten more than the amount measured on the initial radiographic film.

112 There is no role for débridement of open fractures in the emergency room; all should be taken to the operating room for a formal débridement.

113 A fracture gap > 1 cm and a synovial pseudoarthrosis are contraindications.

QUESTIONS

114 What are the deforming forces for this fracture? (*Figure 6-16*)

Fig 6-16

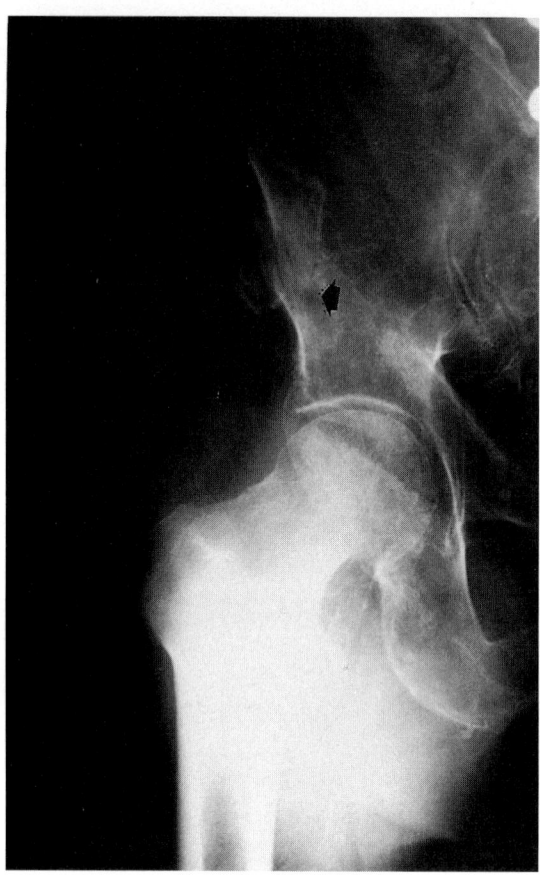

115 How should this patient be treated?

116 Describe the contents of the anterior compartment of the leg?

117 What is the most reliable sign or symptom of a compartment syndrome.

118 Name the ligaments that comprise the ankle syndesmosis.

119 What is the spatial relationship of the medial and lateral malleoli?

ANSWERS

114 This is an avulsion fracture of the anterior pelvis. The sartorius and tensor fasciae latae muscles attach to the anterior superior iliac spine and pull the fragment distal.

115 Early mobilization and weight-bearing ambulation, as tolerated, is the treatment of choice.

116 The extensor hallucis longus muscle, the extensor digitorum longus muscle, the tibialis anterior muscle, the deep peroneal nerve, and the anterior tibial artery and vein make up the anterior compartment.

117 Pain out of proportion to the injury is the most reliable symptom.

118 The anteroinferior and posteroinferior tibiofibular ligaments, the interosseous ligament, and the inferior transverse ligament make up the ankle syndesmosis.

119 The lateral malleolus is posterior and distal to the medial malleolus.

QUESTION

120   Identify the mechanism of injury of this ankle fracture. (*Figures 6-17A and 6-17B*)

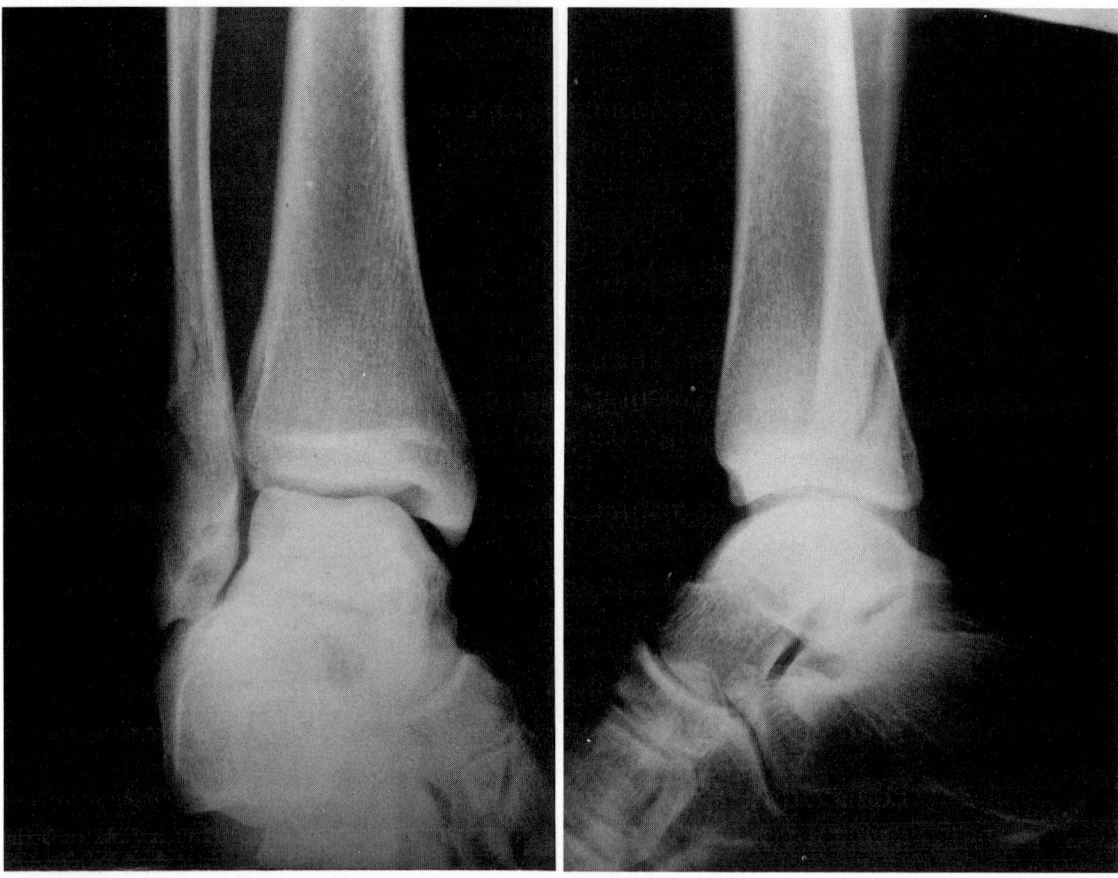

Fig 6-17 **A**   Fig 6-17 **B**

ANSWER

120   This is a supination-external rotation injury. This classification of ankle fractures, based on the mechanism of injury, was described by Lauge-Hansen. In this classification the first word refers to the position of the foot at the time of the injury, and the second refers to the direction of the injury force. The four injury patterns described are: supination-eversion, supination-adduction, pronation-abduction, and pronation-eversion.

QUESTIONS

121   What is the mechanism of this fracture? (*Figure 6-18*)

Fig 6-18

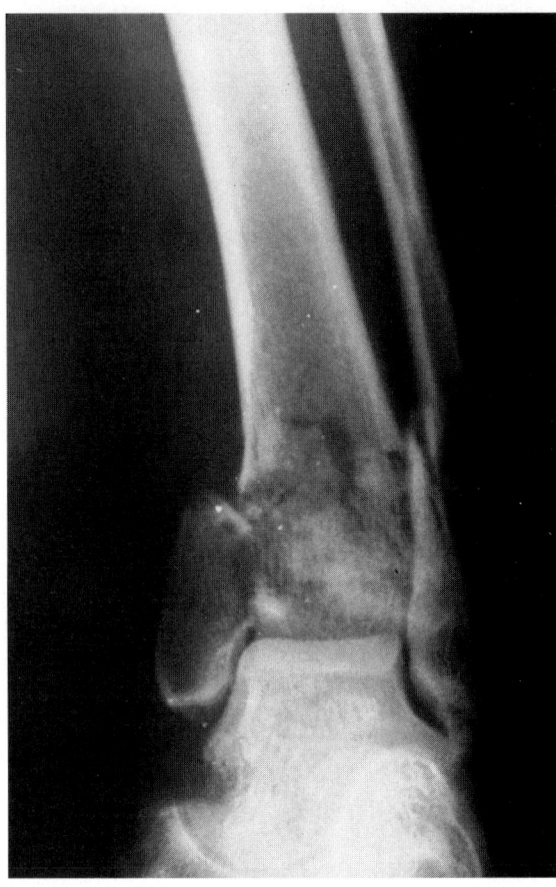

122   What are the treatment principles for operative fixation of pilon fractures according to Allgöwer and Rüedi?

123   What is the usual angular deformity of a tibia fracture with an intact fibula?

124   In a patient with a pelvic fracture, how does one make the diagnosis of an associated urethral injury?

125   What is the acute management of an open pelvic fracture?

ANSWERS

121   Axial loading is the mechanism.

122   1. Establish fibula length.
2. Reduce the articular surface.
3. Bone graft as needed.
4. Stabilize the metaphyseal fracture with use of a medial plate.

123   Varus is the usual angular deformity.

124   An urethral injury should be considered if the patient has inability to void, blood at the urethral meatus, high riding prostate on rectal examination, wide diastasis of the symphysis, or straddle fractures of the pelvis. The diagnosis is confirmed by dynamic retrograde urethrography. In addition, the patient who has hematuria after a pelvic trauma should have an intravenous pyelogram.

125   Irrigation and débridement is the management. A diverting colostomy should be performed if there are buttock or perineal lacerations or a rectal tear. In addition, if there is a rectal tear the retrorectal or presacral space should be drained to prevent abscess formation, and rectal irrigation should be performed. Vaginal lacerations require irrigation, and the fracture site should be irrigated and drained through the space of Retzius. Vaginal laceration < 1 cm should be left open; larger lacerations require repair. The bladder should be drained through a Foley catheter or suprapubic tube, depending on the type of injury. The pelvic fracture should be stabilized at the time of irrigation with either external or internal fixation.

QUESTIONS

126   What is the mechanism of this fracture? (*Figure 6-19*)

Fig 6-19

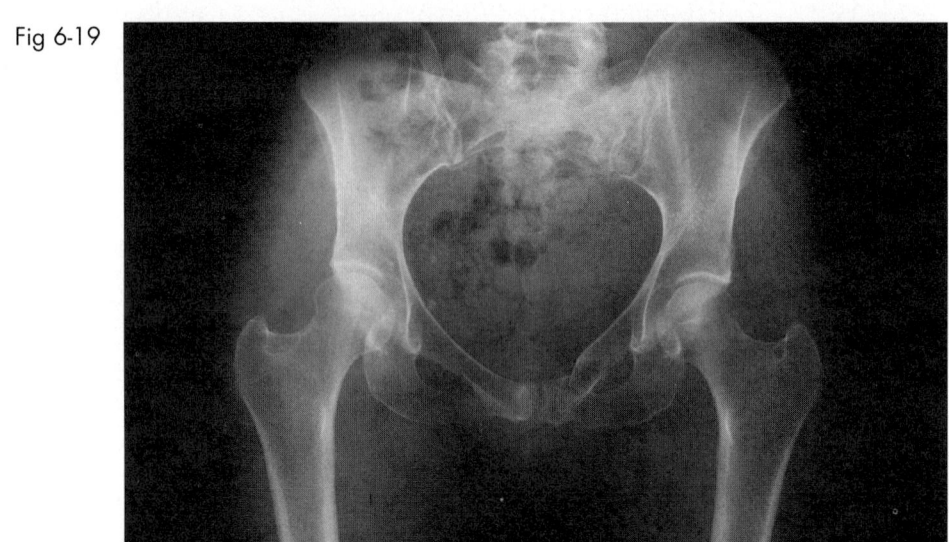

127   What is the management of this fracture?

ANSWERS

126 The mechanism of injury was lateral compression because of the internal rotation deformity of the hemipelvis. According to Tile's classification, this lateral compression is a rotationally unstable, vertically stable pelvis fracture with an ipsilateral anterior and posterior injury.

127 Management is patient mobilization when comfortable with progressive weight bearing as tolerated.

QUESTIONS

128 What is the mechanism of this fracture? (*Figures 6-20A and 6-20B*)

Fig 6-20 **A**

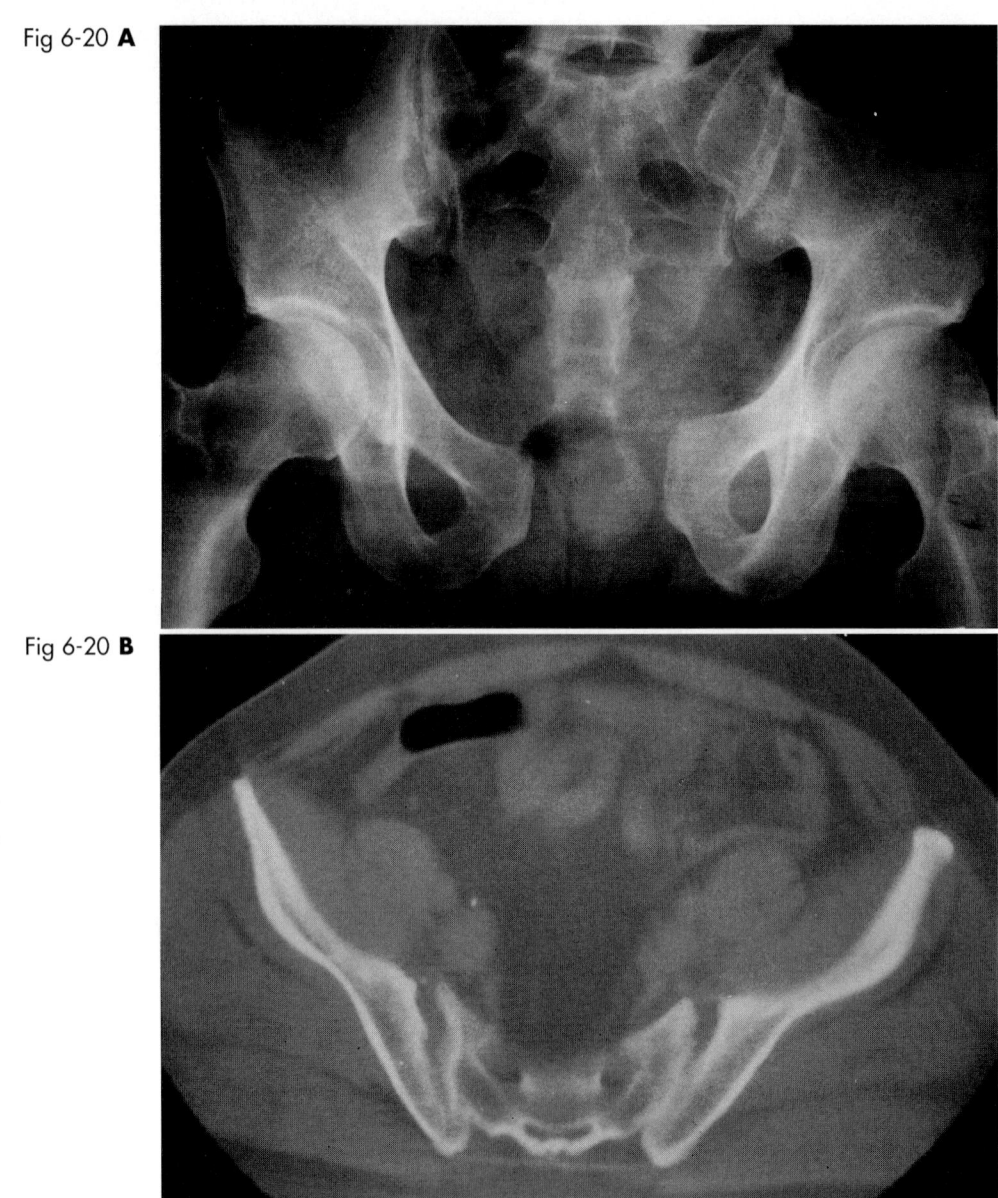

Fig 6-20 **B**

129 What is the acute management of this injury?

130 What is the strongest ligament of the sacroiliac joint?

131 What structure is most at risk during anterior sacroiliac plating?

132 How does one take an inlet and outlet pelvic radiographic film, and what information does it provide?

ANSWERS

128   The mechanism of injury was anteroposterior compression because (1) there is diastasis of the symphysis with a widening of the sacroiliac joints, and (2) the posterior sacroiliac ligaments are intact as demonstrated by the CT scan. According to Tile's classification, this open-book type of injury is a rotationally unstable, vertically stable pelvis fracture.

129   The acute management is closure of the pelvic volume by either internal fixation using symphyseal plate, sacroiliac screws, or external fixation.

130   The posterior sacroiliac ligament is the strongest.

131   The L5 nerve root as it passes over the sacral alae.

132   The inlet pelvic radiographic film is taken with beam directed 45° in a caudal direction, and the outlet radiographic film with the beam directed 45° in a cephalad direction. The inlet radiographic study shows anterior/posterior displacement of the hemipelvis, and the outlet radiographic study shows superior/inferior displacement of the hemipelvis.

QUESTIONS

133 Name the labeled structures *A* through *E*. (*Figure 6-21*)

Fig 6-21

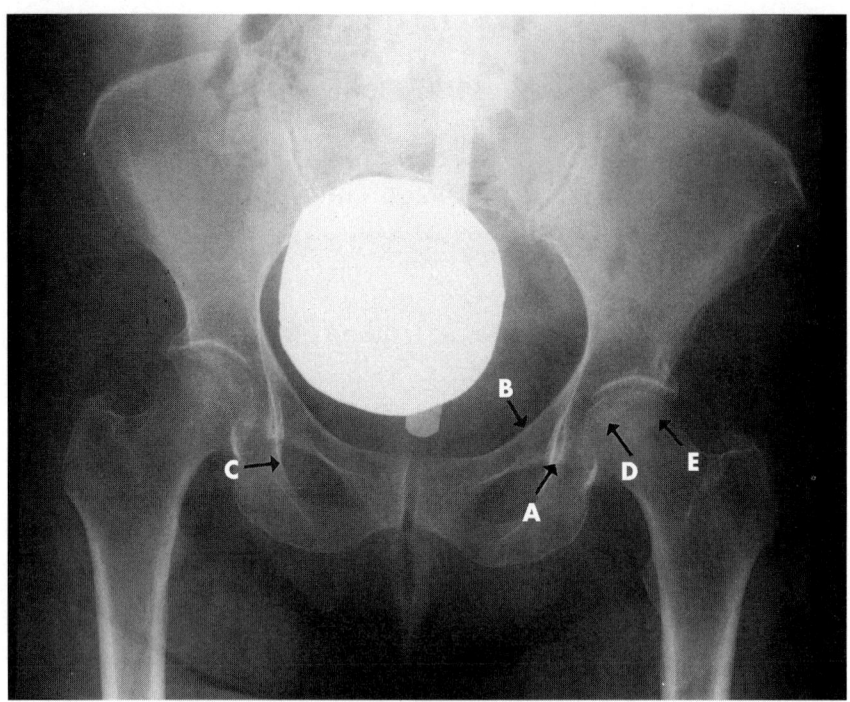

134 What information do the obturator and iliac oblique radiographic films provide as part of the acetabular trauma series?

135 What is the usual source of bleeding in an unstable pelvic fracture?

136 What is the usual source of arterial bleeding in the patient with an unstable pelvic fracture?

137 Describe the Winquist classification of fracture comminution.

138 How should open femoral shaft fractures be treated?

139 What is the incidence of ipsilateral femoral neck and shaft fracture?

140 What is the incidence of ipsilateral femoral shaft and knee ligament injury?

ANSWERS

133 A. The teardrop
B. The iliopectineal line
C. The ilioischial line
D. The anterior acetabular lip
E. The posterior acetabular lip

134 The obturator oblique film provides information about the anterior column and posterior wall of the acetabulum. The iliac oblique film provides information about the posterior column and anterior wall of the acetabulum.

135 Intrapelvic bleeding associated with a pelvic fracture is usually venous in origin. In addition to volume replacement, treatment may include temporary use of military antishock trousers, external or internal stabilization of the pelvic ring, angiography with transarterial embolization, and vascular repair.

136 The superior gluteal artery is the usual source. Angiography of the pelvic arteries should be considered in the patient who does not respond to fluid resuscitation and pelvic stabilization or in whom pelvic stabilization is not applicable. If hemorrhage is from a major artery, surgical repair may be required.

137 The Winquist classification is used to describe comminution of the femoral shaft and is important when contemplating intramedullary femoral nailing.
Type I has a butterfly fragment <25% circumference of the bone.
Type II has a butterfly fragment <50% circumference of the bone.
Type III has a butterfly fragment >50% circumference of the bone.
Type IV has segmental comminution with no contact between the proximal and distal fragments.
Types I and II have axial stability after dynamic intramedullary nailing and will not shorten with fracture rotation.
Types III and IV can shorten after dynamic intramedullary nailing if the fracture rotates.

138 Grade I, II, and IIIA open femoral shaft fractures require emergent irrigation and débridement followed by immediate intramedullary nailing. The care of the patient with Grade IIIB or IIIC fracture should be individualized. All require emergent irrigation and débridement; there is a role for immediate and delayed intramedullary nailing, as well as external fixation.

139 Ipsilateral femoral neck fracture occurs in as many as 5% of all femoral shaft fractures.

140 Ipsilateral knee ligament injury occurs in 5% of femoral shaft fractures.

QUESTIONS

141 Describe the possible factors that can result in a fracture becoming a nonunion.

142 What is the labeled structure in this anteroposterior radiographic film of an infected tibial nonunion? (*Figure 6-22*)

Fig 6-22

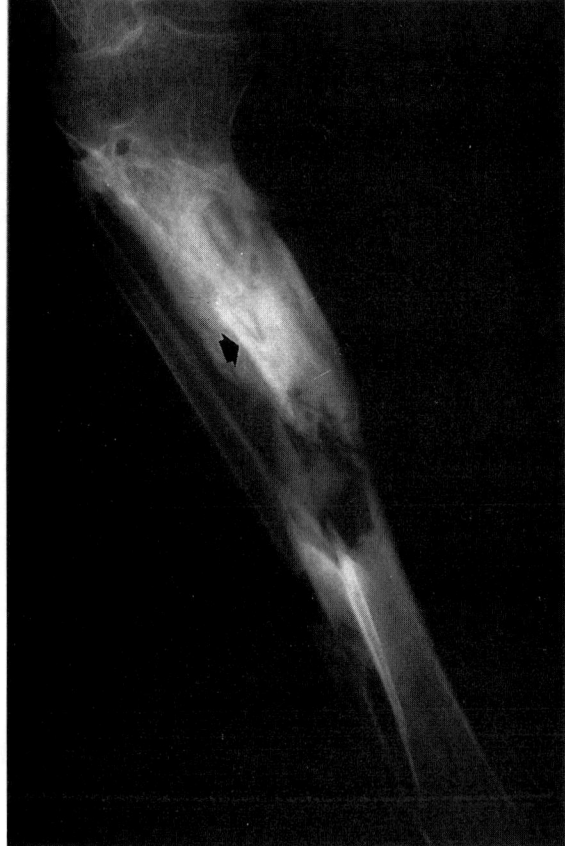

143 What are the treatment principles in the management of osteomyelitis?

ANSWERS

141 The factors that can result in a fracture becoming a nonunion are excessive motion, fracture gap, infection, and failure of revascularization secondary to loss of blood supply.

142 The labeled structure is a sequestrum. A sequestrum is the hallmark of osteomyelitis; it is necrotic bone and is recognized radiographically as an area of sclerosis surrounded by new bone formation (involucrum).

143 Successful treatment of osteomyelitis depends on adherence to several basic principles: the complete débridement of necrotic and infected tissue, the maintenance or creation of osseous stability, the elimination of dead space, and the provision of durable soft-tissue coverage.

QUESTIONS

144   How should this closed tibia fracture be treated? (*Figure 6-23*)

Fig 6-23

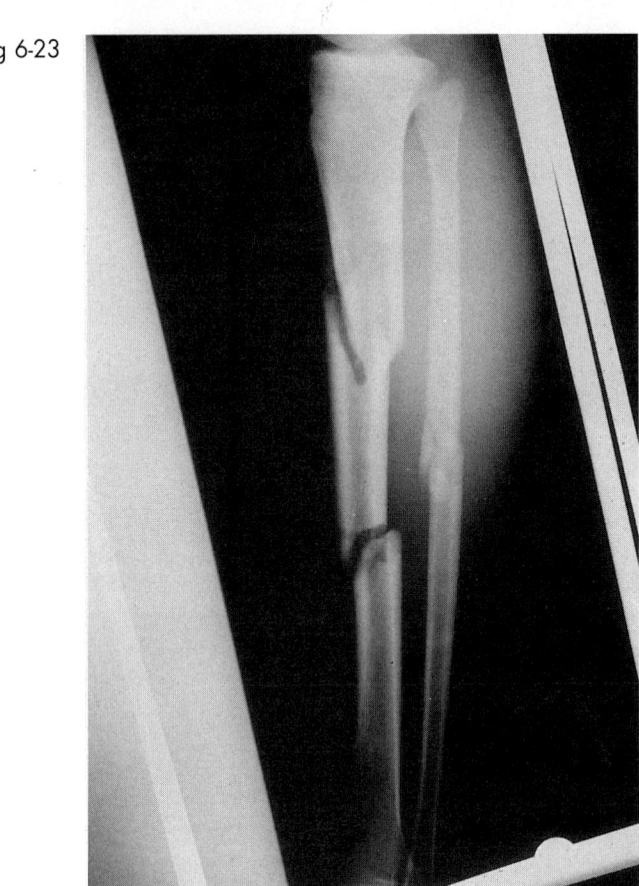

145   Which is the most common type of hip dislocation?

146   Describe the mechanism of injury in posterior hip dislocation.

147   What is the usual position of the extremity with a posterior hip dislocation?

ANSWERS

144   A segmental tibia fracture is an indication for surgical intervention, preferably with an intramedullary nail. One should closely observe the patient for the signs and symptoms of compartment syndrome.

145   Posterior hip dislocations, classified by Epstein on the basis of associated femoral head or acetabular fractures, account for up to 90% of all hip dislocations. Type I is a posterior dislocation with or without an associated minor acetabular rim fracture. Type II has a large posterior acetabular rim fragment. Type III has comminution of the posterior acetabular rim with or without a major fragment. Type IV is a posterior dislocation with a fracture of the acetabular rim and floor. Type V is associated with fractures of the femoral head. Pipkin has subclassified these Type V fracture or dislocations into four separate types as follows:
Type I—A femoral head fracture occurring caudad to the fovea centralis
Type II—A femoral head fracture occurring cephalad to the fovea centralis
Type III—A Type I or Type II fracture with associated femoral neck fracture
Type IV—A Type I, II, or III fracture with associated acetabular fracture

146   Posterior hip dislocations are the result of a force applied to the flexed knee along the axis of the femur.

147   Flexed, adducted, and internally rotated is the usual position.

QUESTIONS

148 Is this an anterior or posterior fracture-dislocation of the hip? (*Figure 6-24*)

Fig 6-24

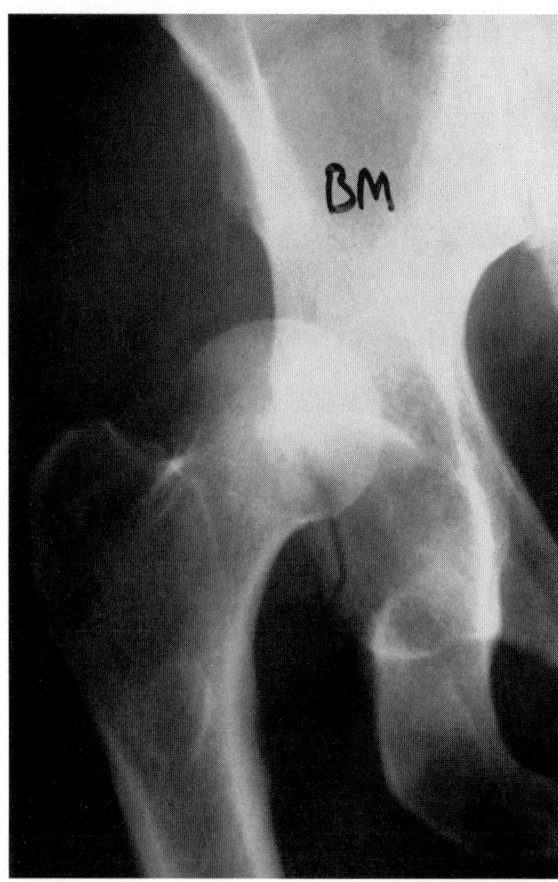

149 What is the appropriate treatment for a hip dislocation?

150 What are the risk factors for osteonecrosis of the femoral head following hip dislocation?

151 Define the three classes of gunshot wounds.

152 What defines the wounding potential of a shotgun blast?

153 What are the treatment principles for a low-velocity gunshot wound?

ANSWERS

148 This is a posterior fracture-dislocation. The lower extremity is adducted and internally rotated; one can tell internal and external rotation by the position of the lesser trochanter.
Because the lesser trochanter is located on the posteromedial aspect of the proximal femur, the lesser trochanter becomes more visible with external rotation; with internal rotation, it becomes less visible.

149 Gentle closed or open reduction, followed by assessment of hip stability and CT evaluation to identify intraarticular fragments or associated fractures, is the appropriate treatment.

150 The risk of osteonecrosis depends on the severity of the injury, time delay to reduction (>6 to 12 hours), and repeated attempts at closed reduction.

151 The three classes of gunshot wounds are:
1. High velocity (>2000 ft/sec)
2. Low velocity (<2000 ft/sec)
3. Shotgun
All handguns are low velocity. All military rifles and most hunting rifles are high velocity.

152 The wounding potential of a shotgun is dependent on:
1. The choke (shot pattern)
2. The load (size of the individual pellet)
3. The distance from the target

153 The patient with a low-velocity gunshot wound can be treated as an outpatient with:
1. Débridement of the entrance and exit wound skin edges.
2. Administration of antibiotic, tetanus toxoid, and antitoxin.
3. Fracture treatment. (Treat as a closed fracture.)
4. Operative débridement if there is
   a. joint involvement (bone or bullet fragment inside joint).
   b. a vascular injury.
   c. a dirty wound.
   d. the bullet is superficial on palm of hand or sole of foot.
   e. a massive hematoma.
   f. foreign material.
   g. excessive tissue damage.
   h. a compartment syndrome.
   i. gastrointestinal contamination.

QUESTIONS

154 What are the treatment principles for high-velocity and shotgun wounds?

155 What are the advantages and disadvantages of military antishock trousers?

156 Which organism(s) is(are) responsible for gas gangrene?

157 What is the treatment for gas gangrene?

ANSWERS

154   High-velocity and shotgun wounds should be treated as high-energy injuries with significant soft-tissue damage and require
1. administration of antibiotic, tetanus toxoid, and antitoxin.
2. extensive operative débridement(s) and irrigation(s).
3. fracture stabilization.
4. delayed wound closure.

155   Military antishock trousers help control bleeding in the patient with a pelvic fracture by decreasing the pelvic volume. They also counteract significant intraabdominal bleeding and help support the systolic blood pressure by increasing the peripheral systemic resistance. Military antishock trousers are simple and quick to apply, reversible, and can be used to splint fractures. The disadvantages of military antishock trousers are:
1. They cause decreased visibility and access of the abdomen and lower extremities.
2. They have been associated with complications such as lower extremity compartment syndrome secondary to prolonged use.
3. They result in decreased lung vital capacity and have caused exacerbation of congestive heart failure.

156   Clostridia are responsible for gas gangrene. Clostridia are anaerobic gram-positive bacteria that produce several exotoxins, which induce local edema, muscle, fat and fascia necrosis, and thrombosis of local vessels. Clostridium perfringens and Clostridium septicum are the two bacteria usually responsible for gas gangrene in humans.

157   A patient with suspected or established gas gangrene should undergo repeated radical débridements and fasciotomies. Antibiotic coverage should include intravenous penicillin or clindamycin (if allergic to penicillin) and a cephalosporin and aminoglycoside to cover other organisms. Hyperbaric oxygen therapy should also be considered.

CHAPTER 7

Foot and Ankle

James J. Sferra
Grant A. Dona
Michael J. Shereff

QUESTIONS

1 A 35-year-old female patient falls after stepping into a hole. She complains of ankle pain with swelling medially and laterally. X-ray films of the ankle reveal a transverse fracture of the medial malleolus. What additional radiographic films, if any, should be obtained and why?

2 A 20-year-old man sustains an inversion injury to his ankle. Radiographic films reveal a displaced fracture of the medial malleolus, an oblique fracture of the fibula extending proximally from the level of the joint line, and a fracture of the posterior lip of the tibia involving approximately 10% of the articular surface. Describe treatment of each fracture in this injury.

3 Describe placement of a syndesmotic screw.

4 While playing racquet ball, a 40-year-old man experiences a sharp pain in his posterior ankle area, accompanied by a loud pop. On examination he is able to actively plantar flex, although weakly. The foot does not plantar flex when the calf is squeezed. What is the diagnosis?

5 Describe presentation of posterior tibial tendon insufficiency.

6 Describe optimum positions for arthrodesis of the ankle.

ANSWERS

1 A radiographic film of the entire leg should be performed to rule out a proximal fibula fracture, frequently accompanied by a rupture of the syndesmosis interosseous membrane up to the level of the fracture (the Maisonneuve's fracture).

2 Operative fixation of this injury customarily would include fixation of the medial malleolus fracture with screws or a screw and Kirschner-wire (K-wire), or possibly tension-band wiring of a small fragment. The lateral malleolus may be fixed with a plate or, possibly, multiple lag screws. Fixation of the posterior lip fracture involving less than 25% of the articular surface is generally not regarded as necessary. Some practitioners will routinely use a screw across the syndesmosis. Alternatively, the integrity of the syndesmosis may be tested after fracture fixation to evaluate the need for a syndesmotic screw. When a bony injury can be fixed medially, the syndesmotic screw may not be necessary.

3 The screw is directed transversely, angulated approximately 25° anteriorly into the tibia, to account for the posterior position of the fibula with respect to the tibia. As the screw is placed, the ankle is dorsiflexed. Lag screw technique is not used; otherwise, excessive narrowing of the ankle mortise will prevent ankle dorsiflexion.

4 This injury likely represents a complete rupture of the Achilles tendon. Although squeezing the calf does not produce plantar flexion (Thompson test), the patient is able to plantar flex by using his tibialis posterior, toe flexors, and possibly the peroneals. This is a common injury in middle-aged athletes.

5 On first presentation, symptoms may be limited to pain posterior to the medial malleolus or along the course of the posterior tibial tendon. As insufficiency progresses, the heel collapses into valgus, the midfoot becomes pronated, with decrease in the height of the longitudinal arch, and the forefoot becomes abducted. From behind, the examiner can visualize more toes on the affected side than are observed on the other limb (i.e., the "too many toes" sign). A single limb heel raise may be painful or impossible.

6 The ankle is best placed in neutral dorsiflexion (some believe slight plantar flexion is acceptable in women), 5° to 10° external rotation (or equal to the contralateral foot), and neutral to 5° valgus (possibly displacing the talus posteriorly on the tibia).

QUESTIONS

7 A 25-year-old man sustains a crush injury to his foot. Two hours later, his foot is severely swollen and painful. He has marked increase in pain with passive dorsiflexion of his toes at the metatarsophalangeal (MTP) joints. X-ray films reveal minimally displaced fractures of the cuboid and lateral cuneiform. Describe appropriate initial treatment.

8 A 25-year-old woman complains of frequent ankle sprains and pain beneath the balls of her feet. She recalls that her mother complained of similar symptoms. Examination reveals bilateral elevated arch, clawing of toes, and mild atrophy of the calves. Describe the most likely diagnosis.

9 A 60-year-old diabetic man complains of spontaneous onset of redness and swelling across his midfoot. He has only mild pain. Describe the likely diagnosis.

10 Describe initial treatment of the condition described in Q9.

11 What is the most common deformity following a Chopart-level (midfoot) amputation, and how may this condition be avoided?

12 What are common sequelae of nonoperatively treated displaced calcaneus fractures?

13 Describe the Hawkins' classification of talar neck fractures.

14 What is the approximate risk for avascular necrosis with each fracture type?

15 What produces Hawkin's sign (subchondral atrophy of the talar dome), and what does this condition imply?

ANSWERS

7 If compartment syndrome is suspected, compartment pressures should be measured. Pain, especially "burning" pain aggravated by passive stretch of involved tissues, may be the first sign of compartment syndrome. The absolute value for compartment pressure release varies between experts, but it is generally 30 mm Hg to 40 mm Hg or 20 mm Hg below diastolic pressure.

8 Although other conditions may produce a similar picture, these symptoms likely represent Charcot-Marie-Tooth disease. In this condition there is cavus foot with plantar flexed first ray, contracted plantar fascia, varus hindfoot, and clawing of the toes. The intrinsics and peroneus brevis are commonly the most weakened muscles. The peroneus longus muscle is usually spared until late in the process, accounting for the plantar flexion deformity of the first ray.

ANSWERS

9   A diabetic with spontaneous erythema and swelling of the foot may have developed a Charcot foot. The foot may or may not be painful. An important differential diagnosis is infection, and differentiating the two may be difficult. Absence of ulceration, normal white blood cell (WBC) count, no elevation in insulin requirement, or elevation of serum glucose are helpful indicators. X-ray films may be normal initially, progressing to subluxation and fragmentation of multiple bones. Labeled WBC bone scan may be the only definitive test.

10   Although improved glucose control may occasionally improve neurologic function, Charcot neuropathic changes are generally not reversible. Therapy during the inflammatory stage is primarily directed at prevention of deformity. Total contact casting, orthotic support, or restricted activities on weight-bearing bones are all recommended to reduce development of collapse and deformity.

11   The most common deformity is equinus deformity. To prevent this, the tibialis anterior should be attached to the talus, and an Achilles tenotomy is commonly performed. This prevents unopposed pull of the Achilles tendon.

12   Displaced calcaneus fractures may develop subtalar and calcaneocuboid arthrosis, subfibular impingement of the peroneal tendons, widening or collapse of the heel, varus malalignment of the hindfoot, and weak plantar flexion as a result of decrease in the tendo Achilles fulcrum.

13 | Type I | Nondisplaced |
| --- | --- |
| Type II | Subluxation of subtalar joint |
| Type III | Dislocation from both the ankle and subtalar joints |
| Type IV | Type III with dislocation of the talonavicular joint |

14 | Type I | 13% |
| --- | --- |
| Type II | 20% to 50% |
| Type III | 83% to 100% |
| Type IV | Virtually 100% |

15   Hawkins' sign, talar subchondral bone resorption, is seen as a radiographic subchondral lucency and implies sufficient preservation of vascular supply to the talar dome. Hawkins' sign may thus be seen any time there is disuse or decreased activities on weight-bearing bones.

QUESTIONS

16 An 18-year-old man complains of heel pain of 3 months' duration. He has recently developed urethritis. What is the most likely cause of these symptoms?

17 Describe the anterior drawer test of the ankle.

18 A 25-year-old woman complains of pain in her anterior tibial area, which begins approximately 15 minutes into each run. Describe work-up of exertional compartment syndrome.

19 How is this syndrome treated?

ANSWERS

16 These symptoms likely represent Reiter's syndrome. The pain in the heel is due to an enthesopathy, and the patient may experience tenderness at the insertion of the Achilles tendon and the calcaneal origin of the plantar fascia. HLA-B27 is positive in approximately 75% of patients with Reiter's syndrome.

17 The ankle is slightly plantar flexed, and the foot is drawn anteriorly from behind the heel by the examiner. With the opposite hand, the examiner holds the tibia fixed and palpates the amount of anterior talar translation in the ankle mortise. This ankle is compared with the opposite ankle. Excessive translation implies injury to the anterior talofibular ligament.

18 This patient experiences pain in the involved compartment initiated by exercise. Physical findings at rest are generally absent. Rest compartment pressures may be elevated (greater than 10 mm Hg), but more reliably, the compartment pressures are consistently abnormally elevated during exercise (greater than 50 mm Hg) and remain elevated longer than normal (less than 30 mm Hg after exercise, returning to baseline in less than 5 minutes).

19 In mild cases, activity modification or modification of shoe wear may be adequate. In severe, persistent cases, fasciotomy of involved compartment(s) may be indicated.

QUESTIONS

Questions 20 to 25.   Identify the structures shown on the medial side of the foot and ankle shown in Figure 7-1.

Fig 7-1

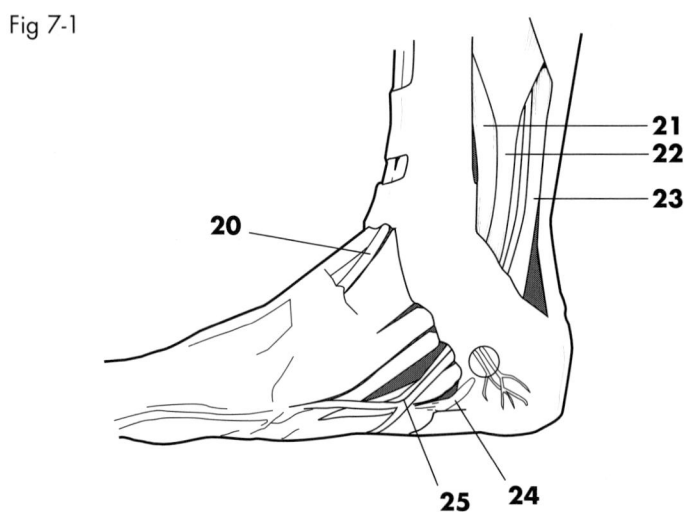

ANSWERS

20 Tibialis anterior tendon, passing beneath the inferior extensor retinaculum to insert on the base of the first metatarsal and the first cuneiform

21 Tibialis posterior tendon, the most anterior of the tendons in the tarsal tunnel, passing behind the medial malleolus, through the tarsal tunnel, and above the sustentaculum tali to insert on the navicular, as well as on the first, second, and third cuneiform, on the cuboid, and, at times, on the base of the fifth metatarsal

22 Flexor digitorum longus (FDL), posterior to the tibialis posterior tendon, crossing superficial to the flexor hallucis longus (FHL), giving rise to the lumbricals before attaching to the phalanges (2 to 5)

23 FHL, the most posterior and lateral of the three tendons, passing inferior to the sustentaculum tali

24 Abductor hallucis, passing superficial to medial and lateral plantar nerves (The fascia surrounding this muscle can act as a site of impingement to these nerves)

25 Posterior tibial artery and nerve, superficial to the FHL, dividing into medial and lateral plantar branches

QUESTIONS

26 The dorsal hallucal nerve (dorsomedial cutaneous nerve), which innervates the dorsomedial aspect of the great toe, is a terminal branch of which nerve?

27 What three structures are released in the first web space when performing a modified McBride soft tissue release during a hallux valgus procedure?

28 What muscle(s) and tendon(s) insert into the first metatarsal head?

29 What are the normal values of the intermetatarsal (IM) angle, the hallux valgus angle, and the interphalangeal (IP) angle on the anteroposterior (AP) radiographic film?

30 A 40-year-old laborer has a painful hallux varus deformity. Radiographic films show an IM angle of 15° and a hallux varus angle of 35°, along with significant arthrosis of the first MTP joint. Conservative measures have failed. What surgical intervention is indicated?

31 A 40-year-old woman has painful moderate hallux varus and keratosis beneath the second metatarsal head along with generalized ligamentous laxity including her first metatarsocuneiform joint. Her IM angle measures 16°. What surgical procedure is indicated?

32 Following the previously described procedure, the patient's transfer lesion beneath the second metatarsal head became more symptomatic. What is the most likely cause of this, and, if conservative measures fail, what surgical intervention is indicated?

33 Following an overzealous bunionectomy procedure, iatrogenic hallux varus is the result, which is symptomatic. What soft tissue procedure is indicated, and what bony procedure can serve as a salvage?

34 What is the most significant stabilizing structure of the MTP joint?

ANSWERS

26 The superficial peroneal nerve divides into a medial and intermediate dorsal cutaneous nerve on the dorsum of the foot. The intermediate cutaneous nerve innervates the lateral side of the third toe and the medial aspect of the fourth toe. The medial cutaneous nerve terminates into lateral, middle, and medial branches. The lateral branch innervates the medial aspect of the third toe and the lateral aspect of the second toe. The middle branch is thin and innervates the first web space, receiving reinforcement from branches of the deep peroneal nerve. The medial branch forms the dorsomedial cutaneous nerve of the great toe. It often anastomoses at the level of the MTP joint with a terminal branch of the saphenous nerve.

ANSWERS

27 (1) The adductor tendon is detached from its insertion into the base of the proximal phalanx and the lateral aspect of the fibular sesamoid.
(2) The lateral first MTP joint capsule is perforated and torn.
(3) The transverse metatarsal ligament is released with caution as the nerve and blood vessels lie immediately plantar to this structure.

28 No muscle or tendon inserts into the first metatarsal head.

29 The normal IM angle is 9° or less. The normal hallux varus angle is less than 15°, whereas the IP angle is normally less than 10°.

30 Significant arthrosis of the MTP joint negates the possibility of carrying out most realignment procedures because stiffness and pain will result. An MTP arthrodesis is the procedure of choice, as it will produce a stable, painless joint that will not deteriorate over time.

31 A subgroup of less than 5% of patients with hallux varus have additional hypermobility of the first metatarsocuneiform joint. When this is accompanied with an increased IM angle, an arthrodesis of the first metatarsocuneiform joint in conjunction with the distal modified McBride soft tissue release is indicated.

32 The first metatarsocuneiform fusion causes some shortening of the first metatarsal, and the metatarsal can be incorrectly placed in dorsiflexion resulting in or exacerbating a transfer lesion. A plantar flexion osteotomy of the first metatarsal is indicated.

33 In the patient with good articular surface and a hallux varus deformity, transfer of the extensor hallucis longus (EHL) can be used to correct the deformity. Half of the EHL is transferred beneath the transverse metatarsal ligament and into the base of the proximal phalanx of the great toe. Some also include fusion of the IP joint of the great toe with this transfer. If the transfer fails, arthrodesis of the first MTP joint is indicated.

34 The plantar plate is formed from the plantar capsule and plantar aponeurosis and serves as the strongest stabilizing structure of the MTP joint. Its major function is resisting dorsiflexion.

QUESTIONS

35 A young woman complains of painful corns on the dorsum of her second and third toe proximal interphalangeal (PIP) joints along with a burning sensation in her forefoot. When standing, hammer toes are present, but when she sits and dangles her feet, no deformity is present. What is the initial treatment for this condition?

36 If conservative measures fail, what surgical options are available?

37 What is the usual cause of a plantar callosity under the IP joint of the great toe?

38 What sign(s) typifies hallux rigidus?

39 What conservative measures can be taken to treat hallux rigidus?

40 Besides a radiographic film, what test best reveals a subluxation of a lesser toe MTP joint?

41 A 35-year-old woman has a painful bunionette deformity with callosity that is unresponsive to conservative treatment. Why must one scrutinize the preoperative foot radiographic films?

42 Her fourth to fifth intermetatarsal angle measures 12° without significant lateral bowing of the distal fifth metatarsal. What is your recommended surgical treatment?

ANSWERS

35 The patient has a flexible or dynamic hammer toe deformity. Conservative treatment consists of wearing roomy, well-fitted shoes with increased width and height in the toe box. This treatment helps avoid direct pressure against a hammer toe, the development of plantar callosities, and resulting metatarsalgia. A metatarsal pad with or without a custom insole or local cushioning over the dorsal callosity can also be added.

36 This deformity seems to be caused by contracture of the FDL tendon, but mere release of this tendon is not usually sufficient for lasting correction. FDL to EDL transfer realigns the toes and enables the FDL to plantar flex the MTP joint and dorsiflex the PIP and dorsal interphalangeal (DIP) joints via the extensor hood. Others prefer to perform a PIP joint arthroplasty in either fixed or flexible hammer toe deformities.

37 A subhallux sesamoid is present at this location in 5% to 13% of people. This accessory bone is located just dorsal to the FHL near its insertion and articulates in the IP joint. It lies in the plantar ligament.

38 Patients with hallux rigidus typically have pain in the first MTP joint associated with limitation of dorsiflexion. Also, plantar flexion can cause pain as a result of traction of the EHL muscle over the dorsal osteophyte on the metatarsal head. Patients tend to shift their weight away from the hallux and toe off on the lateral metatarsal heads.

39 In addition to nonsteroidal antiinflammatory drugs (NSAIDs), shoe modifications that include a wider toe box, an extended steel shank, and rocker-bottom soles are indicated.

40 The vertical stress test is similar to an anterior drawer test at the knee. The examiner holds the metatarsal head down firmly with one hand and grasps the base of the proximal phalanx with the other hand. While holding the phalanx horizontally, a vertical upward stress is applied. If the proximal phalanx translates dorsally, rather than cocking up in a dorsiflexed direction, the test is positive and the joint is subluxable. This subluxation results from insufficiency of the plantar plate.

41 One must carefully assess the AP view to determine if the bunionette is due to an isolated prominent eminence at the fifth metatarsal head, lateral deviation of the distal fifth metatarsal shaft, or rather a significant increase in the fourth to fifth intermetatarsal angle.

42 An intermetatarsal angle greater than 8° is abnormal. With this deformity, a lateral condylectomy does not effectively correct the deformity. Some form of fifth metatarsal osteotomy is necessary.

QUESTIONS

43 Pictured is a cross section through the third metatarsal head(*Figure 7-2*). Identify the structure labeled <u>A</u>.

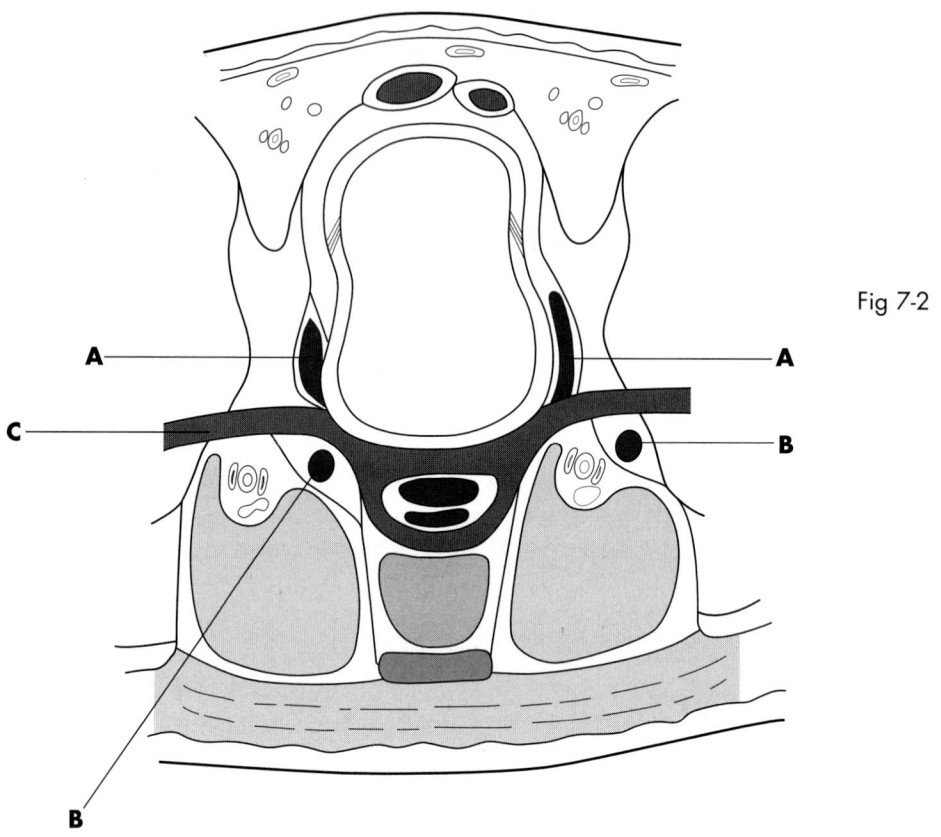

Fig 7-2

44 Identify the structure labeled <u>B</u>.

45 Identify the structure labeled <u>C</u>.

46 What function(s) do the interossei and lumbrical muscles perform?

47 Describe the classic findings in a patient with longstanding rheumatoid arthritis of the forefoot.

48 What is the preferred surgical approach to a patient with rheumatoid arthritis and severe forefoot involvement as described in Q47?

49 One year following the above surgical correction for rheumatoid forefoot involvement, the patient continues to have callosity and bursa formation beneath the fourth metatarsal, which is unresponsive to conservative treatment. What is your approach to this problem?

50 What is the usual cause of first metatarsocuneiform degenerative arthritis, and what is the conservative approach to this problem?

ANSWERS

43 Interossei muscles located in narrow cleft between MTP capsule and extensor aponeurosis.

44 Lumbrical tendon located in its own tunnel on the tibial side of the joint.

45 Deep transverse intermetatarsal ligament.

46 The four dorsal interossei are the abductors of the toes, whereas the three plantar interossei are the adductors. They all pass dorsal to the deep transverse intermetatarsal ligament, whereas the lumbricals remain plantar to this ligament. Nevertheless, the interossei and lumbricals pass plantar to the axis of motion at the MTP joint and dorsal to the axis of motion at the PIP joint. Thus the interossei and lumbricals plantar flex the MTP joints and cause weak extension at the PIP and DIP joints.

47 There is HV with obvious intraarticular involvement of the MTP joints. The lesser toes drift laterally with dorsal subluxation or dislocation. The metatarsal heads are directed more plantarward, the toes show a hammer toe or claw toe deformity, and the protective plantar fat pad is drawn distally, further exposing the metatarsal heads.

48 The preferred surgical approach includes the following:
(1) An arthrodesis of the first MTP joint properly shortened to account for the lesser metatarsal head resections
(2) Correction of the lesser toe IP joint deformities (osteoclasis versus condylectomies)
(3) Release of the soft tissues around the subluxated or dislocated MTP joints with resection of the lesser metatarsal heads taking care to maintain a laterally sloping cascade of metatarsal lengths
(4) K-wires hold the toes and MTPs in the corrected position in the perioperative period.

49 Most likely the laterally sloping cascade of lesser metatarsal length has not been maintained. Either insufficient bone was removed from the fourth metatarsal at the time of the original surgery or regrowth of bone at the resected plantar end of the metatarsal may have occurred. It is important to excise the individual metatarsal heads in an oblique direction, removing more bone from the plantar aspect than dorsally at the time of the original surgery. Revision surgery will require further bone resection.

50 The usual cause is posttraumatic, often the result of Lisfranc's fractures and dislocations. Besides NSAIDs, conservative management consists of total contact orthoses with longitudinal arch support, with or without inflexible rocker bottom soles being added to one's shoes, and appropriate padding of the tongue of the shoes.

QUESTIONS

51 A 30-year-old man has painful dorsal spurs of the first metatarso-cuneiform joint that are resistant to conservative measures. What do your work-up and surgical plans include?

52 What are some technical problems with this procedure?

53 Which metatarsals are not connected via an intermetatarsal ligament between their bases?

54 What is the differential diagnosis for a suspected interdigital neuroma in a 50-year-old woman?

55 A 45-year-old woman allegedly had a third interspace neuroma excision performed elsewhere. On clinical examination, she has intact sensation of her third and fourth toes. Is it possible the neuroma had been completely resected?

56 What is the underlying source of almost all diabetic foot problems?

57 What are the typical complaints of a 50-year-old woman with a 10-year history of insulin-dependent diabetes and a recent onset of neuropathy?

58 Before trimming an excruciatingly painful ingrown great toenail of a 55-year-old insulin-dependent diabetic woman with a long history of peripheral neuropathy, what else should one consider?

59 At her initial clinic visit, a 40-year-old female diabetic is noted to have lost the ability to feel a 5.07 Semmes-Weinstein monofilament on the plantar aspect of her forefoot. No deformity or ulcers are present, but callus is present beneath her metatarsal heads. How do you approach her problem?

ANSWERS

51 Physical examination and a tomogram or computed tomographic (CT) scan should rule out extensive first tarsometatarsal (TMT) articular involvement and other metatarsocuneiform joint involvement. An exostectomy for this painful prominence is indicated and must include a generous amount of bone excision (excavation) because postoperative overgrowth is frequent.

52 In addition to inadequate bony resection, iatrogenic neuromas and residual arthritis may cause morbidity. Adequate postoperative immobilization is required due to the instability arising from this surgery.

53 The first and second metatarsals have no connecting intermetatarsal ligaments. The medial interosseous ligament, or Lisfranc's ligament, arises from the first cuneiform and inserts into the second metatarsal.

54 In all cases of suspected interdigital neuroma, one should consider the possibility of tarsal tunnel syndrome, deficient plantar fat pad, MTP synovitis, subluxation or dislocation, plantar callosity, and lumbar disk disease.

55 Yes, as a result of the degree of overlap that is present in the innervation of this area, approximately 32% of patients still have normal sensation in the web space following complete excision of their interdigital neuroma.

56 Neuropathy, especially sensory neuropathy, in combination with pressure over a bony prominence, is the initiating event of almost all ulcerations and most subsequent infections of the feet in diabetic patients. It is a widely held misconception that diabetic ulcers occur primarily because of circulatory impairment; rather it coexists and contributes to poor healing, but it is not the initiating event.

57 In addition to diminished sensitivity, one describes a burning, searing, tingling, or lancinating dysesthesia, often unrelenting or excruciating in degree. It is often bilateral, symmetric, and worse at night.

58 Patients with a long history of neuropathy are often insensate. Before trimming her nail, her vascular status needs to be assessed. Often these patients experience rest ischemia, which is felt most severely at the most distal point in the extremity. Arteriosclerotic disease is more common and more severe in diabetics.

59 This condition represents the absence of protective sensation. As a result she needs to be educated regarding care and daily inspection of her feet. She should be prescribed appropriate shoe wear and total contact inserts to protect and unweight the high-pressure areas on the plantar surface of her feet.

QUESTIONS

60 Describe the Eichenholtz classification of Charcot's joint arthropathy.

61 What metatarsal is the most commonly fractured?

62 What maximal amount of displacement and angulation can be accepted before an attempt at reduction for an isolated closed metatarsal shaft fracture?

63 Describe expected radiographic findings in a 20-year-old military trainee who is complaining of midforefoot pain after just completing 6 weeks of drills.

64 On a normal AP foot radiographic film, what precise bony alignments are consistently present at the bases of the second and third metatarsals proximally?

65 What radiographic findings are suggestive of an injury to the TMT joint complex (Lisfranc's joint)?

66 What is the procedure of choice for detecting subtle Lisfranc injuries?

67 Describe the detailed anatomic pathology of a grade III "turf toe" sprain in a 22-year-old football player.

68 What tendon(s) insert on the medial and lateral sesamoids?

ANSWERS

60 S.N. Eichenholtz described three stages of the Charcot's joint arthropathy that represent its course from the initial events to eventual healing.
Stage I—*Fragmentation* involves an acute inflammatory process associated with hyperemia and thus swelling, increased heat, and erythema. X-ray films show dissolution, fragmentation and dislocation.
Stage II—*Coalescence* is the diminution of edema, warmth and redness, and the beginning of the reparative process. X-ray films show coalescing new bone formations at the sites of initiating fractures, bone destruction, and dislocations.
Stage III—*Consolidation and Healing (reconstruction)* usually with residual deformity.

ANSWERS

61 The fifth metatarsal is the most commonly fractured. The third metatarsal is the second most commonly injured, followed by the second, first, and fourth metatarsals.

62 This procedure is somewhat controversial; however, most agree that fractures that have angulation of the distal fragment in either plane that is greater than 10° or displacement greater than 3 mm or 4 mm should have attempted reduction.

63 Metatarsal stress fractures are often seen in athletes and military personnel. Although radiographic findings are normal in 10% to 30% of cases, changes may include a hairline fracture through one cortex, reactive bone or localized periostitis, endosteal thickening, intramedullary sclerosis, and resorption at the fracture line.

64 The second metatarsal base aligns with the medial edge of the middle cuneiform. The third metatarsal base aligns with the medial and lateral margin of the lateral cuneiform at the TMT joint.

65 (1) The fleck sign, or fracture, at the base of the second metatarsal often with widening between the first and second metatarsal bases
(2) Compression fracture of the cuboid
(3) Avulsion fracture of the navicular tubercle
(4) Cuneiform subluxation or dislocation
(5) MTP dislocations

66 AP tomograms of the midfoot are most revealing. Also helpful is a CT scan performed in the planes parallel and perpendicular to the metatarsal shaft as they articulate with the tarsal bones.

67 Grade I sprains involve stretching of the capsuloligamentous complex around the first MTP. Grade II sprains have a partial tear of this complex. Grade III sprains involve tearing of the plantar plate from its origin on the metatarsal head-neck junction and impaction of the proximal phalanx into the metatarsal head dorsally. There may be a sesamoid fracture or separation of a bipartite sesamoid in this grade.

68 The medial (tibial) sesamoid serves as a point of insertion for the medial head of the flexor hallucis brevis (FHB) and the abductor hallucis, whereas the lateral (fibular) sesamoid serves as a point of insertion of the lateral head of the FHB and both heads of the adductor hallucis.

QUESTIONS

69 What is the motor innervation of <u>A</u> in Figure 7-3?

70 What is the motor innervation of <u>B</u> in Figure7-3?

Fig 7-3

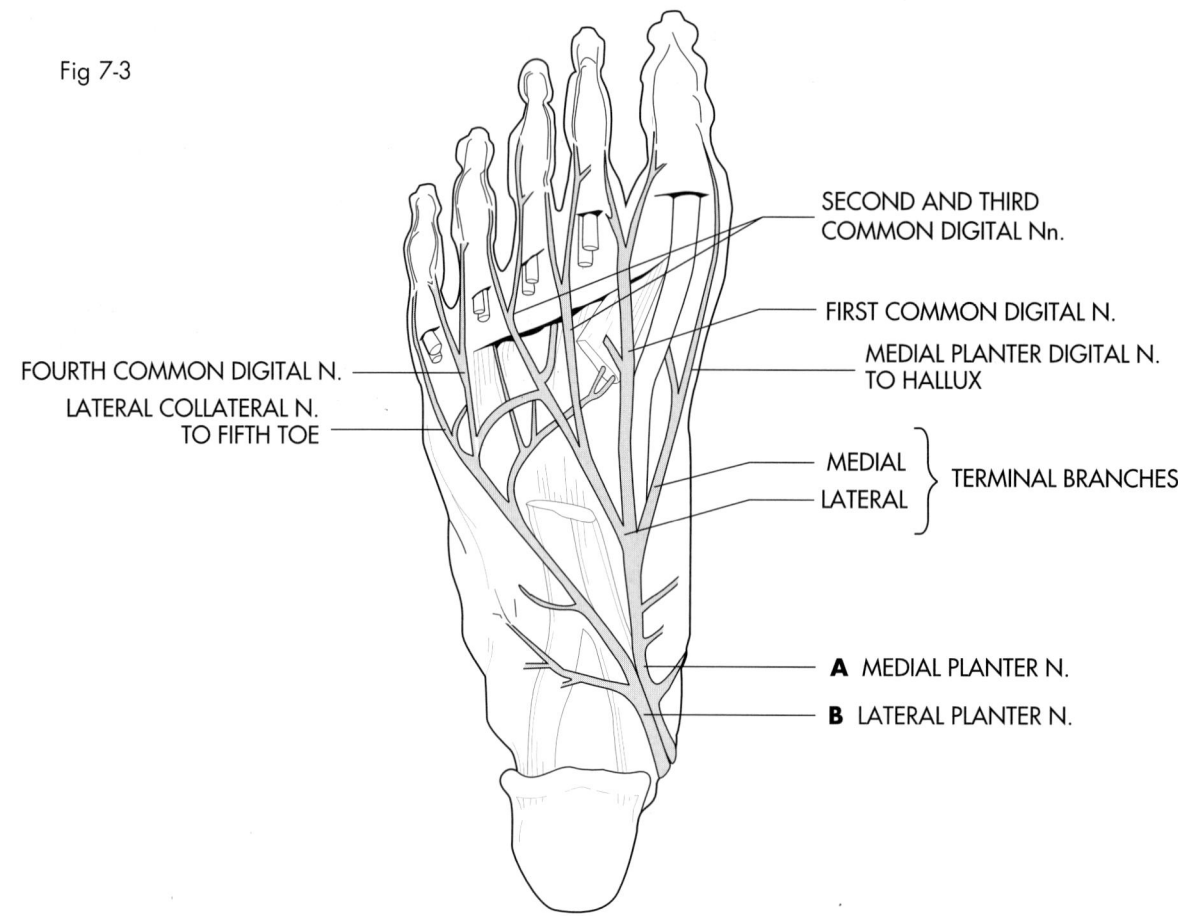

FOURTH COMMON DIGITAL N.

LATERAL COLLATERAL N.
TO FIFTH TOE

SECOND AND THIRD
COMMON DIGITAL Nn.

FIRST COMMON DIGITAL N.

MEDIAL PLANTER DIGITAL N.
TO HALLUX

MEDIAL ⎱ TERMINAL BRANCHES
LATERAL ⎰

A MEDIAL PLANTER N.
B LATERAL PLANTER N.

71 Describe the extraosseous vascular supply of the talus and its clinical significance.

72 Describe the three basic portals in ankle arthroscopy. What structures do they endanger?

73 Describe common osteochondral lesions of the talar dome.

ANSWERS

69 The medial plantar nerve innervates the FHB, abductor hallucis, flexor digitorum brevis (FDB), and first lumbrical muscles.

70 The lateral plantar nerve supplies motor innervation to the quadratus plantae, abductor digiti minimi, flexor digiti minimi, adductor hallucis, all plantar and dorsal interossei, and the second through fourth lumbrical muscles.

71 Approximately 60% of the surface of the talus is covered by articular coverage, rendering a limited available surface for vascular perforations. The talar body is supplied by branches of the posterior tibial, anterior tibial, and peroneal arteries. Of these, the major blood supply is via the artery of the tarsal canal, a branch of the posterior tibial. The artery of the tarsal canal branches in the deltoid ligament to give off the deltoid artery, also an important source of circulation to the talar body. For this reason, the deltoid ligament should be left intact when approaching the talus for fixation of fractures. The tarsal sinus artery is formed from branches of the dorsalis pedis and peroneal artery. This artery forms an anastomosis with the artery of the tarsal canal inferior to the neck of the talus.

72 *Anterolateral* enters the joint between fibula and talus, 0.5 mm to 1.0 cm distal to the joint line. The incision is placed lateral to the peroneus tertius tendon and endangers the superficial peroneal nerve.
Anteromedial enters 0.5 mm to 1 cm distal to the joint line, medial to anterior tibial tendon. The incision endangers the saphenous nerve and vein.
Posterolateral enters 1 cm below the joint line, immediately adjacent to the Achilles tendon and posterior to the peroneal tendon. The incision endangers the sural nerve.

73 Berndt and Harty have classified osteochondral fractures into four stages:
Stage I—an area of compressed subchondral bone
Stage II—a partially detached osteochondral fragment
Stage III—a completely detached osteochondral fracture that remains in situ
Stage IV—a completely displaced osteochondral fragment
The location of the lesion is generally either lateral and slightly anterior on the talar dome or medial and posterior.

QUESTIONS

74 Describe treatment of these osteochondral lesions.

75 A 35-year-old man is seen in your office for ankle pain. He reports he "sprained" his ankle 2 months earlier when he tripped going up a flight of stairs. This was treated with a cast for 4 weeks followed by use of a lace up support. He now notes persistent pain in the lateral ankle area and a painful "popping" sensation when walking. Describe the evaluation and most likely diagnosis.

76 A 20-year-old soccer player complains of posteromedial ankle pain, felt most prominently when kicking the ball. Resisted plantar flexion of the great toe is painful. Describe likely differential diagnosis and further evaluation.

77 Describe treatment of posterior ankle impingement.

78 A 40-year-old man sustains an inversion injury to his plantar flexed foot. Radiographic films reveal a fracture at the tuberosity of the fifth metatarsal with minimal displacement. Describe treatment of this fracture.

ANSWERS

74 Generally, stage I and II lesions are initially treated nonoperatively, by immobilization and restricted activities on weight-bearing bones. If synovitis or significant symptoms persist, operative intervention, usually in the form of removal of the fragment and curettage of the bed of the lesion, is recommended. Stage III or IV lesions are generally treated initially by removal of the fragment and curettage of the base. Pinning, rather than débridement, of the fragment may be considered. Lesions that are less detached and larger, deeper lesions would be more likely considered for pinning.

75 This history is typical for peroneal tendon subluxation or dislocation. The injury is frequently associated with simultaneous peroneal contractions and ankle dorsiflexion. On examination, acutely there is tenderness along the posterior margin of the lateral malleolus. The peroneal tendons may at times be palpated over the lateral malleolus or felt to sublux on ankle dorsiflexion. There may be a popping sensation elicited with ankle motion. X-ray films may show a tiny fragment at the lateral malleolus or the calcaneus, avulsed by the peroneal retinaculum. Acute injuries may be managed by immobilization, although some authors advocate immediate repair of the retinaculum

ANSWERS

to the posterior surface of the lateral malleolus. Patients who exhibit persistent pain and recurrent dislocations of the tendons after closed treatment may be managed with operative repair. This repair consists of three main types of surgical intervention:

Rerouting procedures, which substitutes the calcaneofibular ligament for the incompetent superior peroneal retinaculum.

Groove deepening procedures, which either slides bone blocks or decancellation of the posterior surface of the lateral malleolus and recesses the cortex in this region.

Soft tissue reconstruction or reinforcements, which may involve direct repair of the retinaculum or may use transplanted or local tissues to reconstruct a new peroneal retinaculum.

76   A number of structures may be impinged between the calcaneus and the posterior tibia. The posterior process may sustain an acute fracture, an os trigonum may become symptomatic (i.e., with or without acute separation at the synchondrosis, or impingement pain may exist secondary to a large posterior process on the talus, to a large or a thickened posterior capsule, or to inflamed adjacent tissues caused by posterior process on the calcaneus. Patients may complain of posteromedial or posterolateral ankle pain on plantar flexion. Additionally, coexisting FHL tendinitis may occur, as evidenced by pain on resisted flexion of the dorsiflexed great toe.

The source of impingement may be recognized on a lateral x-ray film of the foot. In some cases, bone scan or CT may be needed to verify the diagnosis.

77   Posterior ankle impingement from whatever cause is generally treated initially nonoperatively, by avoidance of full plantar flexion and rest. A short leg cast may be used if an acute fracture is suspected. If nonoperative treatment fails, excision of the offending structures, as well as FHL tenolysis when indicated, may be performed through a posteromedial or posterolateral incision.

78   This fracture could generally be treated with a short leg cast and non–weight-bearing activities. If a small avulsed fragment does develop a painful nonunion, this may be treated by excision of the proximal fragment with advancement of the peroneus brevis tendon.

QUESTIONS

79 A 20-year-old college basketball player sustains an inversion injury to his ankle when his foot lands on that of another player. On questioning he notes he has had pain in the foot since a similar episode 2 months earlier. X-ray films reveal a fracture at the metaphyseal-diaphyseal junction of the fifth metatarsal bone with intramedullary sclerosis evident in the area. Describe treatment of this fracture.

80 A 30-year-old man sustains a crush injury to his foot. Fractures of the second and third metatarsal necks are treated by a short leg cast for 6 weeks. When seen 3 months after injury, he complains of persistent burning pain in the foot, and he is unable to bear weight. Radiographic films reveal healing of the fractures but marked osteoporosis of the entire foot. Describe the likely diagnosis, work-up, and treatment.

81 Describe the gait disturbance associated with an ankle fusion in excessive ankle plantar flexion.

82 Describe the effect of the position of the subtalar joint on the transverse tarsal joint.

83 Describe the relative benefits and disadvantages of the solid-ankle, cushion-heel (SACH) foot, single-axis foot, multi-axis foot, and flexible-keel-dynamic-response foot prostheses.

84 What are the relative advantages of operative and nonoperative treatment of Achilles tendon rupture?

ANSWERS

79 Fractures at the metaphyseal-diaphyseal junction, which exhibit preexisting stress reaction, are prone to delayed union. Although some authors advocate a trial of treatment with a non–weight-bearing short leg cast, immediate operative intervention in a high-performance athlete is preferable. Intramedullary fixation with a screw and bone grafting has been used with curettage of the sclerotic medullary canal.

80 Reflex sympathetic dystrophy (RSD) is a poorly understood spectrum of symptoms. Hyperesthesias and pain out of proportion to the injury, particularly if it is diffuse and nonanatomic, is typical but not specific for this syndrome. Vasomotor instability may be evident as discoloration, warmth or coolness in comparison with the opposite side, and edema. Diffuse, patchy osteoporosis may provide radiographic film evidence of RSD. Bone scan may show diffusely increased uptake, particularly in juxtaarticular areas. Other diag-

ANSWERS

noses, such as infection, tumor, or unrecognized fracture, should be ruled out. Treatment is controversial, but generally it involves some form of sympathetic blockade, as well as physical therapy emphasizing desensitization, motion, and return of function.

81 Excessive plantar flexion may cause genu recurvatum at heel strike. Additionally, the extremity may rotate externally in an attempt to avoid passing directly over the plantar flexed foot, leading to laxity of the medial collateral ligament (MCL).

82 When the subtalar joint is everted, the axes of the talonavicular and calcaneocuboid joints become parallel, allowing motion at these joints and thus more flexibility. Subtalar inversion causes the axes of the talonavicular and calcaneocuboid joints to diverge, "locking" the transtarsal joint and creating a more rigid foot. For this reason, arthrodesis of the subtalar joint in inversion (hindfoot varus) is to be avoided.

83 The *SACH foot* is low cost, durable, and cosmetic. There is, however, a limited degree of adjustability of resistance to plantar flexion and dorsiflexion. As the heel cushions deteriorate, the prosthesis loses shock absorption.
The *single-axis foot* provides increased knee stability, but it is bulkier and requires somewhat more maintenance than a SACH foot. It is more commonly used as the prosthetic ankle for an above-knee amputation.
The *multi-axis foot* provides more motion than any other prosthetic foot. It is useful for patients who most frequently ambulate over uneven terrain. It is, however, heavy and requires more maintenance than a SACH foot or single-axis foot.
The *flexible-keel-dynamic-response foot* (Flex-Foot, Seattle Foot) allows for not only shock absorption but also some degree of push-off. These prostheses are constructed of extremely lightweight materials. This provides for a more fluid gait and may decrease high-activity energy expenditure. The chief disadvantage is their expense. These prostheses are best suited for the active, high-demand amputee.

84 Operative repair is associated with a lower rate of rerupture (2% to 7%), and allows for better return of plantar flexion strength. Although nonoperative repair is associated with a higher rerupture rate (approximately 15%), it avoids the high-wound complication rate of operative repair (1% infection, 5% wound necrosis). Consideration for treatment includes the activity level of the patient. Additionally, the presence of a large gap between the tendon ends—either palpated or seen on magnetic resosnance imaging (MRI)—is thought by some to be an additional indication for operative repair or reconstruction.

QUESTIONS

85 A 9-year-old boy steps on a nail, which passes through his sneaker and punctures his foot in the metatarsal head area. He is seen in the local emergency room, where his wound is irrigated; he is given a tetanus immunization, and he is provided with a prescription for cephalexin. He comes to your office 3 days later with swelling, redness, and pain in the ball of the foot. Outline possible reasons for persistent infection.

86 Describe evaluation and treatment of the patient in Q85.

87 What types of organisms are commonly found in plantar ulcers in diabetes?

88 In treating comminuted fractures of the tibial plafond, compare limitations of closed and open treatment.

89 Describe surgical approaches to the talus and the limitations of each.

ANSWERS

85 Puncture wounds tend to close over, failing to drain. It is difficult to properly irrigate the wound. A joint, a tendon sheath, or a metatarsal may have been contaminated. Foreign material may have been driven into the wound. Pseudomonas is frequently associated with puncture wounds, particularly when the impaling object passes through a tennis shoe.

86 Physical examination should be directed at excluding joint or tendon involvement. X-ray films should be checked for radiopaque foreign bodies or evidence of bone penetration. Incision and drainage should be performed through the site of the puncture with blunt dissection to the depth of the puncture wound. If there is evidence of joint involvement, the joint should be opened and evaluated with irrigation performed if there is evidence of infection. A similar procedure is performed for any associated tendon sheath infection. Antibiotics should be administered, using antipseudomonas coverage if the wound occurred through a shoe and anaerobic coverage if the wound occurred in a barnyard type of environment.

87 Diabetic plantar ulcers are commonly polymicrobial. Frequently an anaerobe will be one of the organisms cultured from the wound. There is poor correlation between cultures taken from superficial swabs of the wound or from drainage and cultures taken from tissue at the depth of the wound.

88 Closed treatment of comminuted tibial plafond fractures has been associated with a high percentage of poor results, chiefly from post-traumatic arthritis. Although several studies have shown better healing percentages with open reduction and rigid internal fixation, the percentage of poor results is associated with a high rate of wound complications, including infection, skin slough and dehiscence, and osteomyelitis. The frequency and severity of these complications have led some to recommend limited internal or external fixation of the major fragments, with the use of plating on any associated fibula fracture, followed by delayed bone grafting of the metaphyseal defect.

89 The anteromedial approach proceeds between the EHL and the tibialis anterior tendons. Visualization of the fracture is somewhat limited, and it is difficult to place rigid fixation. The anterolateral approach also affords limited visualization of the fracture site. The ability to place rigid fixation, perpendicular to the fracture, is somewhat better, but the superficial peroneal nerve and its branches are at risk, and soft tissue stripping damages the multiple vascular foramina in this region. The posterolateral approach is lateral to the Achilles tendon, placing implants lateral to the lateral process. It provides for the best fixation but does not allow direct visualization of the fracture site.

QUESTIONS

90 What structure is most at risk in the posterolateral approach for talar neck fractures?

91 During what period of time is spontaneous neurologic recovery believed to be possible after a cerebral vascular accident (CVA)? After a closed head injury?

92 What ankle and foot deformity is the most commonly seen after CVA?

93 Describe the gait abnormalities associated with a prosthetic foot placed in too much dorsiflexion.

94 Describe the course of the medial plantar nerve in the foot.

95 Describe the course of the lateral plantar nerve in the foot.

96 Describe vascular study results associated with good healing of an amputation.

97 What nutritional parameters are associated with good healing of an amputation?

ANSWERS

90 The sural nerve is most at risk with this approach.

91 Spontaneous neurologic recovery is expected in 6 to 9 months after a CVA. Spontaneous neurologic recovery is no longer expected 12 to 18 months after a closed head injury. These time periods are of importance in planning corrective surgery for deformity associated with such injuries.

92 An equinovarus deformity, usually with curling of the toes, is the most common deformity that occurs following a CVA.

93 Excessive dorsiflexion causes early and abrupt heel-off with a shortened stride length.

94 The plantar nerves branch from the posterior tibial nerve beneath the flexor retinaculum in the tarsal tunnel. The medial plantar nerve runs forward deep to the abductor hallucis, passing distally in the interval between the abductor hallucis and the FDB and gives off the proper plantar digital nerve to the great toe. At the level of the metatarsal bases, it divides into three common digital nerves. Its distribution may be roughly compared with that of the median nerve in the hand.

95 The lateral plantar nerve arises beneath the flexor retinaculum, passes laterally between the abductor hallucis muscle and the quadratus plantae, and then travels between the flexor digitorum brevis and the quadratus plantae. Its distribution to the digits may be compared with the ulnar nerve in the hand.

96 An ischemic index, or ankle brachial index of 0.35, or 0.45 in diabetes, indicates sufficient perfusion for healing. Calcified, incompressible vessels usually yield a value greater than 1.0 and render the study invalid. Many isotopic tracers have been used, with a correlation shown between skin blood flow level greater than 2.5 mg/100 g/min and healing potential. Transcutaneous oxygen pressure greater than 35 mm Hg at the calf predicts healing of a below-knee amputation. Inhalation of 100% oxygen may increase the accuracy of this test.

97 Although multiple tests have been used, the total lymphocyte count and serum albumin level are most commonly mentioned, primarily because they are inexpensive and readily available. An albumin level of 3.5 and total lymphocyte count greater than 1500 have been noted to predict healing.

QUESTIONS

98 How should the injury shown be treated (*Figure 7-4*)?

Fig 7-4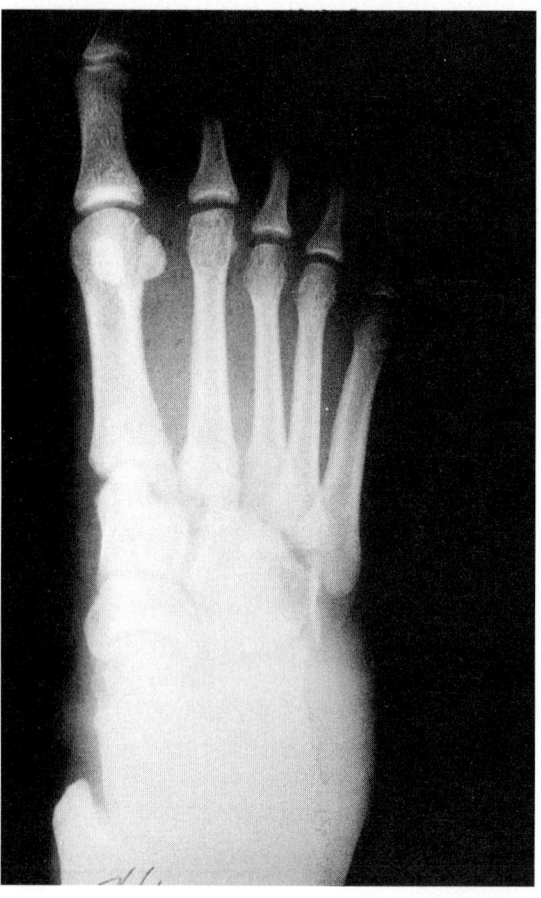

99 What is the mechanism of injury of this fracture, and how should it be treated (*Figure 7-5*)?

Fig 7-5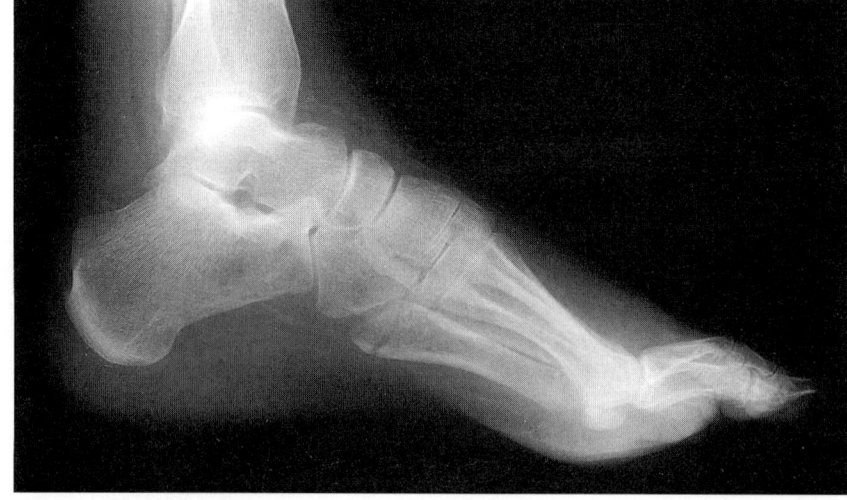

ANSWERS

98 Displaced Lisfranc's fractures and dislocations are optimally treated with open reduction and internal fixation.

99 This avulsion fracture is caused by contraction of the peroneus brevis and should be treated with a short leg walking cast or hard soled shoe.

QUESTIONS

100 How should this fracture be treated (*Figure 7-6*)?

Fig 7-6

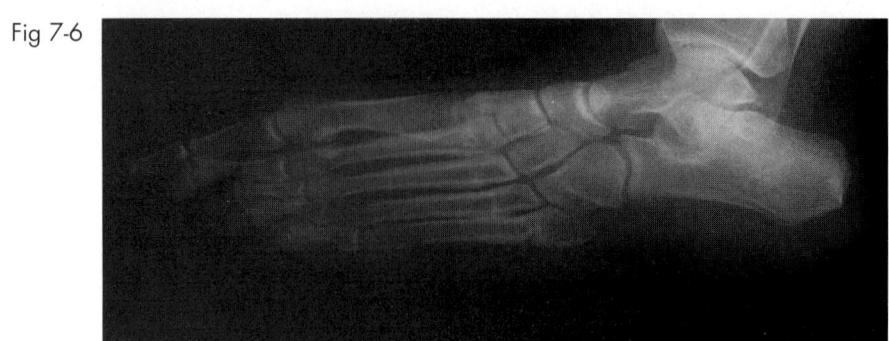

101 How should this fracture be treated (*Figure 7-7*)?

Fig 7-7

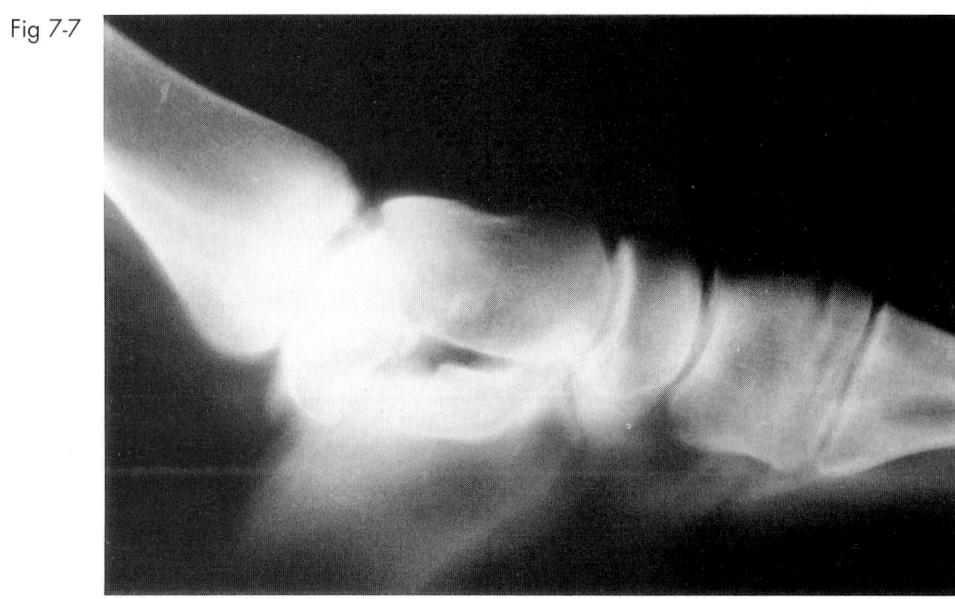

ANSWERS

100 With a short leg cast and non–weight-bearing ambulation for approximately 6 weeks, open reduction and internal fixation is an alternative, particularly for an athlete.

101 This talar body fracture should undergo open reduction and internal fixation using cancellous lag screws.

CHAPTER 8

Spine

Howard M. Place
J. Kenneth Burkus

QUESTION

1   A 21-year-old active man was involved in competitive boxing. He sustained a direct blow to his head and noticed instantaneous total body tingling. He also complained of left-sided facial pain. This resolved within seconds, and he continued with his boxing match. After the match he continued to complain of posterior neck pain and occipital pain. He was found to be neurologically intact. Selected studies are shown in Figures 8-1 through 8-4. (*Figure 8-1*—lateral upper cervical spine; *Figure 8-2*—flexion lateral; *Figure 8-3*—extension lateral; *Figure 8-4*—lateral magnetic resonance imaging [MRI]). What is your diagnosis based upon this history and the radiographic findings?

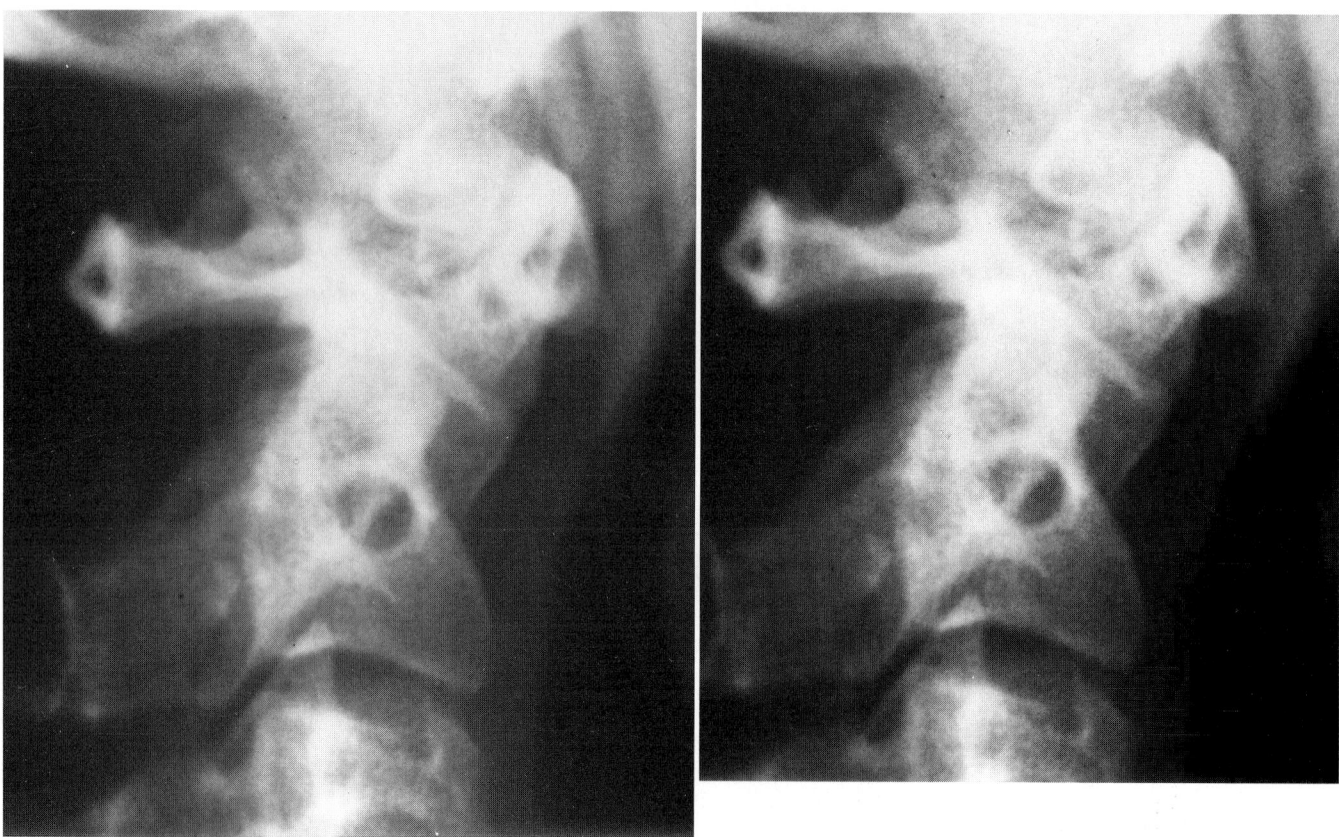

Fig 8-1   Fig 8-2

ANSWER

Fig 8-3

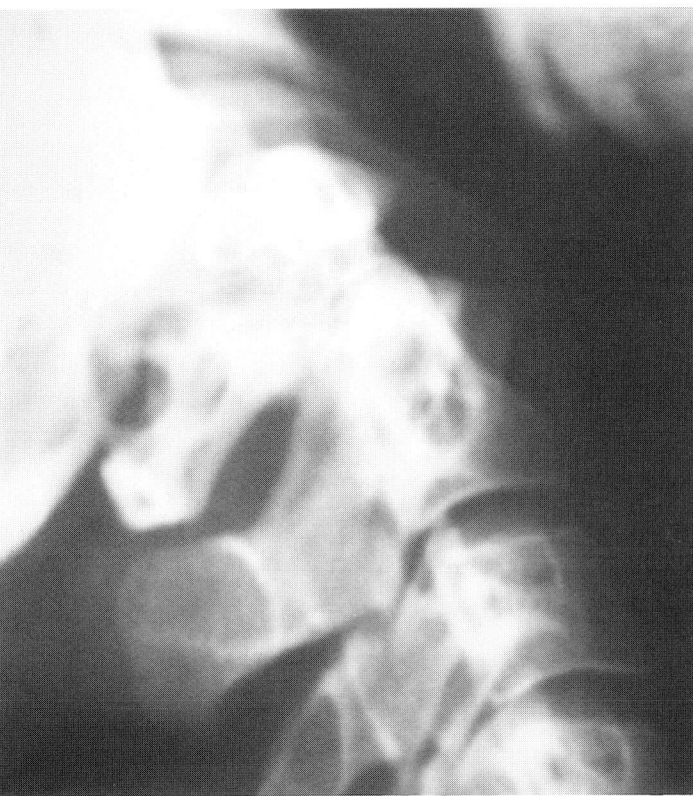

Fig 8-4

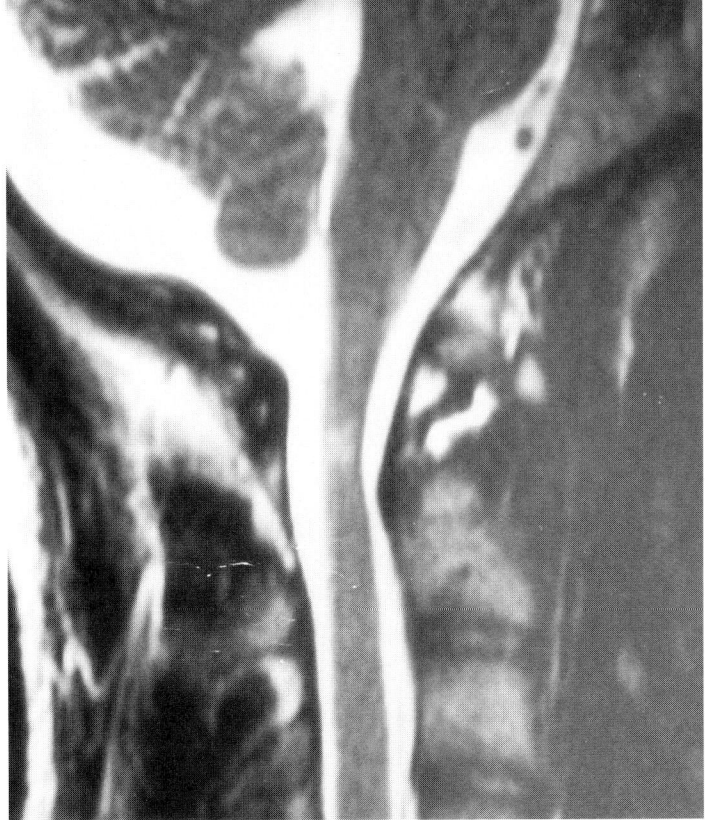

1 The patient's diagnosis is os odontoideum with posttraumatic spinal cord edema.

QUESTIONS

2 What is the etiology of this bony pathologic condition?

3 Does this patient require treatment for his os odontoideum?

4 What are the surgical treatment options for this patient?

5 If this patient had an incompetent ring of C1 (i.e., secondary to fracture or congenital malformation), what would be the best form of surgical treatment?

6 A young active asymptomatic patient has radiographic findings consistent with an os odontoideum. He wants to participate in high school football. What should you recommend?

7 A patient has a type II, odontoid base fracture. Which risk factors need to be considered when deciding on future treatment?

ANSWERS

2 The etiology of os odontoideum is still debated. Some believe that this is a congenital malformation and discuss the five separate primary ossification centers of the axis. Two of these ossification centers are for the odontoid process. Many patients with os odontoideum do not have a history of significant trauma. However, Fielding and associates (*J Bone Joint Surg* 62A(3):376, 1980) believe that this is most likely the result of trauma. He presents a series of patients with os odontoideum, nine of which have a history of significant neck trauma but previously documented normal odontoid processes on radiographic evaluation. It is most commonly accepted at this time that trauma does play some role in the etiology of os odontoideum.

3 Not all patients who have an incidental finding of os odontoideum require surgical treatment. Spierings and Braakman (*J Bone Joint Surg* 64B(4):422, 1982) presented a series of 37 patients, 20 of which were treated nonoperatively and 17 of which were treated surgically. The patients with incidental os odontoideum and local symptoms were treated nonoperatively if it was believed that they had minimal instability. Cord signs, transient cord symptoms, or signs of gross instability recommended for other conditions (rheumatoid arthritis [RA], trauma, Down syndrome) are indications for surgical treatment. This patient meets the criteria for surgical stabilization.

ANSWERS

4 The patient with os odontoideum and no other vertebral anomalies may be treated with posterior wiring and bone grafting of C1-C2. Although there are a number of techniques available, the most common are the Brooks and Gallie fusions. These techniques require postoperative immobilization, usually in the form of a halo orthosis. Some authors are using this technique with C1-C2 transarticular screws. This treatment is believed to significantly increase the torsional rigidity of this fused spinal segment and to decrease the necessity for postoperative immobilization in a halo device. This technique may not be appropriate in children. There has been recent interest in anterior screw fixation of dens fractures. This technique is not indicated where there is significant instability and an established pseudarthrosis present. Regardless of the technique, attention should be directed toward fusing the spine in good alignment.

5 The standard of care for this constellation of findings has been a surgical fusion of the occiput to C2. In children, a posterior flap of periosteum may be elevated off of the occiput with a distal base. This periosteal flap prevents bone from impinging upon the spinal cord from the midline bony defect. An alternative approach employs the posterior placement of C1-C2 transarticular screws. This significantly increases the local rigidity at the C1-C2 level and allows for continued motion at the occipitocervical junction. C1-C2 transarticular screws are not recommended in small children.
There is another alternative to the occiput to C2 fusion. If the C1 defect is not large, this defect may be bone grafted at the time of the C1-C2 fusion. This patient should then be treated in a halo, and re-exploration should be considered.

6 There are no universally accepted criteria to delineate which cervical spine anomalies or injuries preclude a patient from returning to collision sports. There are numerous suggested criteria that evaluate the patient's risk for significant spinal injury. Torg (Operative techniques in sports medicine, 1(3):236, 1993) reports a case of quadriplegia in a football player with a preexisting os odontoideum. It is his recommendation that such anomalies of the odontoid be considered absolute contraindications to participation in contact sports.

7 The reported risk factors for a nonunion in type II odontoid fractures include an older patient, an initial displacement greater than or equal to 6 mm, an angulation of the fracture, a delay in diagnosis, or a posterior displacement of the odontoid.

QUESTIONS

8 What are the surgical treatment options for a 60-year-old man with a 6-mm displaced type II odontoid fracture?

9 A 35-year-old man has a 2-week history of neck pain radiating into his left arm. He states that his left arm pain is worse than his neck pain. There is no history of trauma. His primary care physician evaluated this patient with an MRI and then referred him to you. His physical examination reveals weakness in his triceps and a decreased triceps reflex on the left. He has decreased sensitivity to light touch in his long finger. His MRI is shown in Figures 8-5 and 8-6. What is your diagnosis?

Fig 8-5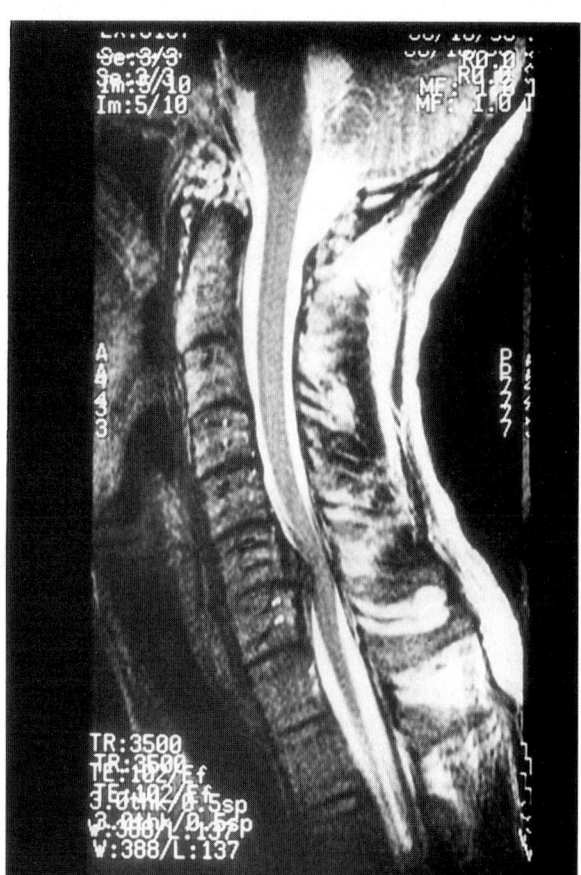

ANSWERS

Fig 8-6

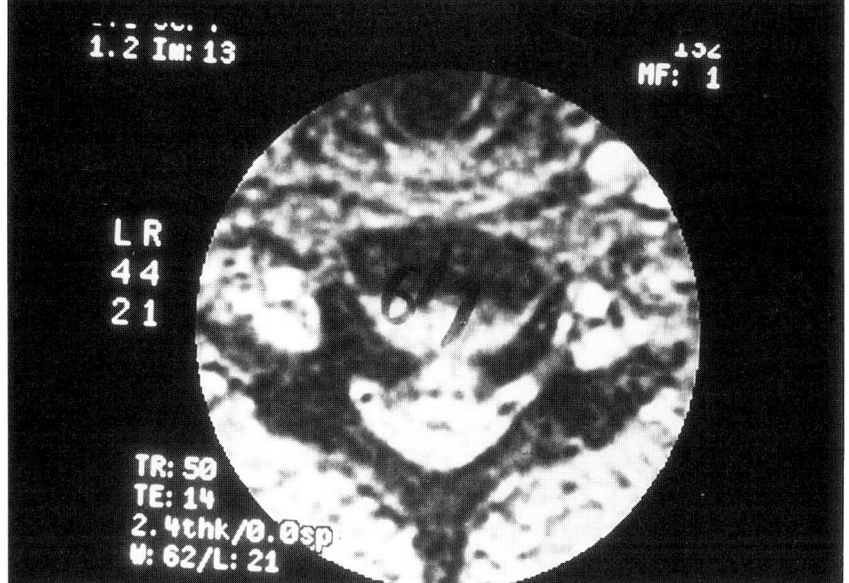

8 The most common surgical treatment for this patient includes an attempted reduction and posterior fusion with a midline wiring technique. Care must be taken to provide the best possible reduction of the fracture and to avoid displacement during the instrumentation portion of the procedure. This is possible with many of the midline wiring techniques by displacing the ring of C1 more posteriorly in relationship to the ring of C2. Other options include transarticular C1-C2 facet screw. This technique is more demanding, though it does have the advantage of providing a more rigid construct. Some centers are also using an odontoid screw placed across the fracture from an anterior approach. This theoretically preserves C1-C2 motion but is technically demanding.

9 This patient has an acute C7 radiculopathy secondary to a C6-C7 herniated nucleus pulposus.

QUESTIONS

10 What is the appropriate initial management of this patient?

11 After 3 months this patient continues to have significant arm pain and weakness. He has failed your prescribed regimen of nonoperative treatment. What are your surgical treatment options?

12 A patient comes to your office with a history of neck pain several months ago, but the pain has since resolved completely. He had no history of radicular symptoms at that time. An MRI was ordered, and it is identical to the MRI shown in Figures 8-5 and 8-6. What is your recommended treatment at this time?

ANSWERS

10 This patient is best managed initially with nonoperative treatment, consisting of short-term immobilization such as in a cervical orthosis, cervical traction, combined with nonsteroidal antiinflammatory agents, and analgesics. Most patients respond to this type of treatment regimen with significant improvement over the next 6 to 12 weeks.

11 The most commonly accepted and reliable surgical approach for this problem is a single level anterior cervical discectomy and fusion. It is indicated principally in the patient with midline or posterolateral disc herniation. A posterior approach via a cervical foraminotomy is considered in the patient who has significant foraminal stenosis or a lateral disc herniation. The series presented by Herkowitz (*Spine*, 1990) suggested a better overall success rate with anterior surgery and fusion as compared with posterior surgery for this condition. Although some prefer a complete anterior cervical discectomy without fusion, most orthopedic surgeons do not because of a significant rate of postsurgical collapse, late kyphosis, and variable recurrence of arm pain attributed to late resultant foraminal stenosis (Abitbol, *Semin Spine Surg*, 1989).

12 The patient is asymptomatic and thus requires no active intervention. The incidence of asymptomatic cervical herniated nucleus pulposus can be as high as 30% (Boden, *J Bone Joint Surg Am*, 1990). Without current radicular symptoms or axial pain, this patient should be treated with continued observation.

QUESTION

13 A 21-year-old rugby player is brought into your emergency room with an inability to move his arms and legs. This problem began 1 hour after injury during the contest. The patient's physical examination reveals flaccid paralysis of his lower extremities, complete absence of motor function in his left upper extremity, and trace firing of his right deltoid muscle. The patient has patchy sensation over the superior lateral aspects of both arms with the absence of sensation below the elbows bilaterally; there is no sensation to light touch or pin prick below the nipple lines bilaterally. Bulbocavernosus reflex is intact. His radiographic films are shown in Figures 8-7 through 8-10. What is your clinical diagnosis?

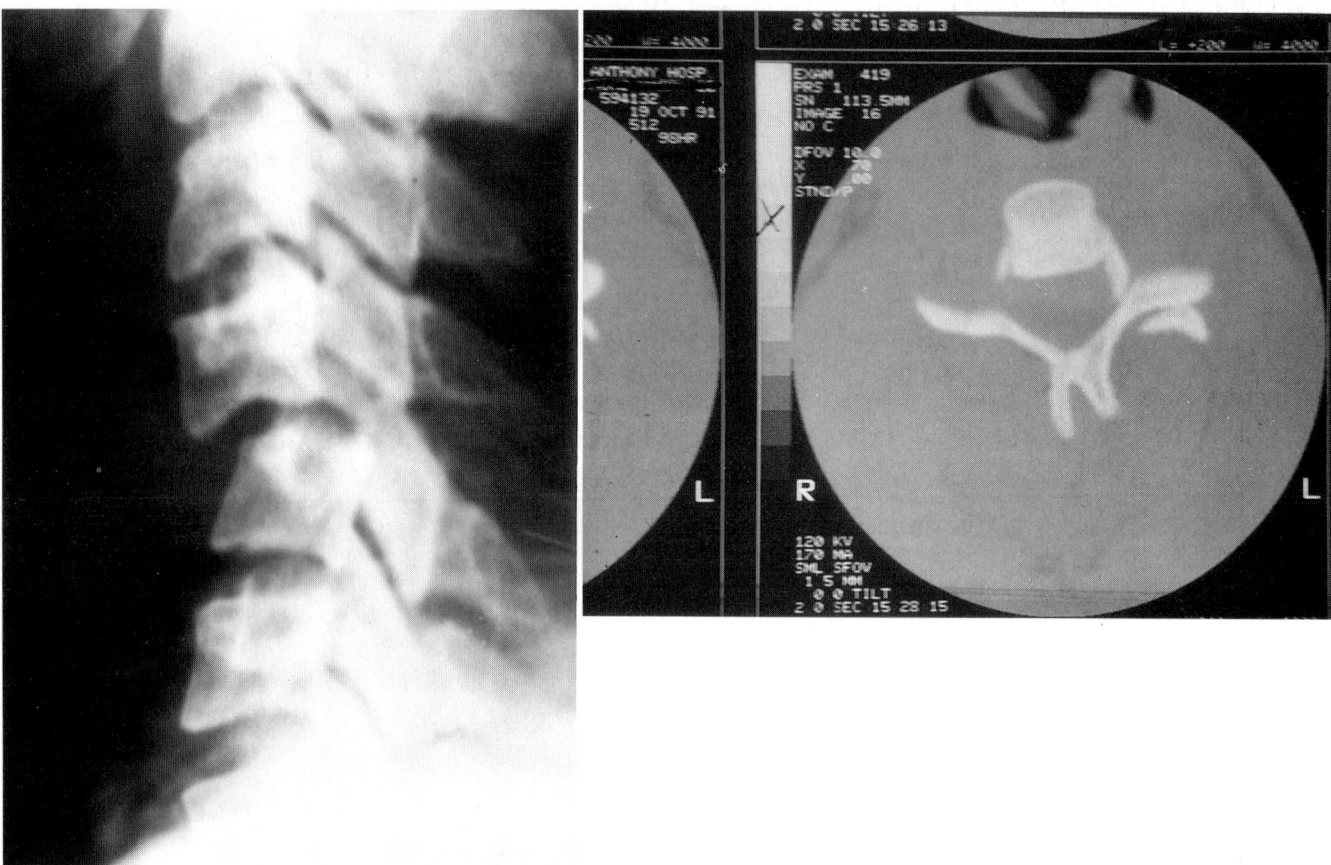

Fig 8-7   Fig 8-8

ANSWER

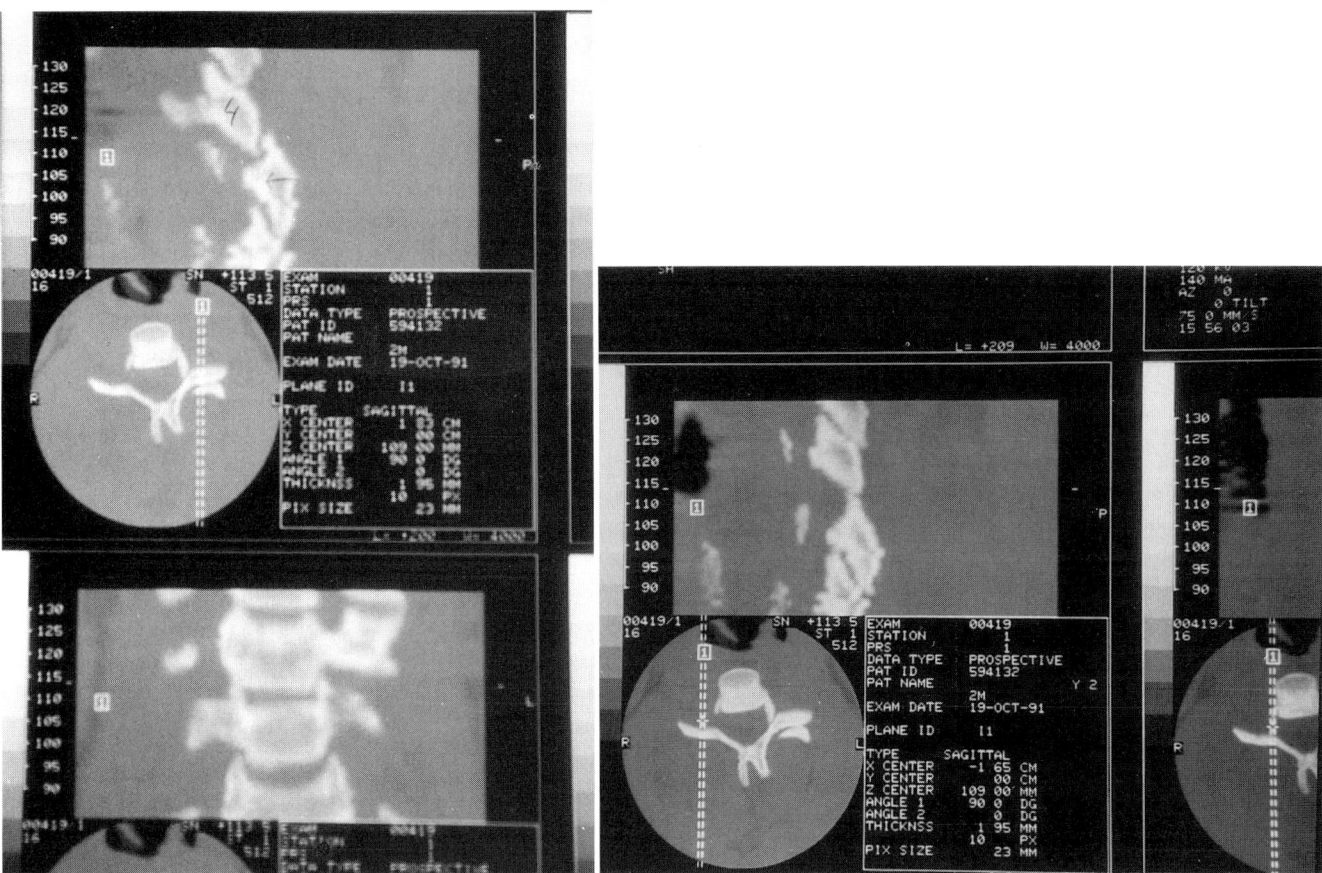

Fig 8-9   Fig 8-10

13   The clinical diagnosis in this patient is C5 quadriplegia secondary to
C5-C6 facet dislocation-subluxation. One can say that this patient has
a complete spinal cord injury because of his physical examination
and the presence of a bulbocavernosus reflex. If this patient were in
spinal shock (i.e., absence of bulbocavernosus reflex within the first
24 hours after the injury), it would be impossible to make the diagnosis of complete spinal cord injury at this time.

QUESTIONS

14   What is the role of steroids in this patient?

15   What is the recommended dose of methylprednisolone in the patient with acute spinal cord injury?

16   What further treatment should be immediately instituted?

17   What is the role of MRI in the patient with this injury?

18   If a patient with similar radiographic studies required operative reduction and his preoperative MRI demonstrated a HNP at the subluxated level, what would be the surgical sequence?

19   In the original patient with a C5 quadriplegia, a closed reduction was performed uneventfully. His neurologic status remained unchanged, and a postreduction MRI showed no evidence of HNP. How should this patient be treated at this time?

ANSWERS

14   Treatment with high-dose methylprednisolone is recommended based upon the study by Bracken and associates (*N Engl J Med*, 1990), which suggested that there was improved neurologic recovery in patients with complete spinal cord injury who were treated with high-dose methylprednisolone within the first 8 hours after their injury. Though the neurologic recovery was small and not always functionally significant, there was a statistically significant improvement in these patients' motor and sensory scores if treated with methylprednisolone as compared with placebo.

15   The patient should receive a bolus of 30 mg/kg of body weight of methylprednisolone within the first 8 hours after injury. This should then be followed by an infusion of 5.4 mg/kg/hr of methylprednisolone for the next 23 hours.

16   In this awake, alert, cooperative patient with an acute complete spinal cord injury, early spinal alignment should be achieved. Numerous studies by Rizzolo (*Spine*, 1994) and others have reported a significant benefit and safety of early cervical traction for reduction of such an injury. There is little to lose and much to gain in terms of potential early neurologic recovery through spinal reduction in the patient with complete quadriplegia by instituting early cervical traction. The functional return of even one root level is significant in this situation.

ANSWERS

17 There has been a great deal of interest recently on the incidence of cervical disc herniation with traumatic subluxation or dislocation of the cervical spine. Eismont and associates (*J Bone Joint Surg*, 1991) presented a series of patients who had significant worsening of their neurologic status after open reduction of their cervical spine alignment. This has led numerous authors to evaluate the role for prereduction MRI. There is clearly a trend toward a greater incidence of cervical herniated nucleus pulposus (HNP) with greater degrees of cervical displacement (Farber et al: *SRS*, 1994). Based upon the reviews by Rizzolo (*Spine*, 1994) and the discussion at the American Academy of Orthopedic Surgeons (AAOS) course on Spinal Instrumentation (1994), MRI evaluation of the spinal axis is not required before reduction of the cervical spine in the alert, cooperative patient. In this patient population, cervical alignment can usually be obtained with cervical traction. During the course of reduction, frequent neurologic examinations must be performed. Should the condition worsen before reduction, the reduction can be halted, and the patient can then evaluated by an MRI to rule out a significant cervical herniated nucleus pulposus. This appears to be true whether the patient had a complete spinal cord injury or no spinal cord injury. However, if the patient does have any degree of altered state of consciousness (i.e., drugs, alcohol, significant head injury, coma), a prereduction MRI is justified. If operative reduction is necessary, a prereduction MRI is recommended.

18 Such a patient would need to be treated initially with an anterior discectomy and fusion followed by posterior open reduction and fusion. If this patient also had a complete spinal cord injury, some centers would consider an anterior discectomy with an instrumented fusion. Postoperative halo immobilization should also be considered.

19 This patient has sustained a significant ligamentous injury. The supraspinous ligaments, interspinous ligaments, and both facet capsules have been completely disrupted. In this instance, nonoperative treatment with immobilization is not recommended, because extensive ligamentous injuries are unlikely to heal. He would be at significant risk for late instability. This patient should be treated with an early single-level posterior or anterior instrumented fusion.

QUESTIONS

20 A 50-year-old woman with significant rheumatoid arthritis is evaluated with a routine screening lateral radiographic film of her cervical spine. This shows 8 mm of anterior atlanto-dens interval, which completely reduces with extension. The patient has no complaint of neck pain and no neurologic signs or symptoms. What is the most appropriate treatment for this patient at the present time?

21 What is the etiology of this patient's cervical instability?

22 What ligamentous structures have been rendered incompetent when the anterior atlanto-dens interval has increased to 12 mm?

23 Which radiologic measurement is most useful in assessing the cervical instability at the atlantoaxial joint with reference to postoperative neurologic recovery in a patient with preoperative myelopathy?

24 What is the appropriate surgical intervention for a patient with fixed atlantoaxial instability, basilar invagination, and subjective weakness and hyperreflexia in their lower extremities?

25 A 20-year-old man is rendered a complete quadriplegic after a gunshot wound to the posterior cervical spine. The patient has the metallic fragment lodged in his spinal canal. What is your recommendation regarding the retained foreign body?

26 A young man is brought to the emergency room with a gunshot wound to his abdomen. He has a bullet lodged in his spinal canal above T12 and has complete paraplegia. He has an obvious perforated viscus. What is the role for fragment removal in this instance?

ANSWERS

20 The natural history of cervical spine disease in rheumatoid arthritis is unpredictable. The course can vary considerably. At this time the patient has no symptoms related to her cervical instability. Not all patients with this degree of atlantoaxial instability will show definite progression. Orthopedically she should be treated with continued observation. Aggressive medical management of her rheumatoid arthritis is recommended to address the underlying etiology of her cervical instability.

21 The dens has a synovial joint both anteriorly between the ring of C1 and the anterior aspect of the dens of C2, as well as a posterior synovial joint between the posterior aspects of the dens and the transverse ligament. In this patient the transverse ligament has been rendered incompetent by the aggressive destructive synovial process related to her rheumatoid arthritis.

ANSWERS

22   When the anterior atlanto-dens interval has progressed to greater than 10 mm, the alar, apical, and transverse ligaments are no longer functional.

23   The preoperative posterior atlanto-dens interval (ADI) in the patient with atlantoaxial subluxation is an important predictor of potential neurologic return after surgery. Boden and associates (*J Bone Joint Surg*, 1993) found that the patient with a posterior ADI of less than 10 mm before surgery had a poor prognosis for a return of motor function after surgery. The patient with a preoperative posterior ADI of 14 mm or more experienced a greater motor recovery after the appropriate surgery.

24   The patient with basilar invagination and long tract signs, such as hyperreflexia and subjective weakness, is best treated with a fusion from the occiput to C2. A simple C1-C2 fusion in this patient population provides no decompression and does not prevent future progression of basilar invagination. Most surgeons would also recommend a C1 laminectomy for upper cord decompression at the time of the occipitoaxial arthrodesis. Further decompression may be necessary by either a suboccipital craniotomy or anterior transoral dens resection. A preoperative flexion or extension sagittal MRI can help further define the need for these two procedures.

25   There is no clear advantage to removal of the retained bullet fragments when lodged in the spinal canal. Waters and Adkins (*Spine*, 1991) presented a review of removal of bullet fragments and found that at the cord level there was no significant improvement in motor recovery. Routine removal of metallic fragments from around the spinal cord is not recommended.

26   Romanick (*J Bone Joint Surg*, 1985) presented a series of similar patients. Of eight patients with a perforated colon, seven developed an infection. This is contrasted to no infections in eight patients with a perforation of the stomach or small bowel. However, Roffi and associates (*Spine*, 1989) found a much lower incidence of infection in a much larger patient population with similar injuries. Their series had only 3 infections in 42 patients. His recommendation for initial treatment is a longer period of broad spectrum antibiotic coverage, no initial spine débridement, and no indication for bullet fragment removal.

QUESTIONS

27   A 35-year-old woman falls down a flight of stairs sustaining a T7 burst fracture. There is no posterior column bony or ligamentous injury. She has no other injuries and is neurologically found to be a complete paraplegic at that level. She has no other skeletal injuries. She is transferred to your facility for definitive care 3 days after her initial injury. What is your treatment recommendation?

28   A 15-year-old teenager sustains a bony flexion distraction injury (Chance fracture) through the body, pedicles, and posterior bony elements of L2. He complains of back pain and is neurologically normal. What type of treatment do you recommend?

29   A 25-year-old woman sustains an L1 burst fracture in a motor vehicle accident. She has substantial weakness in her gastrosoleus and anterior tibial muscles on the right, absent extensor hallucis longus (EHL) function on the left, and patchy sensory deficits in her lower extremities below the knees. Rectal tone, perianal sensation, and bulbocavernosus reflex are normal. Computerized tomographic (CT) scan of her injured vertebra reveals 50% canal occlusion with no posterior laminar fracture. Describe the anatomic location of her deficits (i.e., cord versus conus versus roots).

30   A 50-year-old man is thrown from a horse and lands on his buttocks. He complains of immediate pain in his lower back and initial dysesthesias in his legs. He is found to have an L5 burst fracture with 30% canal compromise. He has no other injuries and has excellent motor function below the knees and intact sensory and sacral function. What is the best treatment option for this patient?

31   What is the most common complication of halo immobilization of the cervical spine?

32   A 46-year-old, otherwise healthy man injures his lower back while lifting a bag of groceries. He has no history of previous back injury and no prior complaint of back pain. His neurologic examination is unremarkable. What is the role of routine radiographic evaluation in this patient?

ANSWERS

27   The treatment of this patient is controversial. In the patient with an isolated burst fracture of the midthoracic spine and complete paraplegia, some authors believe there is no clear indication for operative intervention (Place, Donaldson, Brown et al, *Spine*, 1994). Early mobilization in a brace with a program of spinal cord rehabilitation is recommended. On the other hand, there has been a trend toward early

ANSWERS

surgical stabilization and rehabilitation in a patient with such injury, and many spine surgeons believe this approach facilitates rehabilitation. Others disagree and have demonstrated a somewhat higher complication rate with surgery and possibly a greater delay in achieving independence with activities of daily living compared with nonoperative early mobilization. Thoracolumbar burst fractures may need to be treated differently because of the lack of intrinsic stability at the thoracolumbar junction.

28 In this young patient with a pure bony flexion distraction injury , one can anticipate excellent bony healing after adequate immobilization. Such an injury has minimal soft-tissue disruption, and stability will be obtained once bony union has occurred. This patient should be treated in a hyperextension cast. One can anticipate and strive for normal spinal alignment in the cast. If the patient had evidence of significant ligamentous disruption or a nonreducible kyphotic deformity, a single-level posterior compression arthrodesis is preferred.

29 This patient had a significant nerve root injury. Her spinal cord appears to be functioning adequately because she has maintained conus medullaris function, has no spasticity, and has no discrete functional level. Her patchy sensory deficits, asymmetric weakness, and sacral sparing are suggestive of nerve root compression as opposed to spinal cord compression. This significantly affects the prognosis because root recovery is better than cord recovery after such an injury.

30 Low lumbar burst fractures without neurologic deficit are best managed nonoperatively. Both Court-Brown (*Spine*, 1987) and An (*Spine*, 1991) believe that the patient with a low lumbar burst fracture without neurologic deficit can be satisfactorily treated without surgical intervention. There was a higher rate of persistent low back pain and late kyphotic deformity in the patient who was treated with long posterior constructs.

31 Pin loosening (30% to 60%) is the most common complication of halo immobilization (Botte et al: Operative techniques in orthopaedics, 1993). This is followed by approximately 20% pin site infection rate and other associated complications. The current recommendation for pin tightening in this device includes initial tightening to 8 inch/lb and one retightening at 48 hours. The re-tightened pin must meet resistance within the first two full turns or else it is removed and moved to a nearby site.

32 Plain radiographic films of the lumbar spine are frequently nondiagnostic and not helpful in the evaluation of acute low back pain without trauma. Routine radiographic examination at this patient's initial encounter is not indicated.

QUESTIONS

33   What is the role of MRI in the patient with acute low back pain?

34   What is the incidence of asymptomatic lumbar HNP in an adult population?

ANSWERS

33   MRI is also not indicated in the patient on his initial examination. He has no history of previous back pain and no history of significant trauma. He has a normal neurologic examination and no radicular complaints. Because of its extreme sensitivity, MRI in the lumbar spine is not a good screening tool.

34   Boden and associates (*J Bone Joint Surg*, 1990) suggest an overall incidence of approximately 33% asymptomatic HNP in the lumbar spine. This incidence increases in the patient older than 55 years of age. Greenberg and Schnell (*J Neuroimaging*, 1991) and Jensen and associates (*N Engl J Med*, 1994) also agree with approximately a one-third incidence of asymptomatic HNP. Use of MRI as a screening tool is thus limited because of its high incidence of significant findings in the asymptomatic patient.

QUESTION

35 A 55-year-old man complains of gradually increasing midback discomfort. This began several days earlier after drainage of a dental abscess. The patient complains of persistent midback pain despite activity modification or rest. He has no complaint of leg symptoms. Figures 8-11 through 8-13 are from this patient's initial work-up. What is this patient's working diagnosis at this time?

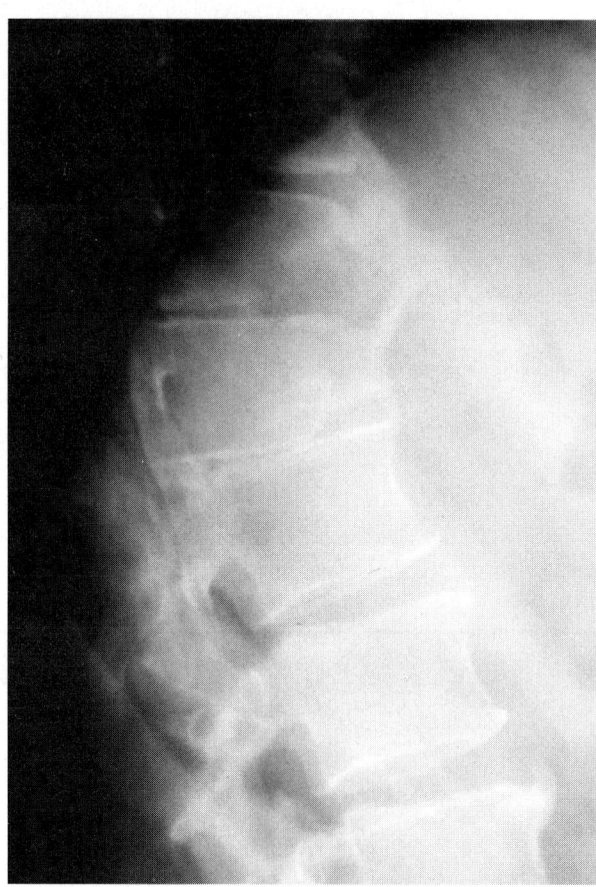

Fig 8-11

ANSWER

35   This patient's history and radiographic examination are consistent with early pyogenic vertebral osteomyelitis of the thoracolumbar spine.

Fig 8-12

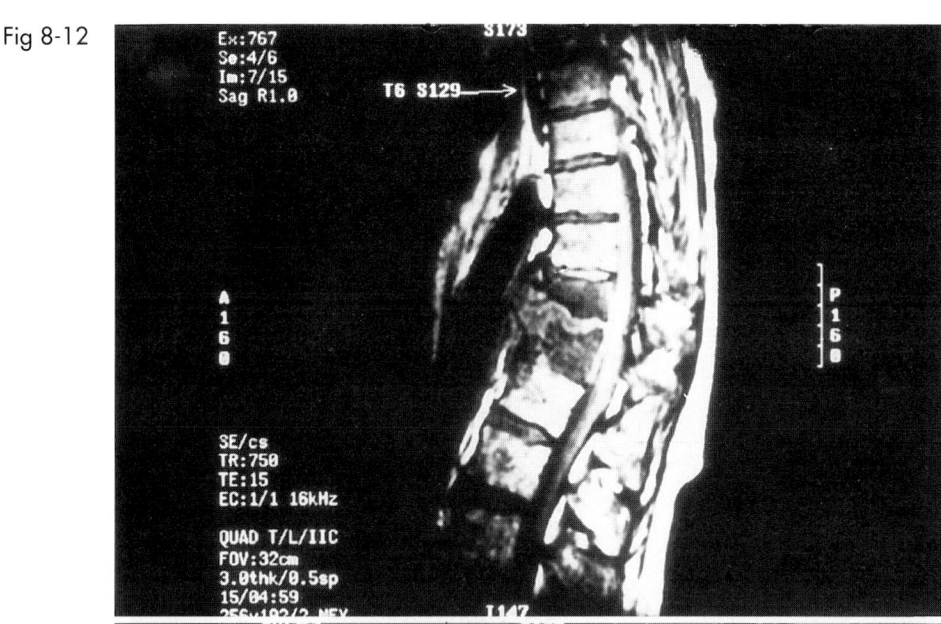

Fig 8-13

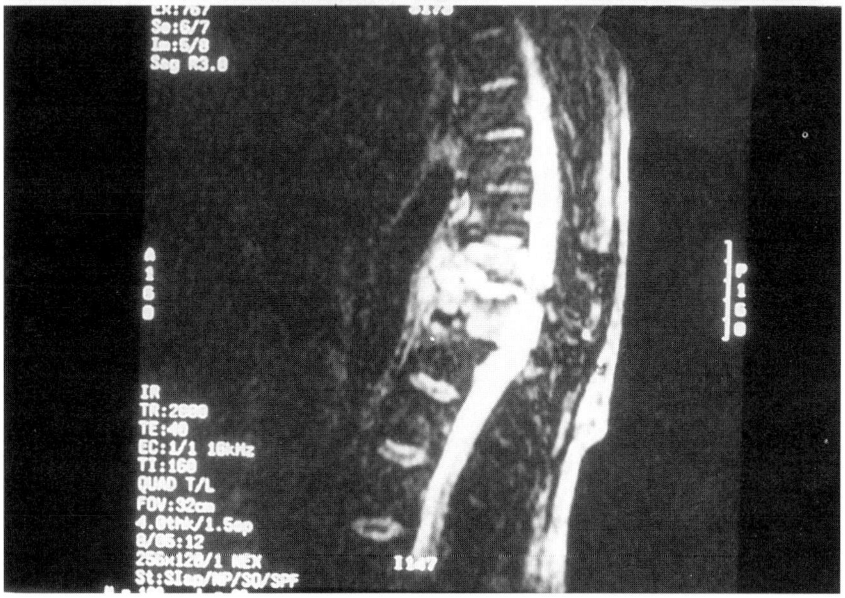

QUESTIONS

36 What radiographic findings are consistent with infection in this patient?

37 How could one differentiate between spinal tumors and spinal infections with the use of MRI?

38 What test should be performed next to aid in the treatment of this patient?

39 What are the indications for surgery in the patient with a pyogenic spinal infection?

40 If the patient were to continue to have symptoms despite adequate antibiotic therapy, what would be the appropriate surgical treatment?

ANSWERS

36 This patient demonstrates loss of disc space height with gross bony destruction. There appears to be loss of endplate clarity and evidence of a soft-tissue abscess. The MRI shows edema in both vertebral bodies without gross vertebral body destruction. The central focus of the pathologic process appears to be the disc space. These findings are all consistent with a vertebral osteomyelitis.

37 According to An and associates (*Spine*, 1991), the most consistent finding in spinal infection is involvement of the disc space and the adjacent vertebral bodies. These vertebral bodies have decreased signal intensity on T1 weighted images and increased signal intensity on T2 weighted images. The disc space is usually spared in spinal destruction because of tumor growth. Irregularities in the vertebral endplates are more common with infection than with tumor growth. Soft-tissue changes are more diffuse with infection, and contiguous vertebral involvement is most consistent with infection.

38 A needle biopsy of the involved disc space should be undertaken to identify the organism involved. Though the yield may be only 70% as opposed to the higher yield of open biopsy (Lestini and Bell: Seminars in spine surgery, 1990), the morbidity is much lower. Organism identification allows for the early initiation of appropriate antibiotic therapy.

39 Indications for surgery are continued symptoms despite adequate antibiotic treatment, vertebral body collapse, and neurologic deficit. Some authors (Blumberg and Balderson: Seminars in spine surgery, 1990) suggest that the presence of a paravertebral abscess is also an indication of surgery.

40 In the patient with an isolated discitis and contiguous vertebral body involvement, an anterior procedure for decompression of the abscess and disc space would be indicated. Débridement of obviously necrotic bone should be performed, and an attempt at stabilization should be made with an interbody strut graft. Given the fact that this is a one-level process and that there is not significant bony destruction in the contiguous vertebral bodies, a tricortical iliac crest bone graft would be appropriate. The role of instrumentation in the patient with an active infection is at best unclear and is not indicated.

QUESTIONS

41 The patient in Figures 8-14 and 8-15 has had 12 weeks of persistent left lower extremity burning pain and weakness. What physical findings would you expect upon examination of this patient?

Fig 8-14

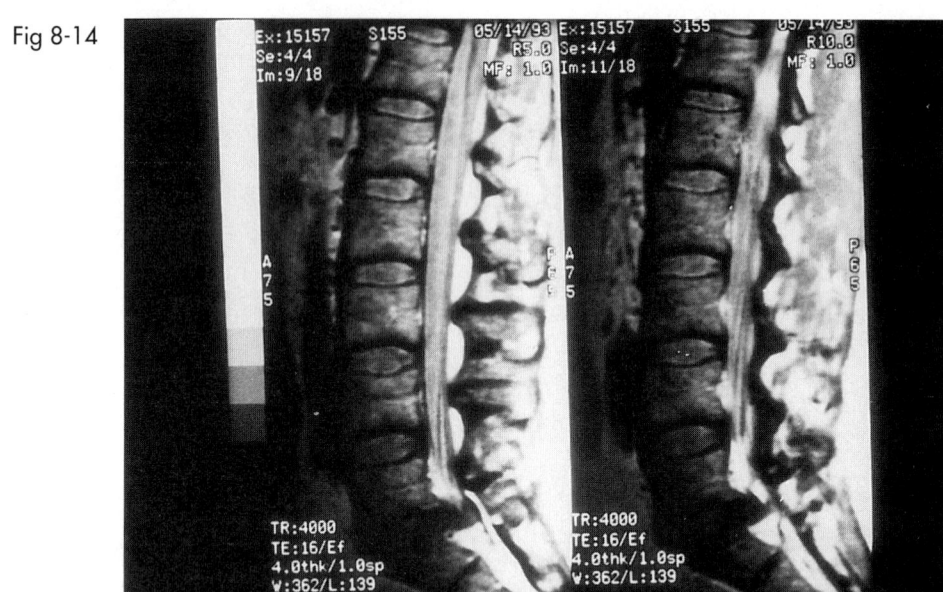

Fig 8-15

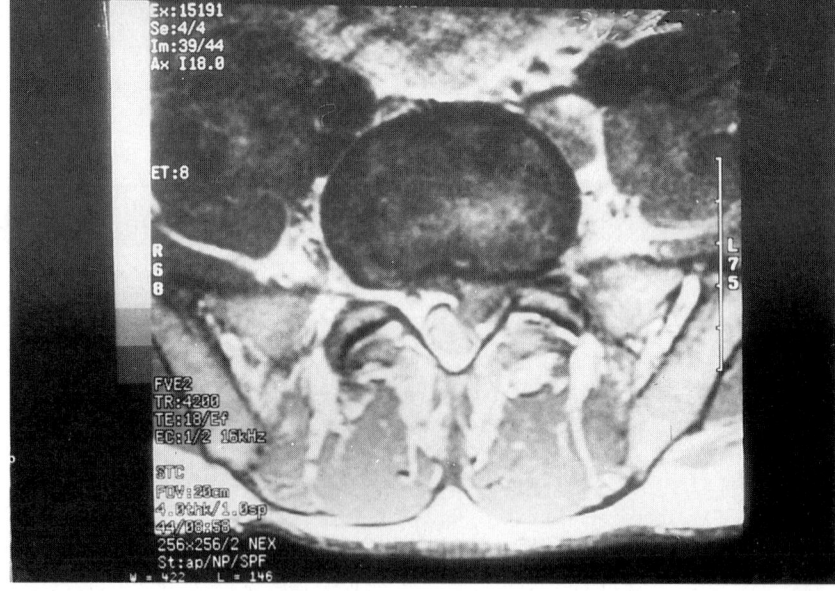

42 What is the appropriate initial management of this patient?

43 What is the role of lumbar fusion in the patient with an acute S1 radiculopathy refractory to nonoperative therapy?

ANSWERS

41 The patient in Figures 8-14 and 8-15 has a left-sided paracentral L5-S1 herniated nucleus pulposus. A herniated disc at this location most commonly involves the nerve root for the level below the disc space involved. This would therefore involve the S1 nerve root on the left. A left S1 radiculopathy would most likely demonstrate a weakness in his gastrosoleus muscle group and a decreased or diminished ankle jerk on the left side. A positive straight leg raise with pain radiating below the knee and into the foot may also be expected.

42 This patient should be initially managed with limited activity and analgesics. Prolonged bed rest is felt to be detrimental. Deyo and associates demonstrated no additional improvement from bed rest for longer than 2 days. Numerous mechanical interventions such as traction, posture modification, and manipulation are controversial and not clearly beneficial. The benefit of exercise is also questioned. A McKenzie exercise program may have a prognostic value. The patient who is able to obtain normal lumbar extension is frequently able to be successfully treated nonoperatively as opposed to the patient who cannot obtain normal lumbar extension (Kopp et al, *Clin Ortho*, 1986). Your attention should be directed toward prevention of back disability with appropriate activity modification and an early return to work with appropriate work restrictions (Dillin, *Semin Spine Surg*, 1989).

43 A lumbar fusion is not indicated in the initial treatment of the patient with leg pain secondary to a herniated nucleus pulposus. White and associates (*Spine*, 1987) showed no improvement in their prospective series of excision versus excision and fusion. The fusion group had an overall less satisfactory rate and higher complication rate. First-time lumbar herniated nucleus pulposus is best treated with disc excision without fusion.

QUESTIONS

44   Two weeks after an uncomplicated lumbar disc excision a patient develops increasing back pain, including pain at rest and increased pain with activity. He has no radicular symptoms. On physical examination he has a well-healed wound and limited motion with flexion and extension of his lumbar spine. He has tenderness to deep palpation in the area near his incision and has a negative straight leg raise. The erythrocyte sedimentation rate (ESR) is 42. What is this patient's diagnosis?

45   Intraoperative spinal cord monitoring is currently commonplace in many centers. What parameters of change should present a serious concern for potential significant neurologic injury?

ANSWERS

44   This patient most likely has a postoperative deep wound infection versus a disc space infection. Postlaminectomy disc space infections typically develop in a slightly delayed fashion. They can occur without wound drainage, and the most significant finding is frequently persistent back pain. The ESR is extremely sensitive in diagnosing a deep infection after lumbar spine surgery (Jonsson et al, *Spine*, 1991). After 2 weeks the ESR values have typically returned to normal in the majority of normally healing postoperative patients.

45   According to Nash and Brown (*J Bone Joint Surg*, 1989) an increase in latency of 10% or more and a decrease in amplitude of greater than 50% are changes that are indicative of serious neurologic injury.

QUESTION

46   A 28-year-old man has an 18-month history of midback and buttocks pain with activity. He has difficulty running because of pain, which radiates down his lower extremity. He has noticed a certain "jumpiness" in his lower extremity over the last 6 months. He has no difficulty with bowel or bladder control. Physical examination reveals hyperreflexia in his lower extremity and no motor weakness. Sensory examination is within normal limits. The patient's studies are shown in Figures 8-16 and 8-17. What is your diagnosis?

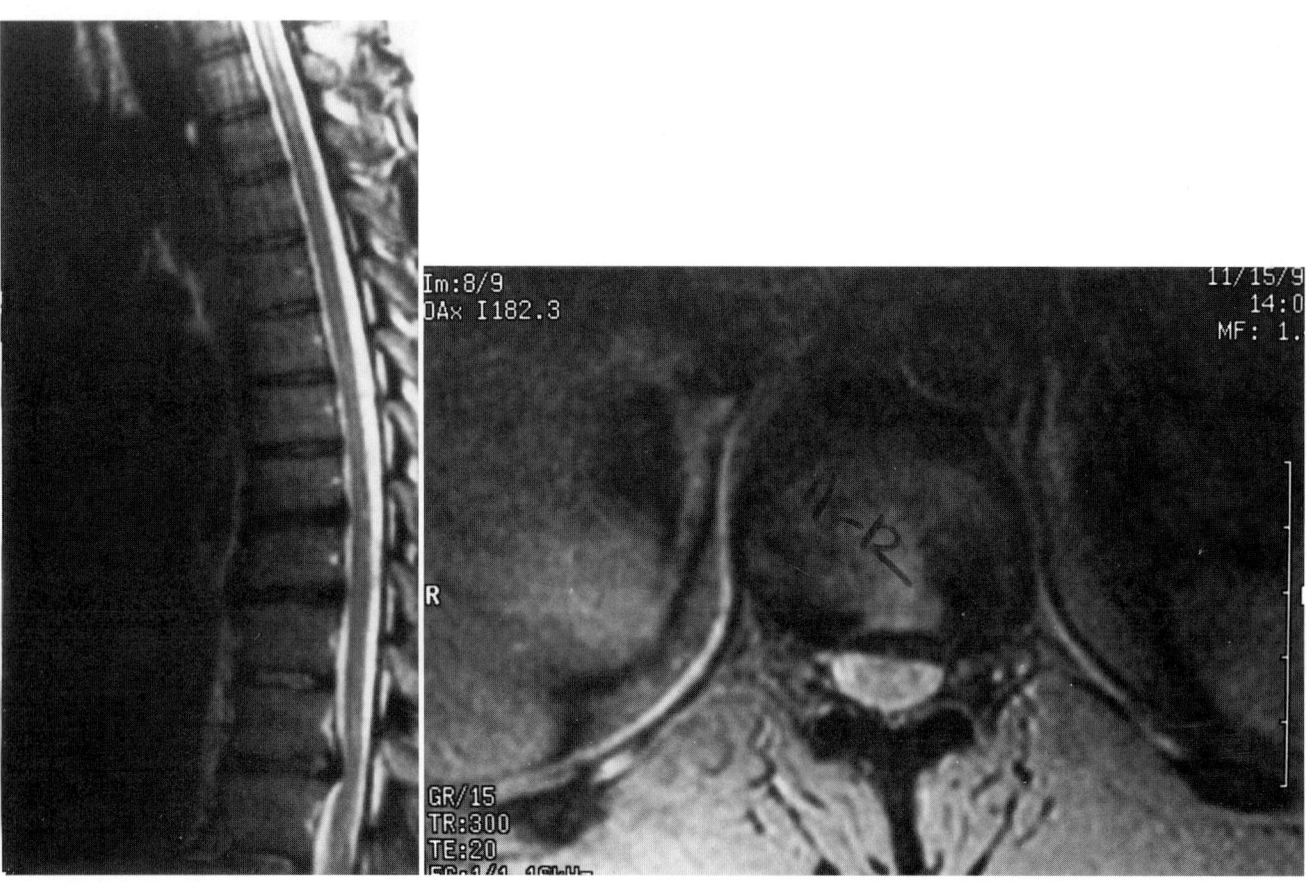

Fig 8-16   Fig 8-17

ANSWER

46 This patient has a T11-T12 herniated nucleus pulposus with resultant myelopathy.

QUESTIONS

47 What is the best form of treatment for this patient?

48 What is the safest approach for the surgical treatment of this lesion?

49 A patient is diagnosed with a sacrococcygeal chordoma. It appears to involve most of the middle to lower sacrum. What is your recommended treatment?

ANSWERS

47 This patient has a history of prolonged back and buttocks pain with activity. He has failed previous nonoperative therapy for his back pain. His condition has continued to worsen, and he has demonstrated spinal cord involvement by his increased spasticity and hyperreflexia. This patient should be treated surgically at this time. Not all patients require surgical treatment for thoracic disc herniations (Brown et al, *Spine*, 1992). However, the patient with persistent pain refractory to nonoperative treatment and any significant neurologic deficit should be treated surgically.

48 A standard anterior approach with thoracotomy has the least risk for neurologic injury. The highest likelihood for significant postoperative neurologic decline is in the patient treated with a posterior approach via laminectomy (Brown et al, *Spine*, 1992). A costotransversectomy could be considered in this patient; however, the ability to stabilize the spine at the thoracolumbar junction and visualize across the entire canal is more limited with this approach as compared with a transthoracic approach. Thoracoscopic disc excision is gaining in popularity and may be the best answer in the future.

49 Chordoma is a malignant tumor most commonly found in the spinal axis. Its cell type of origin is from the remnant notochord. According to Samson and associates (*J Bone Joint Surg*, 1993) these tumors are best treated by a wide resection. This is most frequently performed via a posterior approach. Bowel and bladder function can usually be maintained if the second sacral root can be preserved.

QUESTION

50 A 54-year-old active woman complains of back pain and leg pain. She states that her back is bothersome at most times and that her legs bother her after standing 10 minutes or walking farther than one block. This pain is relieved by sitting. Her symptoms have been getting gradually worse over the last 6 months despite bracing, physical therapy, and nonsteroidal antiinflammatory agents. Her studies are shown in Figures 8-18 and 8-19. What is your diagnosis?

Fig 8-18

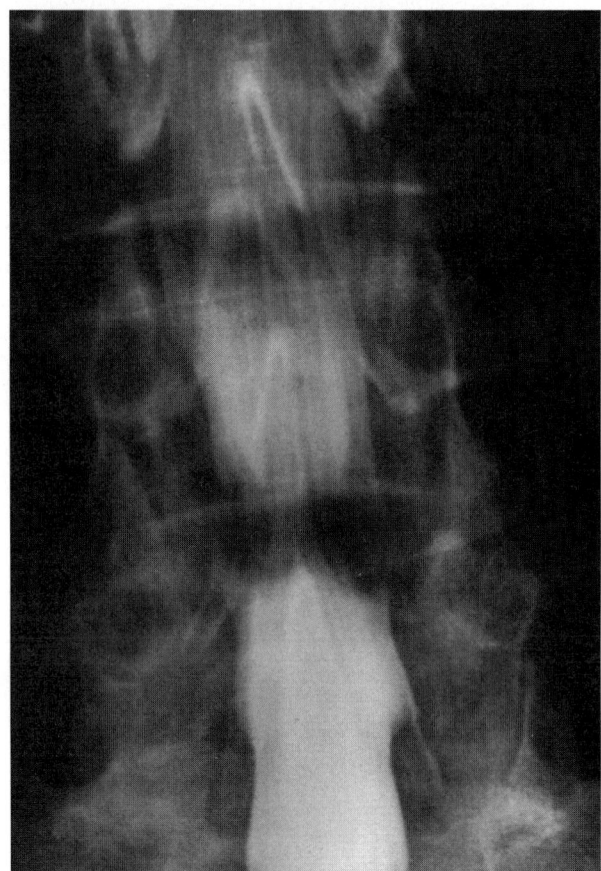

ANSWER

50 This patient has a high-grade spinal stenosis associated with a degenerative spondylolisthesis of L4 and L5.

Fig 8-19

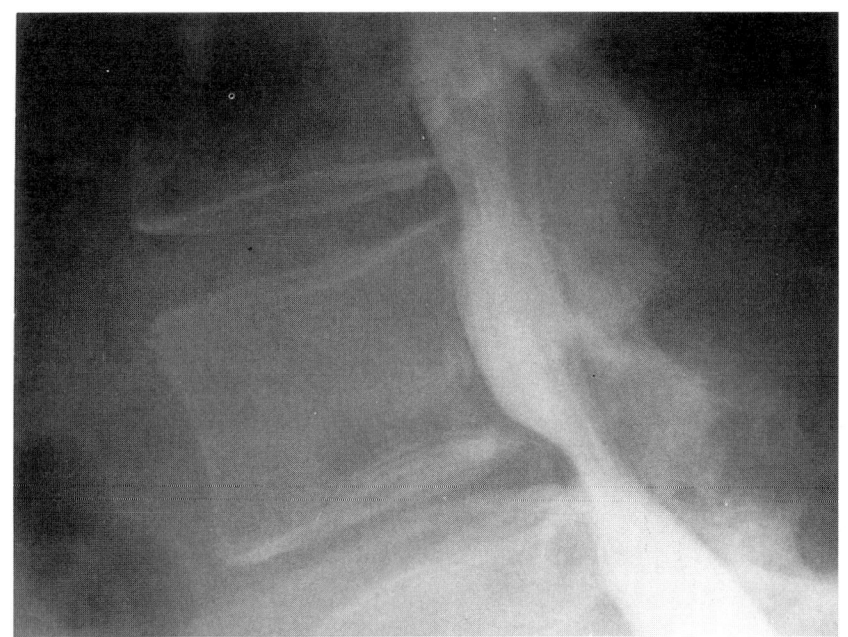

QUESTIONS

51 What is the etiology of this skeletal deformity?

52 What is the best treatment for this patient?

53 What is the role of pedicle screw instrumentation in this treatment scheme?

ANSWERS

51 Degenerative spondylolisthesis is a result of segmental spine degeneration. The studies show no mechanical malformation (i.e., abnormal facets) as in type I dysplastic spondylolisthesis or bone defect as in type II isthmic spondylolisthesis. In this condition the posterior elements are found to be intact, and there is believed to be gradual remodeling of the facet joint and increased motion caused by disc degeneration (Taillard, *Clin Ortho*, 1976). The associated disc space collapse and forward subluxation of L4 on L5 result in narrowing of the spinal canal thus leading to spinal stenosis.

52 This patient should be treated by a lumbar decompression at the involved level with a single segment posterior fusion. Herkowitz's prospective study (*J Bone Joint Surg*, 1991) has suggested that the patient treated with decompression and a posterior arthrodesis has less limiting back and leg pain and a better functional result than decompression without fusion.

53 Pedicle screws can significantly enhance the satisfactory results in the surgical treatment of this condition. Bridwell and associates (*J Spinal Disord*, 1993) have suggested improved results with an instrumented posterior fusion in these patients. This is also clearly the case in the North American Spine Society retrospective cohort series on the use of pedicle screws in degenerative spondylolisthesis. Given this patient's age, diagnosis, and bone quality, pedicle screw instrumentation should be considered.

QUESTION

54 A 33-year-old man complains of low back pain that radiates into his buttocks and down the posterior aspect of his legs to the posterior thigh. He states that the pain in his legs occurs mostly with vigorous activity, such as running or heavy lifting. He complains of a relatively constant ache in his lower back, which has been significantly worsened by some recent heavy lifting. The physical examination reveals some midline lumbosacral tenderness with a slight palpable step-off in the area of the lumbosacral junction. He has normal reflexes and no appreciable motor weakness. His radiographic films are shown in Figures 8-20 and 8-21. What is the radiographic diagnosis?

Fig 8-20

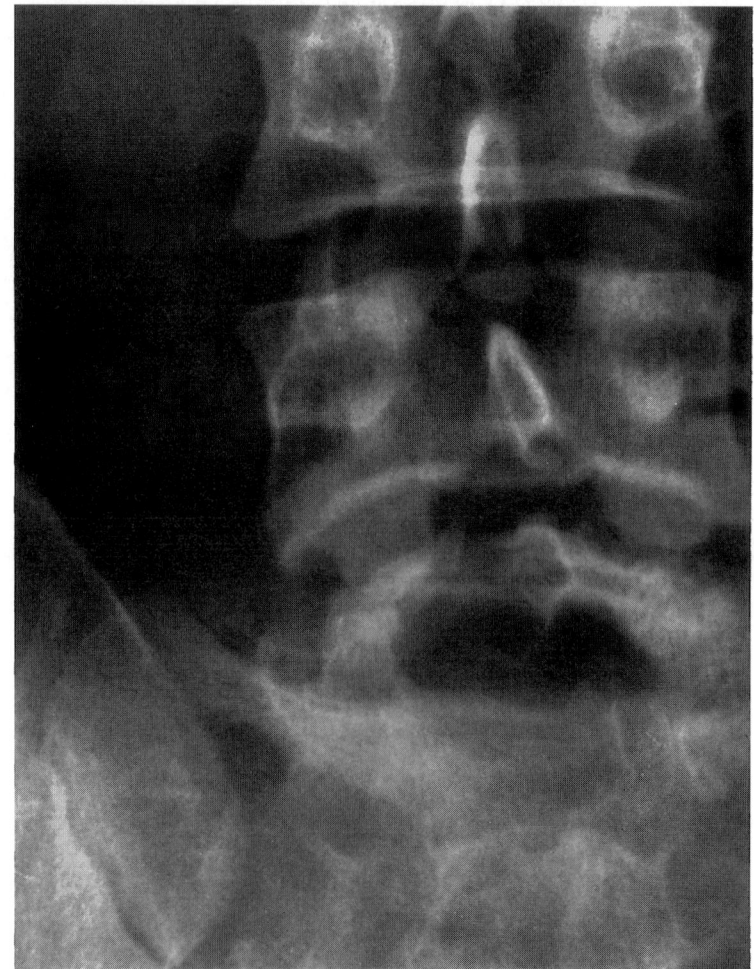

ANSWER

54 This patient has a grade I, L5 on S1 spondylolisthesis. This appears to be the isthmic type.

Fig 8-21

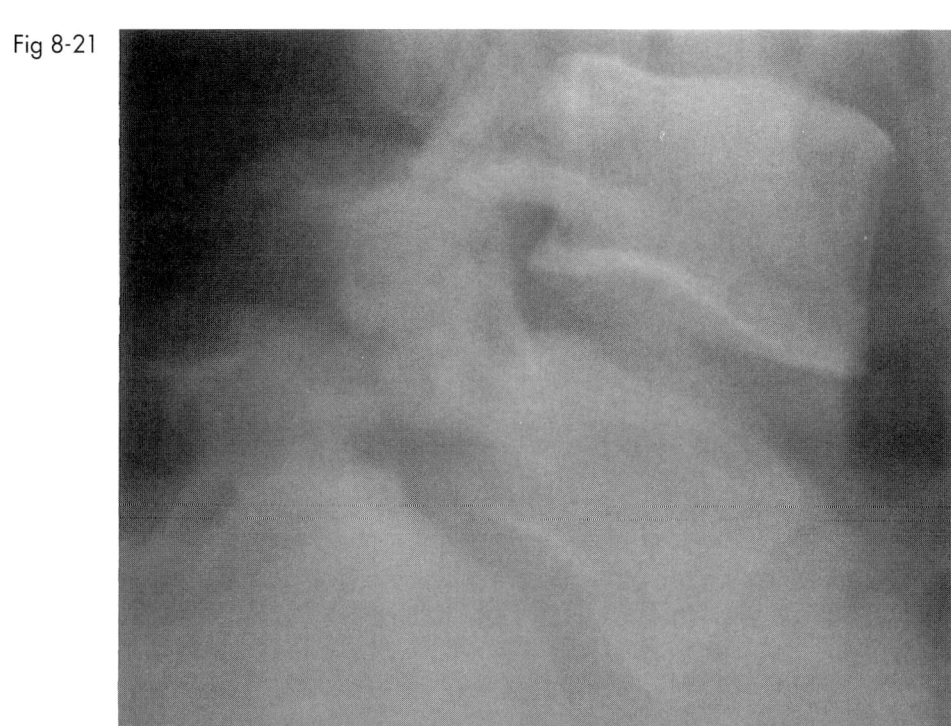

QUESTIONS

55 What are the five types of spondylolisthesis according to Wiltse?

56 What is the approximate incidence of spondylolisthesis in the U.S. population?

57 What is the most common nerve root that is irritated with an L5 on S1 spondylolisthesis?

58 What is the role of lumbar decompression in this patient?

59 What is the best form of surgical treatment for this patient?

60 Adolescent idiopathic scoliosis is associated with what risk factors for progression?

61 Infantile idiopathic scoliosis occurs more commonly in which sex?

62 What are the age limits that define infantile idiopathic scoliosis?

63 In what region of the spine do most patients with infantile idiopathic scoliosis develop their curve?

64 What are the risk factors for progression of the curve in children with infantile idiopathic scoliosis?

65 How is the rib-vertebral angle difference measured?

66 How is the apical vertebra of the curve identified?

ANSWERS

55 The five types of spondylolisthesis are type I (dysplastic), type II (isthmic), type III (degenerative), type IV (traumatic other than pars), type V (pathologic). Some include type VI (postsurgical instability).

56 The best natural history study was performed by Frederickson and associates (*J Bone Joint Surg*), which reported the overall incidence of spondylolisthesis to be approximately 6%. This percentage is the approximate incidence found at the end of adolescence. There does not appear to be a significant number of new cases of isthmic spondylolisthesis that develop after adolescence.

57 The L5 nerve root is the most commonly irritated nerve root in an L5 on S1 spondylolisthesis. The L5 root is impinged by the hypertrophic nonunion at the pars associated with residual foraminal and lateral recess stenosis. In addition, there is some pressure applied by the L5 pedicle as the L5 vertebral body descends into the pelvis with the higher grade spondylolisthesis slips.

ANSWERS

58 The role of simple lumbar decompression (Gill procedure) is clear. Such procedures tend to destabilize the spine and thus increase overall low back discomfort. Aggressive midline decompression by a procedure such as the Gill procedure is to be avoided as the only form of surgical treatment unless a fusion is also performed.

59 The most common procedure for this single-level, low-grade spondylolisthesis is a posterior instrumented spinal fusion using pedicle screw type of instrumentation and posterior decompression. Pedicle screw fixation at this level typically provides the best purchase with incompetent posterior elements. Though considered experimental, the recent Food and Drug Administration (FDA) cohort study suggests that at least in degenerative spondylolisthesis the use of pedicle screws has a significantly higher success rate than uninstrumented fusions. An uninstrumented fusion is possible in this patient, though a drastic increase in the type and length of postoperative immobilization would need to be considered. The role of anterior strut grafting and posterior stabilization is not yet clearly delineated for this condition. Some authors believe that grafting and stabilization are beneficial because both provide a better structural support for the lumbosacral junction before final incorporation of the fusion mass. Others believe that this treatment is not indicated with proper contouring of the lumbosacral spine. The most common procedure for this condition at this time is a single-level instrumented posterior spinal fusion with decompression.

60 Age, maturity, sex, magnitude of the curve, and curve pattern are the associated risk factors.

61 Infantile idiopathic scoliosis occurs more commonly in the male gender.

62 The age limits that define infantile idiopathic scoliosis are the appearance of the spinal curve between birth and 3 years.

63 The thoracic spine is the region where infantile idiopathic scoliosis most often develops.

64 A rib-vertebral angle difference of Mehta of greater than 20° and rib phase 2 are the risk factors.

65 The apical vertebra is identified. The difference in the angle of the head of rib to the vertebral body is measured. The difference between the angular measurements is the rib-vertebral angle difference.

66 It is the vertebral body in the midportion of the curve that is laterally translated farthest from the midline. Its vertebral endplates are parallel to the vertebral bodies outside of the curve. It is commonly the most rotated vertebra of the curve.

QUESTIONS

67 The apex of a typical curve in idiopathic infantile scoliosis has its apex to which side?

68 How is the phase of the rib determined?

69 How is the phase of the rib associated with progression of the curve in infantile idiopathic scoliosis?

70 An 18-month-old male child is seen with a 25° left thoracic scoliosis extending from T4-L2. The rib vertebral angle difference of the apical vertebral is 15°. The ribs are in phase 1. How would you treat the child?

71 The patient in Q70 is unable to keep his follow-up appointment and returns to see you at age 3. His curve has increased to 35°. What is your treatment?

72 The patient in Q71 returns at age 5 with a 60° curve. What is your treatment plan?

73 A 16-year-old female patient is seen for the first time with a 36° right thoracic scoliosis. She is a Risser 4 and a Tanner 4. What is your treatment plan?

74 How is juvenile idiopathic scoliosis defined?

75 What percentage of patients with idiopathic scoliosis develop curve patterns in the juvenile period?

76 In juvenile idiopathic scoliosis curve patterns that involve the thoracic spine, the apex of the curve projects to which side?

77 When should brace treatment be instituted in the patient with juvenile idiopathic scoliosis?

78 An 8-year-old child is seen in the clinic for the first time with a right thoracic curve of 18°. What treatment plan do you recommend?

79 The patient in Q78 returns in 6 months with an increase in the curve to 25°. What is your treatment plan?

80 The patient in Q79 does not wear her prescribed brace and returns to see you at age 10 with a 46° curve. She is premenarcheal and a Tanner 2. What is your treatment plan?

81 What is the prevalence of adolescent idiopathic scoliosis in the United States?

ANSWERS

67 Its apex is to the left side.

68 The apical vertebra is identified. The heads of the rib do not overlap the apical vertebral body in phase 1. There is overlap of the rib head with the vertebral body in phase 2.

69 Progression of the curve is associated with rib head vertebral body overlap—phase 2.

70 Observation with radiographic follow-up in 4 to 6 months is the treatment of choice.

71 Milwaukee brace is the treatment of choice.

72 Subcutaneous rod and continued bracing program is the treatment.

73 Observation is the treatment plan. A brace should not be used because she has minimal future skeletal growth given her Risser and Tanner scores.

74 Juvenile idiopathic scoliosis is defined as a curve that is first diagnosed between 3 and 10 years of age.

75 The percentage is 12% to 16%.

76 The apex of the curve projects to the right.

77 When a scoliosis curve has reached 20 to 25°, radiographic documentation of progression of 5° or more is an indication for brace treatment.

78 Observation of the curve pattern with radiographic follow-up in 4 to 6 months is the recommended treatment.

79 A bracing program is the treatment.

80 Posterior spinal fusion with instrumentation is the treatment plan. One must be aware that this patient is quite immature, and a crankshaft phenomenon is possible. A preoperative anteroposterior pelvic radiographic film should be obtained to examine this patient's triradiate cartilage. There is some support to suggest that the patient treated posteriorly only and who has an open triradiate cartilage is at the greatest risk for a later crankshaft deformity.

81 In the U.S. population, 2% to 4% have curves of 10° or more.

QUESTIONS

82   Underarm thoracolumbosacral orthosis (TLSOs) are best used for which curve patterns in adolescent idiopathic scoliosis?

83   When is a patient weaned from a brace for adolescent idiopathic scoliosis?

84   Has electrical surface stimulation been shown to be an effective treatment to control the progression of adolescent idiopathic scoliosis?

85   How are the major and minor compensatory curve patterns established by radiographic criteria?

86   How are bending films taken?

87   How is the stable end vertebra established to stop the fusion in idiopathic scoliosis?

88   What percentage of patients with Duchenne's muscular dystrophy will develop scoliosis?

89   When does the scoliosis curve pattern progress in the patient with Duchenne's muscular dystrophy?

90   What is a contraindication for surgery in this patient?

91   What is a Jefferson fracture?

92   Is a Jefferson fracture a stable injury pattern?

93   What is the treatment of an unstable Jefferson fracture?

94   Following a difficult vaginal delivery, you are asked to see a newborn child because of the infant's inability to move the lower extremities. Your examination reveals that the patient has paraplegia with no evidence of trauma or spinal deformity. Radiographic films of the spine were within normal limits. What is the most likely cause of this paraplegia in the newborn?

95   How could this patient sustain a spinal cord injury with negative radiographic evidence of injury?

96   What imaging technique might be helpful in confirming the diagnosis of SCIWORA?

ANSWERS

82   TLSOs are best used for curves with an apex at or below T8.

83   When there has been no increase in height for a 4-month period and when the Risser sign is at least 4, the patient can be weaned from the brace.

84   No.

85   The major curves are larger and less flexible on side bending films. The apical vertebra is also farther laterally translated from the midline.

86   The patient must be supine for accurate bending films.

87   The stable end vertebra is usually neutrally rotated and bisected by the center sacral line (King et al, *J Bone Joint Surg* 65A:1302, 1983).

88   Eighty percent of patients with Duchenne's muscular dystrophy will develop scoliosis.

89   When the patient stops walking and becomes wheelchair bound, the scoliosis curve pattern is in progress.

90   A preoperative vital capacity of less than 30% is associated with respiratory failure following surgery.

91   A Jefferson fracture is a four-part fracture of the ring of the atlas (C1).

92   The stability of the fracture pattern is based on the integrity of the transverse ligament. The fracture pattern is unstable if the lateral masses of the atlas are displaced by more than a total of 7 mm over the edges of their articulation with the C2 body on an anteroposterior open mouth view of the atlantoaxial complex.

93   Application of a halo vest is the recommended treatment.

94   Birth trauma can result in spinal cord injury without radiographic abnormality (SCIWORA). This represents the most likely cause of this child's paraplegia.

95   The bones and ligamentous support of the spine in an infant can tolerate four times as much stretch as the spinal cord. It has been demonstrated that the infant cervical spine can elongate up to 2 inches without radiographic evidence of injury. Unfortunately the less elastic cervical cord has much less capacity to elongate before sustaining damage.

96   MRI may show evidence of cord injury secondary to cord stretch, trauma from a spontaneously reduced vertebral dislocation, or vascular injury in the absence of radiographic changes.

QUESTIONS

97 At what age does the thoracolumbar spine in a child become biomechanically similar to that seen in an adult?

98 A 7-year-old child comes to the emergency room following a motor vehicle accident as a restrained passenger in the rear of the vehicle; the child is without loss of consciousness but complains of abdominal pain. Physical examination demonstrates evidence of a 2$^{1}/_{2}$-inch strip of ecchymosis over the anterior abdomen and pain over the midlumbar spine. What problems does one need to rule out in the presence of "lap belt sign?"

99 The 7-year-old patient from question 98 was found to be neurologically intact with no intraabdominal pathology. Radiographic studies showed an L3-4 Chance fracture or dislocation. How should this patient be treated?

100 A 9-year-old child has compression fractures of T2 through T4 following a motor vehicle accident. Should this patient be worked up for a metabolic bone disease because of multiple fractures as a result of this trauma?

101 How should the patient described in Q100 be treated with anterior wedging of 10° at each level, totaling 30° from the thoracic vertebral body fractures?

102 At birth the conus medullaris can be variable. When does it reach the typical adult level (L1)?

103 A 13-year-old boy sustains an abdominal injury from blunt trauma after being struck by a car. The patient developed midthoracic level paraplegia 2 hours after the accident while preparing for abdominal surgery in which a ruptured spleen was removed. He had a normal spine series taken on admission. What is the cause of this neural deficit?

104 What caused injury to this artery?

105 How can this diagnosis be confirmed?

106 What is the prognosis for improvement through immediate decompression of the spinal cord in the patient described in question 103?

107 Four hours after admission, a previously neurologically intact 10-year-old with an unstable L2 fracture-dislocation notices loss of feeling in the legs and weakness in attempts at moving the legs. Your examination confirms these findings. Further evaluation fails to demonstrate any thoracic, abdominal trauma, or hypotensive episodes. What should be done?

ANSWERS

97   At 8 to 10 years of age, a child's thoracolumbar spine is biomechanically similar to that of an adult.

98   One must be aware of injuries at the level of the "lap belt sign." Specifically, one must look for spinal and neurologic injuries and retroperitoneal and intraabdominal pathology.

99   Most children with a Chance dislocation are candidates for nonoperative treatment in a cast. Because many of these injuries are associated with an intact posterior element periosteal tube, or nonossified vertebral element fractures, many will heal with cast immobilization.

100   In children, spinal trauma frequently results in multiple levels of vertebral injury as a result of increased elasticity of the pediatric spine. This elasticity allows for distribution of force to multiple levels. The metabolic work-up is not indicated.

101   Recommended treatment is bed rest until comfortable, then extension casting and bracing of the spine. The Heuter-Volkmann principle, which favors remodeling of the spine in response to applied forces through the open endplates, facilitates correction of wedging.

102   Conus medullaris reaches L1 by about the third month after birth.

103   In contrast to cervical paraplegia noted in infants and newborns associated with SCIWORA, delayed midthoracic paraplegia in a teenager with normal spine films is suggestive of a vascular insult to the cord in the watershed area served by the artery of Adamkiewicz.

104   Vascular injury is usually associated with blunt chest or abdominal trauma, severe hypotension from a ruptured spleen, or retroperitoneal hematoma.

105   MRI is the best imaging option.

106   The prognosis for neurologic improvement is poor. In this patient, paraplegia from a vascular injury to the cord is usually permanent and complete. Surgical decompression is not indicated.

107   The problem is a deterioration in neurologic status in a previously neurologically intact patient. In the absence of findings suggestive of an isolated vascular injury to the cord, the patient should be taken to the operating room to align the spine and decompress the cord. Immediate intravenous administration of steroid has advocates as a preoperative measure to decrease edema around the cord.

Figure Credits

Chapter 5

5-24   Redrawn from Reckling FW: *Orthopaedic anatomy and surgical approaches*, ed 1, St Louis, 1990, Mosby.

5-25   Redrawn from Reckling FW: *Orthopaedic anatomy and surgical approaches*, ed 1, St Louis, 1990, Mosby.

Chapter 6

6-2 A, C, D   Redrawn from Wasielewski RC et al: Acetabular anatomy and the transacetabular fixation of screws, *J Bone Joint Surg* 72-A: 503, April 1990.

6-2B   From Wasielewski RC et al: Acetabular anatomy and the transacetabular fixation of screws, *J Bone Joint Surg* 72-A: 503, April 1990.

6-3   Redrawn from Failure of femoral components, *Clin Orthop* 141: 19, June 1979.

6-5   Redrawn from Moreland JR, Hanker GJ: Lower extremity axis alignment of normal males. In Dorr LD, editor: *The knee*, ed 9, Presented at the First Scientific Meeting of the Knee Society. Baltimore, 1985, University Park Press.

6-6   Redrawn from Crowninshield et al: Cement stresses in THA, *Clin Orthop* 146: 72, Jan-Feb 1980.

Chapter 7

7-1   Redrawn from Reckling FW: *Orthopaedic anatomy and surgical approaches*, ed 1, St Louis, 1990, Mosby.

7-2   Sarrafian SK: *Anatomy of the foot and ankle: descriptive, topographic, functional*, ed 2, Philadelphia, 1993, Lippincott.

7-3   Redrawn from Reckling FW: *Orthopaedic anatomy and surgical approaches*, ed 1, St Louis, 1990, Mosby.

Index

Page numbers in italics indicate illustrations.